Fundamentals of
Orthopedic Radiology

Feb 14, 2005

To Dear ████████

    Thank you for being
an inspiration with your
dedication to Physical Therapy
+ patient care!

        Best wishes,
        Lynn McInnis
        Philadelphia, PA

**Contemporary Perspectives
in Rehabilitation**

Steven L. Wolf, PhD, FAPTA
Editor-in-Chief

PUBLISHED VOLUMES

Electrotherapy in Rehabilitation
Meryl Roth Gersh, MMSc, PT

Dynamics of Human Biologic Tissues
Dean P. Currier, PhD, PT, and Roger M. Nelson, PhD, PT

Concepts in Hand Rehabilitation
Barbara G. Stanley, PT, CHT, and Susan M. Tribuzi, OTR, CHT

Cardiopulmonary Rehabilitation: Basic Theory and Application, 2nd Edition
Frances J. Brannon, PhD, Margaret W. Foley, MN, Julie Ann Starr, MS, PT,
and Mary Geyer Black, MS, PT

Rehabilitation of the Knee: A Problem-Solving Approach
Bruce H. Greenfield, MMSc, PT

Burn Care and Rehabilitation: Principles and Practice
Reginald L. Richard, MS, PT, and Marlys J. Staley, MS, PT

Wound Healing: Alternatives in Management, 2nd Edition
Joseph M. McCulloch, PhD, PT, Luther C. Kloth, MS, PT,
and Jeffrey A. Feedar, PT

The Biomechanics of the Foot and Ankle, 2nd Edition
Robert A. Donatelli, PhD, PT, OCS

Pharmacology in Rehabilitation, 2nd Edition
Charles D. Ciccone, PhD, PT

Thermal Agents in Rehabilitation, 3rd Edition
Susan L. Michlovitz, MS, PT, CHT

Fundamentals of Orthopedic Radiology

Lynn N. McKinnis, PT, OCS
Private Practice
Butler, Pennsylvania

 F. A. DAVIS COMPANY • Philadelphia

F. A. Davis Company
1915 Arch Street
Philadelphia, PA 19103

Printed in the United States of America

Last digit indicates print number: 10 9 8 7 6 5 4 3 2 1

Publisher, Allied Health: Jean-François Vilain
Developmental Editor: Crystal Spraggins
Production Editor: Glenn L. Fechner
Cover Designer: Louis J. Forgione

As new scientific information becomes available through basic and clinical research, recommended treatments and drug therapies undergo changes. The author and publisher have done everything possible to make this book accurate, up to date, and in accord with accepted standards at the time of publication. The author, editors, and publisher are not responsible for errors or omissions or for consequences from application of the book, and make no warranty, expressed or implied, in regard to the contents of the book. Any practice described in this book should be applied by the reader in accordance with professional standards of care used in regard to the unique circumstances that may apply in each situation. The reader is advised always to check product information (package inserts) for changes and new information regarding dose and contraindications before administering any drug. Caution is especially urged when using new or infrequently ordered drugs.

Library of Congress Cataloging-in-Publication Data

McKinnis, Lynn N., 1959–
    Fundamentals of orthopedic radiology / Lynn N. McKinnis
        p.   cm.—(Contemporary perspectives in rehabilitation)
    ISBN 0-8036-0139-5
    1. Radiography in orthopedics.   I. Title.   II. Series.
    [DNLM: 1. Musculoskeletal Diseases—radiography.   2. Fractures—
radiography.   3. Bone and Bones—radiography.   WE 141 M4785 1997]
    RD734.5.R33M35 1997
    616.7'107572—DC20
    DNLM/DLC
    for Library of Congress   96-33387
                                                                                    CIP

The publishers have made every effort to trace the copyright holders for borrowed material. If they have inadvertently overlooked any, they will be pleased to make the necessary arrangements at the first opportunity.

This book is dedicated with love
  to my Mom, who finds joy in her work
  to my Dad, who takes pride in his work
  to my husband, Dave, who lives his work
  and to our children, Jesse and Ann
  for whom I wish all these things.

Foreword

In caring for patients with musculoskeletal disorders, rehabilitation specialists have relied on diagnoses and, at times, specified "orders" as a basis for treatment. Over the past two decades, however, the emerging interest in manual therapies and the more autonomous roles assumed by many physical and occupational therapists have resulted in a need to better understand normal and pathological biomechanics and the musculoskeletal system. Through such understanding, physicians and rehabilitation experts have enhanced their communications and trust. This excitement over increasing physician-therapist collaborations, however, has not resulted in readily available materials designed to help the rehabilitation clinician better comprehend the pathologies for which treatment is rendered. We all invariably learn about radiographs and imaging techniques from transient communications or "hand me down" informatics, not from our own reference resources. In fact, three years ago when we first approached Lynn McKinnis to transfer her vast knowledge base from lecture materials to the written word, we were somewhat stunned by the realization that a text for rehabilitationists to better comprehend radiographic anatomy in a manner that is relevant to treatment simply was nonexistent. As a result, *Fundamentals of Orthopedic Radiology* was born.

This text has been painstakingly nurtured so that its contents will have importance for students and clinicians. The text has been developed from several premises. First, we have assumed that all rehabilitation clinicians would wish to become more familiar with the fundamentals underlying radiographic techniques. Second, we believed that all clinicians and students would wish to confirm their abilities to clearly differentiate soft tissue structures from bony ones and become adept at observing not only differences between fractures and intact bone, but, more significantly, in identifying factors associated with osteoporosis, infection, degenerative joint disease, rheumatoid disease, and tumors. Third, clear differences in the presentation between normal and pathological images in both children and adults seemed relevant and important. Next, we felt that all students and experienced clinicians would want clarification on identifying fractures, their causes, and means for fixation. Collectively, these premises form the basis for the first three chapters of this text.

Thereafter, Lynn has carefully examined the anatomy, pathology, and special considerations of each anatomical region, beginning with the spine and ending, nine chapters later, with the distal extremity. In each of these content areas, the same methodical approach that has characterized past books in the *Contemporary Perspectives in Rehabilitation* series has been followed. The reader is encouraged to think and problem-solve as greater familiarity with the pathology explored in each chapter is achieved. The purpose in this approach is twofold. First, we wish this text to be used as a guide to greater knowledge and understanding of musculoskeletal pathology for students. Second, we wish clinicians to gain greater insights into changes they see in their clients as they communicate with referring orthopedic specialists. In so doing, the text should become a ready reference source. Familiarity with it should facilitate an ability to write about improvements resulting from interventions. Such transcriptions should transcend the typical description of treatment techniques and standard reports on changes in impairments. Further knowledge about how time and treatment are impacting the actual pathology, *vis-à-vis* a better understanding of pathological changes, forms the basis for expanding communications so that inclusion of these changes can be related to improved function. In short, transcending verbal and written communications from the exclusive construct of rehabilitation treatment and into the realm of interactions between treatment, outcome, and changes in radiographic anatomy form the cornerstone for enhanced credibility in a marketplace where reimbursement decisions may be imparted by nonclinicians seeking information in these three latter domains.

This book was written with this contemporary perspective in mind. We invite your comments so that future editions will meet the greatest needs for the largest number of users. Provision of information in a user-friendly manner where such information was not available is always a challenge. Every effort has been made to meet that challenge. In the process we hope to have made a small contribution to the collective mission of elevating rehabilitation science to even greater recognizable heights—not only by rehabilitationists, but by our interdisciplinary colleagues and health care providers as well.

Steven L. Wolf, PhD, FAPTA
Series Editor

Preface: To The Reader, A Non-Radiologist

Traditionally the field of radiology has been considered to be the domain of the physician. Ancillary clinicians (physical therapists, occupational therapists, athletic trainers, or other rehabilitative clinicians) involved directly in the physical evaluation, treatment, and rehabilitation of the patient have generally excluded themselves from interaction with radiology. This self-built professional boundary evolved from the misconception that information gained from viewing films was pertinent only to medical diagnosis and therefore pertinent only to the physician. Because most allied-health curricula have minimized exposure to radiology, simply reading the radiologist's "x-ray report" has become accepted as sufficient. We have convinced ourselves that even if radiographs hold a wealth of information to enhance patient treatment, we are incapable of finding it on our own. Fortunately, development of medical imaging courses at the university level and in professional continuing education courses are now giving both new graduates and experienced clinicians the confidence to dialogue with radiologists, gain relevant information from the radiologist's report, and most significantly, *view films with their own eyes.*

While it is logically accepted that clinicians need to be aware of the patient's medical diagnosis, it is a novel idea for some that there is something to be gained in the patient's care if clinicians view films themselves. And, for others, the idea is more than novel—it can be threatening if it is mistakenly perceived by physicians as a move toward diagnosis or second-guessing the diagnosis, or if it is mistakenly perceived by clinicians as either an opportunity or a responsibility to do just that. Professional collaboration to enhance quality of patient care is the singular most important goal.

Why do clinicians need to view films? Although there are as many examples as there are patients, the following two reasons seem to summarize the general idea and should be easily appreciated by both physicians and clinicians:

1. *A more comprehensive evaluation is obtained.* The success of rehabilitation depends on the effectiveness of the clinician's evaluation. The more thorough the evaluation, the more substance the clinician has to build the rehabilitation program on. Many of the clinician's evaluation tools—observation, palpation, goniometry, manual muscle testing, ligamentous stress testing, joint end-feels, joint mobility testing—are dependent on the clinician's own perceptive skills and have an inherent degree of subjectivity and limitation. Radiology can provide an objective, visual aspect to the evaluation that makes the expertise of the clinician more comprehensive. Supplementing the initial evaluation and re-evaluations with musculoskeletal radiological images increases the clinician's awareness of the patient in an added dimension. The clinician's knowledge of functional anatomy becomes more dynamically effective by allowing direct

visualization of the processes of growth, development, healing, disease, and dysfunction.

2. *The information the clinician seeks is often of a different nature than the information the physician seeks and of a different nature than may be described in the radiologist's report.* For example, a physician needs to know if a fracture in the distal radius that has united with a malunion deformity is clinically stable; if so, the cast can be removed and the patient can be sent to therapy for rehabilitation. The therapist, however, needs to know not only that the fracture is healed but also the severity and configuration of the malunion deformity. By viewing the patient's films, the therapist becomes aware of the degree to which adjacent joint mechanics of the hand, wrist, forearm, and elbow have the potential to be affected by the deformity. The therapists's treatment goals may thus be modified from striving to obtain full premorbid range of motion to obtaining a lesser degree of motion, adequate for function but minimizing the abnormal joint mechanics that may accelerate degenerative changes in the joints.

These are the starting points for the relatively new idea of a frequent intersection between the fields of rehabilitation and radiology. The future holds potential for many other crossroads that advance the scopes of both fields. For example, the goal of accurately correlating and quantifying palpable joint motion findings with radiological evidence would require the collaborative expertise of both manual orthopedic physical therapists and orthopedic radiologists. Collaborations require an understanding of what each party has to offer.

The extensive knowledge of anatomy that most clinicians possess is prerequisite to but not sufficient for understanding radiographic images. The clinician needs an organized introduction to the fundamentals of radiology to appreciate the content of radiological images, including both possibilities and limitations. The goal of this text is to serve that purpose—to be a primer for clinicians who are just beginning to approach radiology. Accordingly, the focus of this text is the plain-film radiograph—the beginning of radiology.

This author is not a radiologist, and this text does not pretend toward diagnosis. The references to radiologic signs that are diagnostic for certain pathologies are made with the intent of highlighting the characteristic appearance of such pathologies, correlating radiologic signs with pathological progression, explaining the ability or inability of certain imaging modalities to identify different stages of disease, or simply for professional interest's sake. In general, I have made a best effort at providing the reader with (1) a broad, general awareness of the capabilities of plain-film orthopedic radiology, (2) enough technical and vernacular background to comprehend the information presented by the radiologist, and (3) sufficient anatomical examples and tracings to confidently view films and recognize what has been previously diagnosed. Because this territory has been predominantly uncharted for the benefit of the clinician, it was at times difficult to find a middle ground between too much diagnostic detail and enough detail to provide a clear picture. For any transgressions or omissions this author apologizes and provides her address at the end of this preface for welcome criticisms that may enhance any future revisions.

So who is your author? A practicing physical therapist who sought to find the answers for questions that were too basic to be found in any radiology text and too embarrassing to be asked out loud (i.e., "is it still a right leg if the R marker is backward?"). The opportunity to design an imaging course in a graduate physical therapy program was the impetus to find those answers, and writing and lecturing to therapists across the nation subsequently followed. It was some comfort to find that so many clinicians were similarly mystified by radiology, and as frustrated that the information on their patients' films and radiology reports were in part inaccessible to them because of unfamiliarity with radiographic technology, language, and anatomy images. In keeping with the idea of a primer for nonradiologists then, this text was developed with the idea of answering some of those first questions in the minds of radiographic novices, such as, "What do the shades of gray represent? What structures can be seen? What structures can't be seen? What other imaging studies may or may not be appropriate in this case?"

For the reader who has never viewed films before, this text hopefully reads like learning to swim in the shallow end of the pool instead of being thrown into the deep. It is therefore desirable to wade through these chapters in the order intended. In Chapter 1, "General Principles of Orthopedic Radiology," the shades of gray are logically accounted for and will render subsequent viewing of plain films more meaningful. Chapter 2, "Radiographic Evaluation of Normal Versus Pathologic Bone," illuminates the analytical process used by radiologists in diagnosing pathology. Chapter 3, "Radiographic Evaluation of Fracture," defines the language used in the radiologic report to describe trauma, healing, and complications of healing. The remaining nine chapters each cover a body segment and follow a common format. The goal of each of these anatomy chapters is to exist for the clinician as a radiologic reference point for viewing their patients' films.

Each anatomy chapter begins with an osseous anatomy review to refamiliarize the reader with anatomical landmarks that will aid in viewing plain films of that region. A brief review of ligamentous anatomy is presented to assist in understanding the mechanics of common traumas evaluated on plain films, such as avulsions or sprains. Muscular anatomy, although important in appreciating joint stability and injury potential, was simply beyond the scope of the text. Similarly, the brief explanations of joint mobility were intended as reminders of joint function and to acknowledge terms frequently associated with radiographic description, such as inversion, eversion, flexion, and extension. Discussions of arthrokinematics in normal and dysfunctional states are easily found in other texts. Growth and development is presented to make the reader aware of the vast differences in the radiographic images of the immature skeleton in infants, children, and teenagers contrasted to the mature, ossified skeleton of adults.

The routine radiographic evaluation comprises the heart of each anatomy chapter. Normal films of young to middle-aged adults are used throughout the text. Tracings of the films, with anatomy labeled, accompany each radiograph. Ideally, readers will take the time to make their own tracings of the radiographs by using a transparency sheet and erasable marker, and then compare their results with that of the printed tracing. Drawing is an invaluable intellectual exercise for teaching anatomy and will certainly enhance the reader's perception of plain-film anatomy. To that end, the illustrations other than the tracings were purposefully kept as line drawings, in two dimensions like plain films. The idea is to assist the reader in making the mental leap from viewing the illustration to viewing the plain film.

The remainder of each anatomy chapter includes brief discussions and film examples of trauma and/or disease processes commonly seen at that body segment. The choice of pathologies presented was arbitrary and by no means comprehensive. Factors included statistical frequency, variety between chapters, rehabilitative potential, clinical interest, and intriguing appearance on film. At times, examples of imaging studies other than plain films are presented as ancillary studies or when representing the diagnostic imaging modality of choice.

Examples of skeletal anomalies, or deviations from the norm, are presented in some anatomy chapters. While certain examples may have important clinical significance, such as a cervical rib that compresses the neurovascular bundle and causes radiating symptoms in the patient's arm, other examples may have little known clinical significance, such as a spina bifida occulta at a lumbar vertebra, which is often an incidental finding. Whatever the amount of clinical significance assigned, the examples of anomalies remind the reader of the infinite variations in "normal," or what we try to define as normal.

The summaries of the chapters are organized into easily accessible lists of practical points that highlight the clinical aspects of the chapter content.

Self-tests using "unknown" radiographs are presented at the end of every chapter to challenge the reader's visual interpretation skills. Answers are found in the back of the book.

It is the wish of this author that in this text the reader find satisfaction in gaining a new vision with which to see anatomy and the potential for developing a skill that makes viewing plain films a valuable tool that contributes to the rehabilitation of patients and individual professional growth.

Lynn N. McKinnis PT, OCS
119 Kemar Drive
Butler, PA 16001

Acknowledgments

For providing the patient films that made this book possible, and also for their personal generosity, support, and encouragement during the development of this book, I am deeply indebted to the following radiologists and hospital radiology staffs: Arthur Nussbaum, MD, Peter Fedyshin, MD, and Sarah Hample, RTR, at North Hills Passavant Hospital, Pittsburgh, PA; Jeffrey Towers, MD, Associate Professor of Orthopedic Radiology, University of Pittsburgh, at Montefiore Hospital, Pittsburgh, PA; Lance Cohen, MD, Pediatric Fellow at Children's Hospital, Pittsburgh, PA; and Linda Barto, RTR, at Butler Memorial Hospital, Butler, PA.

Many thanks to Margie Brindl, Administrator of Undergraduate Medical Education in Radiology at the University of Pittsburgh, for guidance in the radiology library and for sharing her expertise in this area.

Special thanks to Steve Wolf for giving me this opportunity to write, and to the staff of F. A. Davis for their dedication to this book, especially Jean-François Vilain, Publisher, Allied Health, and Crystal Spraggins, Developmental Editor.

Grateful appreciation is extended to the manuscript reviewers, Paul Beattie, J. Gregory Bennett, Charles Ciccone, Richard Nyberg, Russ Paine, and Bjorn Svendson, for their expert advice.

Special thanks to my colleagues at Keystone Rehabilitation Systems and Concordia Lutheran Home for their flexibility, which enabled me to fit this text into my work schedule. The moral support of these friends was truly appreciated.

As always, thank you to my friend and mentor Charles W. Etter, PT, who teaches by example what it is to be your best.

On the home front, this book was possible because of the loving care provided by our parents, Mary Elizabeth McKinnis and Frank and Berniece Nowicki, and our friend, Debi Anthony, for our toddler, Jesse, and our new baby, Annie.

And heartfelt gratitude to my best friend and husband, David Lindsey McKinnis MEd, PT, who taught me how to teach and how to write. His most tangible contribution to this book was in creating and drawing all of the art. These original illustrations often simplified difficult material and greatly enhanced the practical use of the text. His most intangible contribution was in giving me the belief in myself that I could write it.

Reviewers

Paul F. Beattie, PhD, PT, OCS
Assistant Professor
Ithaca College/University of
Rochester
Department of Physical Therapy
Rochester, New York

J. Gregory Bennett, MS, PT
Director
Rehabilitation Services
Dominion Physical Therapy/Inova
Health System
Fairfax, Virginia

Charles Ciccone, PhD, PT
Professor
Department of Physical Therapy
Ithaca College
Ithaca, New York

Richard Nyberg, PT, MMSc, OCS
Instructor
Emory University
Division of Physical Therapy
Atlanta, Georgia

Instructor
Institute of Physical Therapy
St. Augustine, Florida

Russ Paine, PT
Director
Healthsouth-Houston
Houston, Texas

Bjorn Svendson, DHSc, PT, AMPT
Adjunct Assistant Professor
Health Science, Program in Physical
Therapy
Oakland University
Lansing, Michigan

Contents

General Principles of Orthopedic Radiology

Radiology is the branch of medicine concerned with radioactive substances including x-rays, radioactive isotopes, and ionizing radiations and the application of this information to prevention, diagnosis, and treatment of disease.[1] Physicians specializing in radiology are called *radiologists*.

In recent decades the advent of sophisticated imaging technology has revolutionized medical diagnosis and the field of radiology itself. Many subspecialties now exist within radiology. Although most imaging studies are produced by ionizing radiation, nonionizing studies, such as diagnostic ultrasound and magnetic resonance imaging (MRI), are used extensively. Additionally, the ability to image areas of the body that had previously been inaccessible to nonsurgical evaluation has made interventional and biopsy procedures possible, using diagnostic imaging for guidance. Virtually all systems of the body can be evaluated by the tools of radiology. This expanded scope of practice has spawned new descriptors to encompass the growth of radiology, and designations such as *medical imaging* or *diagnostic imaging* are thus becoming more commonplace.

Orthopedic radiology is the area of radiology that specializes in the radiologic diagnostic evaluation of one system of the body, the musculoskeletal system.

The fundamental tool of the orthopedic radiologist is conventional radiography, or *plain-film radiography*. Although many advanced imaging modalities are now commonly used in orthopedic radiology, plain-film radiography remains the most effective means of demonstrating a bone or joint abnormality.[2] Additionally, plain-film radiography screens for a significant portion of pathologies, with little risk to the patient and with extreme time and cost-effectiveness. Thus, *plain-film radiography is the first-order diagnostic study, or the first imaging procedure to be done following the clinical examination.* The results of the plain-film studies may direct treatment or nontreatment of the patient, or may serve as a departure point for additional studies that may be necessary to complete the diagnosis. Plain-film radiographs have been a staple of medical management over the past century and most likely will continue that role into the next century.

The goal of this chapter is to provide the clinician with the basic knowledge necessary to visually comprehend the plain-film radiograph. Perceiving the translation of three-dimensional human anatomy into two-dimensional line images and shades of gray requires a foundation that combines anatomy with the science of radiography. Establishing this foundation thus involves an understanding of multiple factors, including the production of x-rays and radiographs, the properties of radiodensity, the densities of the human body, the effects of angles of projection over straight and curved planes, the perception of a third dimension, familiarity with common body positioning, recognizing anatomic markers on radiographs, correct methods of viewing radiographs, and an awareness of image-quality factors that may alter the radiographic image.

An additional goal is to introduce and describe briefly some imaging modalities other than plain films commonly used in orthopedic radiology. Throughout the text, reference will be made to these modalities when they are the imaging modality of choice in certain diagnostic investigations.

WHAT IS A RADIOGRAPH?

A *radiograph* is an x-ray film containing an image of an anatomic part of a patient (Fig. 1–1). The terms "x-ray" and "radiograph" are often incorrectly used interchangeably. X-rays themselves are invisible to the human eye, and the x-ray film is the physical material on which the image is exposed. Radiographs include both the x-ray film and the anatomic image contained on it.[3] *Plain-film* or *conventional radiograph* designates a radiograph made without contrast enhancement or other modifications. Production of a plain-film radiograph requires three materials: (1) the x-ray beam source, (2) the patient, and (3) the x-ray film. The process begins with the generation of *x-rays*.

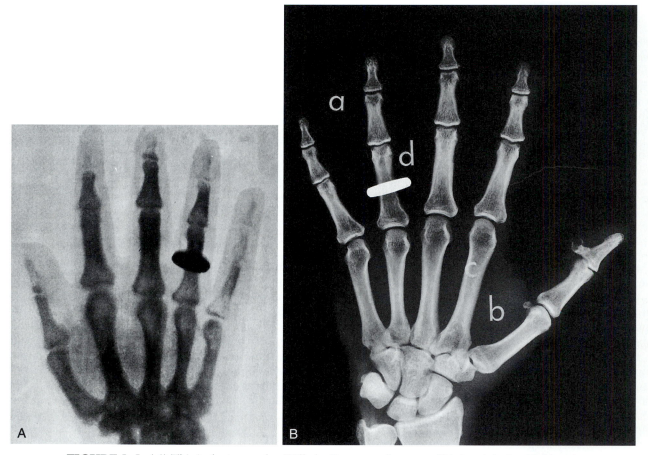

FIGURE 1–1. (*A*) This is the image that Wilhelm Roentgen first saw of his hand during his historic experiments with a primitive x-ray tube and fluorescing cardboard in his laboratory in 1895. Six years later, Roentgen won the first Nobel Prize in physics for his discovery of x-rays. By that time, this remarkable scientist had explored most of the basic physical and medical applications of this newly discovered radiant energy form. (*B*) This is a modern radiograph of a hand. *a*, Blackened area of the film represents that area where only air is interposed between the beam source and the film. *b*, Soft tissues absorb part of the beam before it reaches the film and the shadow is gray. *c*, Calcium salts in bone absorb more x-rays than the soft tissues and expose the film only lightly, thus the shadow of bone is mostly white. *d*, The dense metal of the wedding ring absorbs all of the x-rays, and so no area of the film is exposed underneath it and the image is solid white. Note that in contrast to the historic x-ray in Figure 1–1, this is a doubly reversed print. This is what the clinician sees when he or she views radiographs on film or when radiographs are printed for publication. (From Squire and Novelline,[7] pp. 2–3, with permission.)

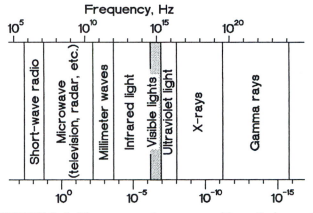

Frequency, Hz

FIGURE 1–2. Electromagnetic spectrum. (From Carlton and Adler,[5] p 36, with permission.)

X-rays are a form of electromagnetic radiation similar to visible light but of shorter wavelength. The various forms of radiant energy are grouped according to their wavelengths in what is called the "electromagnetic spectrum" (Fig. 1–2). The shorter the wavelength in the electromagnetic spectrum, the higher the energy of the radiation. The relatively high energy of x-rays allows them to penetrate dense substances and to produce ionization (loss of electrons) of atoms and molecules. Thus, x-rays are a form of *ionizing radiation.*[4] The penetration of the body by x-rays and the ionization of the silver atoms on film results in the gray images of the radiographs.

The *x-ray tube* is the device in which x-rays are generated (Fig. 1–3). The tube consists of a cathode and an anode enclosed within a glass envelope, which is then encased in a glass housing.[5] Production of x-rays begins with a high-voltage current passing through a vacuum. Electrons are driven from the cathode and strike the anode, creating x-rays via an energy conversion. X-rays are beamed through a series of lead shutters and travel out of the tube in divergent rays to the patient. The patient's body absorbs various amounts of radiation from the beam, depending on the densities of the tissue the beam has passed through.[6] As the x-ray beam emerges from the body, different areas of the beam contain different intensities of radiation. This remainder of the beam reaches the x-ray film. X-ray film is a type of modified photographic film that is sensitive to light and radiation. The various intensities of x-rays left in the beam cause chemical reactions with the silver emulsion coated on the film, producing various shades of gray. Thus, the *final image is a representation of the radiodensities of the anatomic structures the x-rays have passed through.*

What Is Radiodensity?

The term "radiodensity" refers to those physical qualities of an object that determine how much radiation it absorbs from the x-ray beam. An object's *radiodensity* is determined by a combination of (1) its composition (or atomic weight) and (2) its thickness.[7] *The greater an object's composition or thickness, the greater its radiodensity.* The terms "radiopaque" and "radiolucent" are commonly used to describe greater and lesser degrees of radiodensity, respectively.[8]

An inverse relationship exists between the amount of radiodensity of an object and the amount of blackening on the x-ray film. The more radiodense or radiopaque an object is, the more radiation it absorbs, resulting in less of the x-ray beam reaching the film. This causes developed images to be whiter. Lead, for example, is so radiodense or radiopaque that it is used as a radiation shield, casting a white image on the radiograph. In contrast, a *less* radiodense or radiolucent object absorbs *less* radiation and thus more of the beam reaches the film, rendering a blacker image. Air is the best example of a radiolucent substance, as seen on the black background of the radiograph.

There are four major physical densities in the human body; thus there are four major shades of gray, or *radiographic densities,* on the radiograph (Fig. 1–4 and

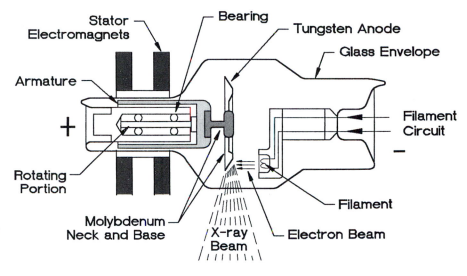

FIGURE 1–3. A rotating anode x-ray tube. (From Carlton and Adler, 1992, p. 141, with permission.)

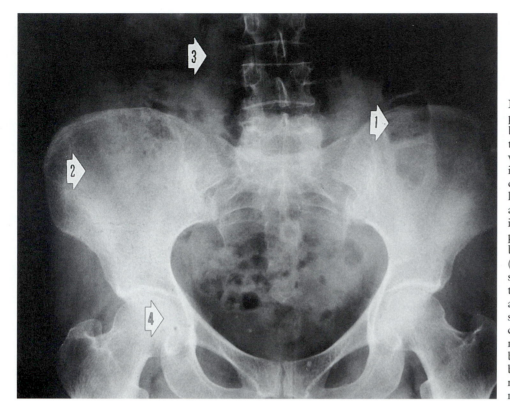

FIGURE 1–4. The four major physical densities of the human body are demonstrated on this anterior or posterior view of the pelvis. (1) Air gas—This is seen in the intestines. (2) Fat—Fat is seen as a dark streak representing the fatty layer next to the peritoneum in the abdominal wall. This stripe, which is the fold of the fat layer as it turns posteriorly toward the patient's back, is known as the flank stripe. (3) Water—Muscles and soft tissues share the same density as water. The psoas muscle extends along the borders of the lumbar spine. (4) Bone—The osseous components of the proximal femur, pelvis, sacrum, and spine are best demonstrated on radiograph because bone possesses the greatest radiographic density of the four natural densities.

Fig. 1–5).[9] Identification of tissues is based on the radiographic contrast between the radiographic densities of the images:

1. **Air—black.** Air is the least-radiodense substance in the human body, being present in the lungs, stomach, and digestive tract, and it represents the black surrounding background of the radiograph.
2. **Fat—gray-black.** Fat is more radiodense than air. It is present subcutaneously, along muscle sheaths, and surrounds organs. Fat images as gray-black.
3. **Water—gray.** Water-based substances are more radiodense than fat. All the fluids and soft tissues of the body including blood, muscle, cartilage, tendons, ligaments, nerves, and fluid-filled organs share approximately the same density. These substances image as medium gray.
4. **Bone—white.** Bone is the most radiodense substance occurring naturally in the human body and casts the whitest image of the four densities. The teeth image the whitest of all bone because of their high calcium content.

Two additional substances are often added to this list because of their common usage in medicine (Fig. 1–6).

5. **Contrast media—bright white outline.** Contrast media such as the barium sulfate used in upper and lower gastrointestinal studies will image as a bright white outline in contrast to the normal radiodensity of bone.
6. **Heavy metals—solid white.** Heavy metals used in teeth fillings, in prosthetic devices such as total joint replacements, in pins and wires used in fracture fixation, or in the lead shields used for gonad protection image as uniformly solid white.

Listing the effective atomic number and volume density of each of the foregoing substances further illustrates the definition of radiodensity as a function of composition (Fig. 1–5).[10]

Note that whereas air has a higher effective atomic number than fat or water, it has significantly lower

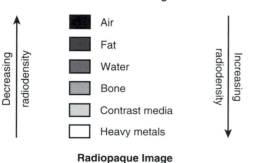

FIGURE 1–5. Radiographic density (shades of gray) as related to object radiodensity. (From Richardson, JK, and Iglarsh, ZA: Clinical Orthopaedic Physical Therapy. WB Saunders, Philadelphia, 1995, p 630, with permission.)

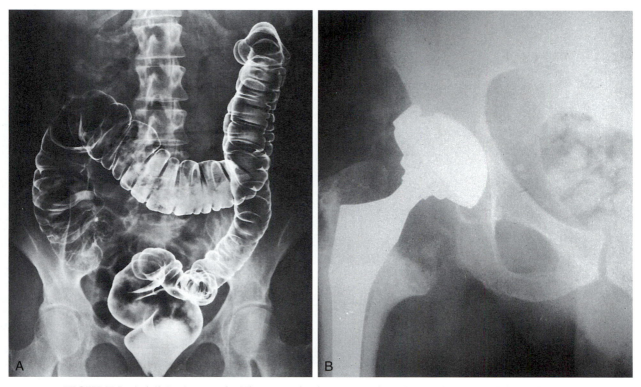

FIGURE 1–6. (*A*) Barium study. This normal colon is coated inside with barium and distended with air. Contrast media such as barium sulfate are used in gastrointestinal studies to contrast with the normal radiodensity of the bone. The bright white outline caused by the media allows detailed visualization of structures not normally visible on plain radiographs. (From Squire and Novelline,[7] p 159, with permission.) (*B*) Total hip arthroplasty. The heavy metals used in the prosthetic components of this joint replacement absorb all the x-rays and cast a solid white image on the radiograph. Any anatomic structures behind the prosthesis are obscured. (From Richardson and Iglarsh, p 673, 1994, with permission.)

tissue density. As a result, air will absorb fewer x-rays than fat and will image blacker.

As stated previously, an object's radiodensity is also determined by its thickness. Simply speaking, *the thicker a substance is, the more radiodensity it possesses relative to a thinner portion of the same substance.* Figure 1–7 illustrates how a stepwise increase in thickness produces progressively lighter shades of gray on the radiograph. So, although an object may be of homogeneous composition, its thicker portions will absorb more x-rays than its thinner portion, and its thicker portions will image lighter.[11] The numerous shapes and irregular surfaces of the bones in the skeleton present many different thicknesses for the x-ray beam to pass through. As a result, the radiographic images of bone have variations in the shades of white and are not uniformly white.

How Many Dimensions Can You See?

Understanding how composition and thickness determine an object's radiodensity is part of the foundation for understanding the images of the radiograph. Now consider the contribution of *form* to the radiographic image. The form or shape of an anatomic image will depend on the *angle of projection* of the x-ray beam. That is, the direction that the x-ray beam passed through the body part will determine its silhouette on film and also alter its radiographic density.[12] To illustrate:

Look at the three radiographs made of the wedge of wood (Fig. 1–8). The different angles of projection created three very different silhouettes and radiographic densities:

- When the wedge is placed flat on its broad side on the film plate, the resulting triangluar image is of uniform radiographic density because the x-ray beam traveled through equal thicknesses at all points on the solid wedge.
- When the wedge is placed upright on its base, the resulting rectangular image shows greater radiodensity present at the center of the image, where the x-ray beam traveled through the greatest thickness from the top of the wedge down to the base.

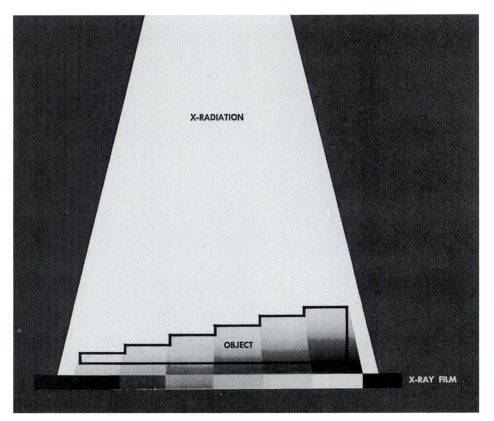

FIGURE 1–7. Radiodensity as a function of thickness of the object. Here the object filmed is of homogeneous composition and has a stepwise range of thickness. The thicker the object, the greater amount of radiation it absorbs; so the radiographic image is a lighter shade of gray. (From Fundamentals of Radiography, Eastman Kodak, 1980, with permission.)

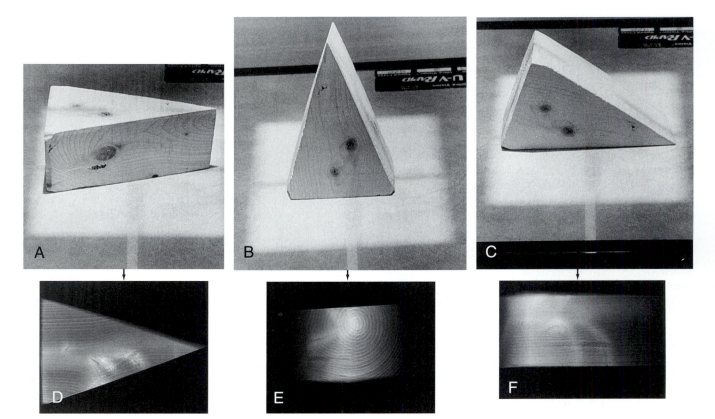

FIGURE 1–8. (A–F) A wedge of wood radiographed from three different angles produces three distinctly different radiographic images with varying radiographic densities. (Note the whorls representing seasonal growth, and the knot in the wood. These present an increased density because of more tightly packed wood cells.)

- When the wedge is placed on its long side, the resulting rectangular image shows a gradual decrease in radiographic density from the thick end to the thin end of the wedge.

If the viewer had no prior knowledge of the form of the object, information regarding the straight planes, dimensions, and whether the object was hollow or solid could easily be deduced by viewing all three images and noting the variations in outline and radiographic density.[13]

Curved surfaces, however, are slightly more complex than straight planes. Curved surfaces radiograph *tangentially* as a series of planes. In this instance it is helpful to imagine a curved plane as being at some points either relatively parallel to the film or relatively perpendicular to the film. The portion of the curved plane that is parallel to the film will be relatively thin with little radiographic density. The part of the curve that is perpendicular to the film will absorb more of the beam and image with greater radiographic density. To illustrate:

Look at the two radiographs of a hollow plastic pipe (Fig. 1–9).

- The first image is made with the pipe stood on its end on the film plate. The image is of a circle of equal radiographic density, as the x-ray beam travels down the same length of pipe at all points. The radiographic density of the center matches that of the surrounding air, indicating the pipe is hollow. The length of the pipe is not possible to determine on this one radiograph.

- The second image is made with the pipe lying on its side on the film plate. *The center of the image is the least radiodense area because the x-ray beam only traversed a thickness equal to the sum of two sides. The image of two very radiodense lines on either margin is a result of the x-ray beam traveling over a greater cumulative distance of the relatively perpendicular curved plane sides of the pipe.* This image is consistent for hollow tubular structures, like the long bones of the skeleton.

It is plain to see from these examples that more than one projection is required to gain useful information about a structure. A single radiograph provides only two dimensions—length and width. The third dimension, depth, is compensated for by viewing a second radiograph projected at a 90-degree angle to the first image. Thus, the old adage "one view is no view" is a pertinent reminder that critical diagnostic information is missing if only one film is available for evaluation. *At least two images, as close to 90 degrees to each other as possible, are required to view all three dimensions* (Fig. 1–10).[13]

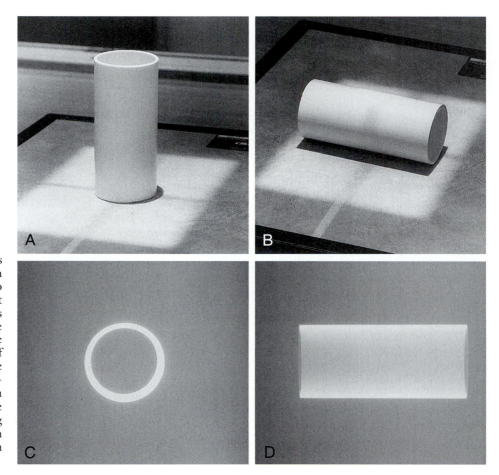

FIGURE 1–9. (A–D) Radiographs made of a hollow plastic pipe from two different perspectives yield two entirely different images. The first image (C) reveals that the pipe is hollow but tells nothing about the length of the pipe. The second image (D) reveals the length dimensions of the pipe. Without having seen the first image, it is still possible to deduce that this object is tubular with a less dense center by observing the densities of the margins contrasting with the density of center. (From Richardson and Iglarsh, 1994, with permission.)

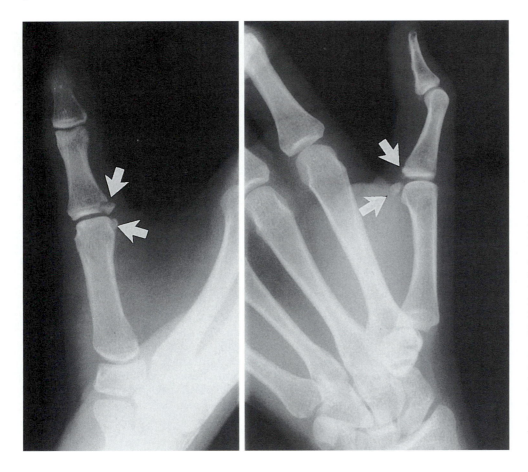

FIGURE 1–10. These two films of the thumb demonstrate the necessity of viewing two images, as close to 90 degrees to each other as possible, in order to gather accurate diagnostic information. On the dorsoplanar image on the left, the arrows point to what may be either two bone fragments or two sesamoid bones. On viewing the lateral film, it becomes obvious that the fragment seen at the base of the proximal phalanx was indeed a fracture, whereas the object seen at the head of the metacarpal was a sesamoid bone.

Thinking Perceptually

In evaluating medical radiographs, two projections made at right angles will provide the viewer with the factual dimensions of length, width, and depth. It is up to the viewer's mind's eye, however, to *reconstruct form* while looking at the two projections. Knowledge of anatomy in great detail is the heart of the radiologist's science. No matter how advanced the machinery of imaging becomes, the interpretation of the data is still dependent on the viewer's *perceptual* foundation of anatomy.

The three radiographs of the finger illustrate this concept (Fig. 1–11).[14,15] The first radiograph is a plain film of a finger, projected in an anteroposterior direction. In the next radiographs, the finger has been coated with barium and radiographed in an anteroposterior and a lateral position. In 1–11A the soft tissues image as a faint gray outline. In 1–11B and 1–11C the barium has collected in the crevices of the skin and the nail, and the illusion of depth is easily perceived by the novice.

The perception of the third dimension in the evaluation of plain films is critical. The radiologist views

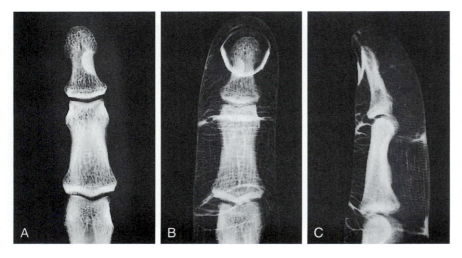

FIGURE 1–11. (*A*) Plain film radiograph of a finger. (*B,C*) Plain film radiographs of a finger that has been coated with barium. (From Richards, A: *Medical Radiography and Photography*, p 28, with permission.)

most radiographs in this manner, perceiving three dimensions and reconstructing form via a knowledge base of anatomy.

A ROENTGEN ROSE

Squire[16] eloquently summarized the fundamentals of radiodensity, form, and perception by describing radiographs not as pictures but as "composite shadowgrams representing the sum of the densities interposed between beam source and film." Squire illustrated her point with this radiograph of three roses (Fig. 1–12). Evaluating a radiograph of something familiar allows the viewer to confidently apply the new concepts and terms just presented. Consider the following:

1. Thinking perceptually, the viewer supplies the third dimension by recognizing form and identifying the image as three actual roses, in different stages of bloom.
2. Density and thickness principles are evident in the greater radiographic density of the overlapping petals of the tightly closed bud versus the open petals of the rose that is in full bloom.
3. The single petal is the most radiolucent structure on the image.
4. The leaves are slightly more radiodense than the single petal.
5. The veins of the leaves are denser than the leaves themselves. This is due to the more tightly packed cell structure of the veins, and also to the added density of the fluid in the veins.

6. The stems are thicker than the other structures, evidenced by their increased radiographic density.
7. The form of the stems can be deduced as tubular by noting the increased density of the margins of the stems versus the less dense centers of the stems. The margins have greater density because they represent curved planes radiographed tangentially.
8. Like the veins on the leaves, fluid adds density to the hollow tubular stems.
9. The form of the leaves can be deduced as thin, broad, and flat by noting the dimensions of a leaf flat on the film and another leaf positioned at 90 degrees to the film.
10. The variations in curved plane densities are evident in comparing the radiographic density of the leaf lying flat on the film (parallel to the film) versus a leaf curling up (relatively perpendicular to the film). The flat leaf is radiolucent. The curled leaf has relatively greater radiographic density.

ANALYZING THE IMAGE

A foundation for understanding how different structures produce different images has been presented. Further comprehension of medical radiographs is gained by understanding *body positioning*, being fa-

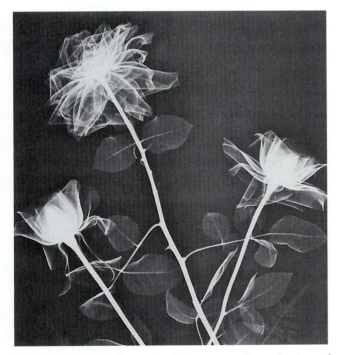

FIGURE 1–12. Radiograph of three roses. (From Squire and Novelline,[7] p 9, with permission.)

TABLE 1–1 Primary Radiographic Projections and Body Positions

Projections	Positions
AP	*Body positions*
PA	
Lateral	Upright
AP oblique	Seated
PA oblique	Recumbent
Axial	Supine
AP axial	Prone
PA axial	Trendelenburg
AP axial oblique	
PA axial oblique	*Radiographic positions*
Axiolateral	
Axiolateral oblique	Right lateral
Transthoracic	Left lateral
Craniocaudal	Right posterior oblique (RPO)
Tangential	Left posterior oblique (LPO)
Inferosuperior	Right anterior oblique (RAO)
Superoinferior	Left anterior oblique (LAO)
Plantodorsal	Right lateral decubitus
Dorsoplantar	Left lateral decubitus
Lateromedial	Ventral decubitus
Mediolateral	Dorsal decubitus
Submentovertical	Lordotic
Verticosubmental	
Parietoacanthial	
Orbitoparietal	
Parieto-orbital	

Source: Ballinger, PWB: Merrill's Atlas of Radiographic Positions & Radiologic Procedures, vol 1, ed. CV Mosby St. Louis, 1995, p 50, with permission.

miliar with *identification markers*, and appreciating the factors that determine *image quality*. The person responsible for controlling all of these variables is the *radiographer*, who interacts with the patient and actually produces the radiograph.

Most radiographers are *radiologic technicians (RTs)*. These nationally registered professionals are schooled in the areas of anatomy, photography, and physics. Radiography has been described as being both an art and a science, and RTs may take the credit for that.

Positioning for Routine Radiographs

Over the years radiologists and radiographers have developed specific positioning for "routine" radiographic assessment of the individual bones, joints, and tissues.[17] The purpose of routine (or standard or basic) projections is to provide the most visualization possible with the minimal number of radiographs, and thus expose the patient to minimal radiation. *Routine radiographs serve as a basic assessment tool and screen for a significant portion of pathologies.*

The choice of positioning and the number of projec-

tions composing a routine radiographic examination of the joints has recently become standardized in the United States. In 1989, a survey of 520 hospitals affiliated with Radiologic Technology Educational Programs was undertaken to determine a national norm for all radiographic positioning.[18] Accomplished by this survey was the establishment of routine projections for all common radiographic procedures and the determination of the most common optional or extra projections taken to better demonstrate specific anatomic parts or pathologic conditions. The routine and optional projections presented in the anatomy chapters of this text conform with these national norms, as documented by Bontrager.[19] The physical reference for all positioning terms used in naming projections is the *anatomic position*.

Anteroposterior, Lateral, and Oblique Projections

The most common projections in routine radiographic assessment of bones and joints are the *anteroposterior (AP), lateral, and oblique projections* (Table 1–1)

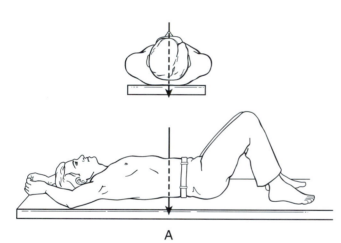

A

Anteroposterior (AP) projection

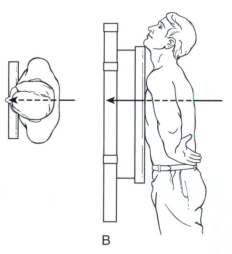

B

Posteroanterior (PA) projection

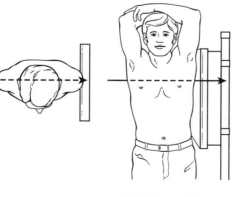

Left lateral projection

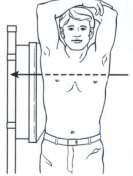

Right lateral projection

C

FIGURE 1–13. Examples of the most common radiographic projections.

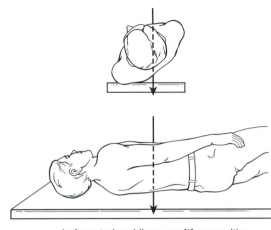

Left posterior oblique **position** resulting
in an AP oblique projection

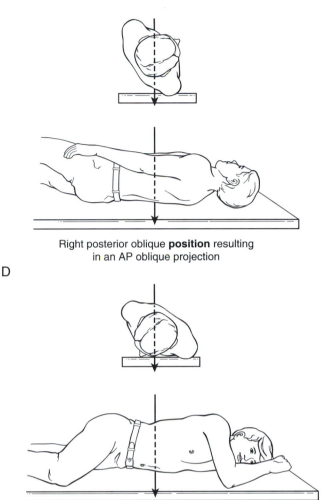

Right posterior oblique **position** resulting
in an AP oblique projection

D

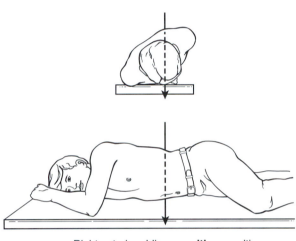

Right anterior oblique **position** resulting
in a PA oblique projection

Left anterior oblique **position** resulting
in an AP oblique projection

E

(Fig. 1–13). As stated previously, at least two radiographs made at right angles are necessary to provide adequate information about the dimensions of a structure. It follows, then, that the routine radiographic assessment of any part of the skeletal system includes at least an AP and a lateral projection. Oblique projections are additionally included in the routine assessment of many joints for the purpose of greater visualization of complex anatomic structures.

An AP projection means the x-ray beam has traveled through the body in an anterior-to-posterior direction. All joints are evaluated by an AP projection, with the exception of the hand.[20] The hand is normally radiographed in a *posteroanterior (PA) projection*. That is, the hand is placed palm down on the film, and the beam is projected through the back of the hand toward the film.

A lateral projection means the x-ray beam has traveled through the body at right angles to the AP or PA projection.[21]

An oblique projection involves rotation of a body part so that the beam traverses the body part at an angle somewhere between the AP and lateral projections.[22] The degree of obliquity varies depending on the anatomic structure being visualized.

The precise positioning of a body part in an AP, lateral, or oblique projection is the responsibility of the radiographer. Accurate positioning guarantees that the body part *will be visualized exactly as planned*. For example, a *true lateral projection* of the cervical spine will directly superimpose the right- and left-side facet joints, allowing clear visualization of the joint surfaces. A correctly positioned *oblique projection* of the cervical spine will permit visualization of the intervertebral foramen of one side of the spine (Fig. 1–14). The opposite is true in the thoracic and lumbar spines, however. In these spinal regions the lateral projection best demonstrates the intervertebral foramina, while the oblique projection best demonstrates the facet joints. See Chapters 5 and 6 for routine radiographs of these spinal regions and Table 1–2 for a summary of these points.

Viewing Radiographs

Radiographs are analyzed on *view boxes*, also called *illuminators*. The radiographs are clipped to the view box surface and illuminated from behind (Fig. 1–15). Additional wattage is used in the form of "hot lights"

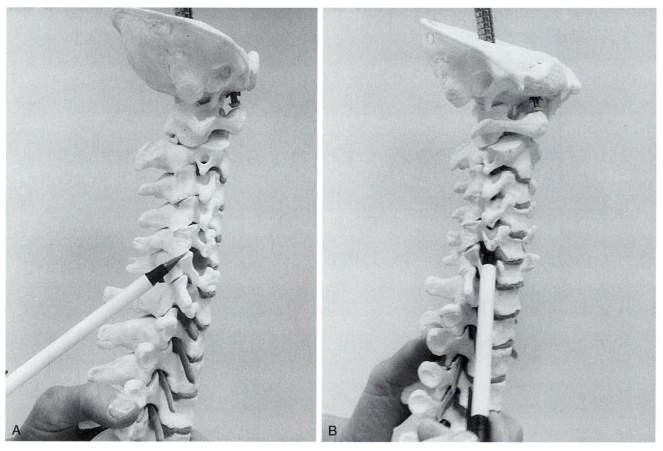

FIGURE 1–14. (*A*) The lateral projection of the cervical spine best demonstrates the *facet joints,* indicated by the point of the pen. (*B*) The oblique projection of the cervical spine best demonstrates the intervertebral foramina. The tip of the pen is the C5–6 right intervertebral foramen.

to focus attention on areas of the image that may not be adequately illuminated on the view box (such as the subacromial region in a routine AP radiograph of the shoulder. See Fig. 1–16).[23]

Because radiographs are transparent, they may be viewed from either side. The custom, however, is to place the radiographs on the view box as if the patient were *facing* the person viewing the films.[24] This is possible with all AP and PA projected radiographs. Lateral radiographs are generally viewed in the same direction that the path of the beam traveled. Radiographs of the hands and feet are usually viewed through their dorsal aspects, with the digits pointing up.

TABLE 1–2 Summary of Radiographic Positions That Best Visualize Intervertebral Foramina Versus Zygapophyseal Joints

	Cervical Spine	Thoracic Spine	Lumbar Spine
Intervertebral foramina	Oblique 45°	Lateral	Lateral
Zygapophyseal (facet joints)	Lateral	Oblique 70°	Oblique 45°

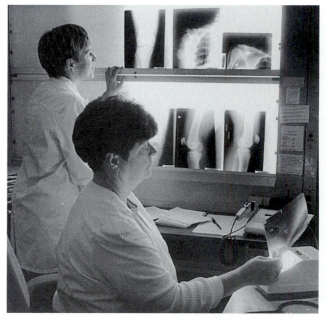

FIGURE 1–15. Radiographs are analyzed on view boxes, also called illuminators. Additional wattage gained from "hot lights" focuses attention on areas that may not be adequately illuminated on the view box.

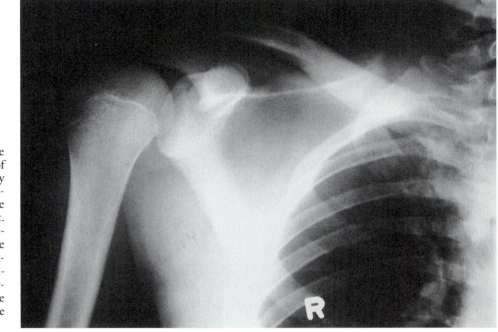

FIGURE 1–16. Because of the varying thicknesses and densities of the body, not all areas of anatomy are adequately exposed on one radiograph. Each radiograph is made to expose the focal area of interest. Thus, in the routine anteroposterior projection of the shoulder, the glenohumeral joint is properly exposed, whereas the acromioclavicular joint is underexposed. In order to adequately demonstrate the acromioclavicular joint, a separate radiograph is made.

Some potentially misused terms in discussing positioning are *projection* and *view*. "Projection" refers to the path of the x-ray beam. "View" is not a positioning term but is used in discussing the radiograph or the image. As a reminder, the patient's *x-rays* are not viewed (x-rays are invisible to the human eye), but rather the patient's *radiographs* or *films* are viewed.

Film Markers

A minimum of two markers are usually imprinted in the emulsion of every radiograph.[25] These are *patient identification* and *anatomic side* markers. Markers are placed on the film during the procedure, rather than afterward, to avoid potential mismarkings.

The patient identification information usually includes the patient's name, age, case number, date, and institution.

The anatomic side markers are radiopaque letters correctly indicating the patient's right or left side of the trunk, or right or left limb. These may be either the words *"right"* or *"left"* or just the initials *"R"* or *"L."* The letters may sometimes appear backward or upside down on the developed films. *Do not* orient the radiograph to obtain a correctly positioned letter. *Always view radiographs as if viewing the patient in anatomic position.* Thus, an AP film of the patient's left lower extremity would be placed on the view box with the fibula on the viewer's righthand side (Fig. 1–17).

Some additional markers that may be used are[26]:

internal or INT: indicates that a limb has been rotated internally.
external or EXT: indicates that a limb has been rotated externally.

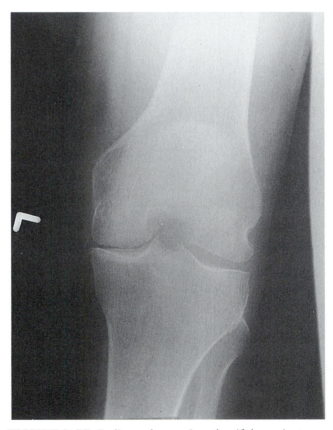

FIGURE 1–17. Radiographs are viewed as if the patient were standing in front of the viewer in anatomic position. This radiograph of the lower extremity is positioned properly. The L marker tells us this is the patient's left leg, so the film is placed on the view box with the fibula to the viewer's right-hand side.

erect or upright: indicates that the patient was vertical for the examination. This may also be indicated by a special mercury ball marker wherein the ball drops down if the patient is upright.

weight bearing or WTB: indicates the patient was standing for the examination.

decubitus or decub: indicates the patient was recumbent.

inspiration (INSP) and expiration (EXP): used in comparison films of the chest indicating the state of respiration.

radiographer's initials: the initials of the radiographer are generally placed on the R or L markers to identify the individual responsible for that examination.

IMAGE QUALITY FACTORS

The factors by which one evaluates the quality of a radiograph are termed *image quality factors*. The four image quality factors are *density, contrast, detail,* and *distortion.*[27] Density and contrast are *photographic properties* that control visibility, whereas detail and distortion are *geometric properties* that control clarity.[28] Although it is the radiographer who monitors the technical aspect of these factors, the viewer too must have an appreciation of how these factors contribute to or alter the image.

Radiographic Density

Radiographic density can be defined as the amount of blackening on the radiograph.[29] The radiographer adjusts radiographic density by varying *milliamperage* and *exposure time,* which regulate the amount of x-rays emitted from the x-ray tube during an exposure. Milliamperage and time are referred to in combination as *milliampere seconds (mAs).* Additionally, *distance* affects radiographic density according to the inverse square law. For example, twice the distance from the beam

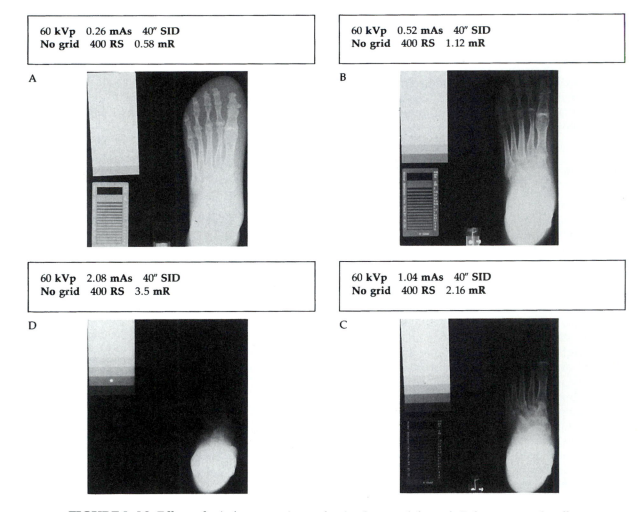

FIGURE 1–18. Effects of mA changes on image density. Images *A* through *D* demonstrate the effect of increasing mAs. Each image is double the density of the previous one. (From Carlton and Adler,[5] p 363, with permission.)

source will reduce density on the film by one fourth. Standard distances are usually used in medical radiography, however, so radiographic density is primarily controlled by mAs. The radiographer uses his or her knowledge of human densities, part thickness, and positioning to select appropriate mAs for each radiograph. An underexposed (too little radiographic density) or overexposed (too much radiographic density) radiograph will not accurately visualize the anatomy being sought (Figs. 1–18, 1–16).

Radiographic Contrast

Radiographic contrast is the difference among various adjacent radiographic densities.[30] Great variation among densities produces high contrast, and less variation produces low contrast. High or low contrast is not necessarily good or bad in itself. The purpose of contrast is to make anatomic detail more visible. So, in a chest radiograph, for example, low contrast is desired to visualize the very fine lung markings and the many shades of gray of the soft tissues of the heart and lungs (Fig. 1–19). In a skeletal film, however, high contrast is often required to clearly visualize cortical margins of bones. The primary controlling factor for contrast is *kilovoltage (kVp)*. The higher the kVp, the greater the energy of the x-ray beam, so that penetration occurs more uniformly through all tissue densities. The result is less variation in tissue absorption and low contrast among the radiographic densities on film. Conversely, the lower the kVp, the greater the variation in tissue absorption and the higher the contrast appears on the film image.

Kilovoltage is also a secondary controlling factor for

density. Higher kVps result in a corresponding overall increase in density, decreasing the need for mAs. The relationship of mAs and kVps is balanced by the radiographer with the goal of reducing patient exposure to radiation while obtaining the best possible results in a radiograph. A general rule states that the highest kVp and lowest mAs that yield sufficient diagnostic information should be used on each radiographic examination.[31]

Recorded Detail

"Recorded detail" is defined as the geometric sharpness or accuracy of the structural lines recorded on the radiograph.[32,33] Recorded detail is also referred to as *definition*, *sharpness*, *resolution*, or simply *detail*. Lack of detail is known as *blur* or *unsharpness*. The primary controlling factor of detail is motion. Motion affects recorded detail because it does not allow sufficient time for an image to form. Unwanted motion may result from voluntary processes such as patient movement or breathing, involuntary processes such as the heartbeat or intestinal peristalsis, or vibration in the equipment (Fig. 1–20).

Other factors influencing detail are the *distances* between the beam source, patient, and film, and the *focal spot (or beam source) size*. X-rays obey the common laws of light and projection, so the variables critical to the projected image are the beam source diameter, the distance between the beam source and patient, and the distance between the beam source and film. These variables are adjusted to reduce as much as possible the geometric blurring of the image. With regard to the effect of distance on positioning, the viewer must be

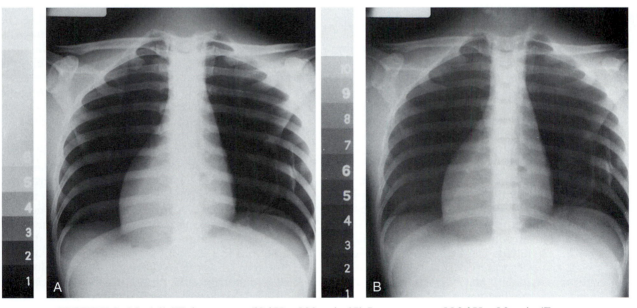

FIGURE 1–19. (*A*) High contrast, 50 kVp, 800 mA. (*B*) Low contrast, 110 kVp, 10 mA. (From Bontrager,[3] p 33 , with permission.)

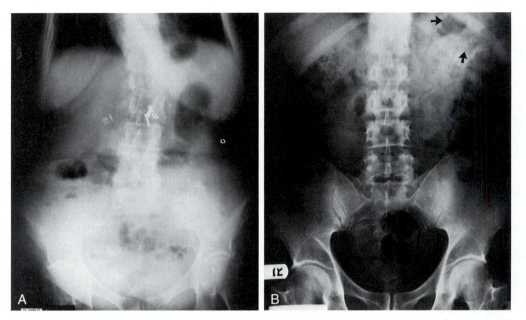

FIGURE 1–20. (*A*) Voluntary motion caused by breathing. (*B*) Involuntary motion from peristaltic action in the upper left abdomen. (From Boutrager,[3] p 34, with permission.)

aware that the *closer an object is to the film plate, the more sharply it is defined*. The chest radiograph, for example, is routinely done in a *PA* projection because the lungs are located more anterior in the thorax, so this projection will place the lungs closest to the film plate. The lumbar spine, however, is routinely projected in an *AP* direction, as this places the patient's spine closest to the film plate. Additionally, the *portions* of the spine closest to the film are most sharply defined, so the spinous processes are imaged with greatest clarity.

Radiographic Distortion

Radiographic distortion is the difference between the actual object being examined and its recorded image. This misrepresentation can be classified as either *size* or *shape* distortion (Fig. 1–21).[34,35] Size distortion involves both elongation and foreshortening of the image. The primary factors controlling distortion are the distances between beam source, patient, and film, the alignment of the body, and the position of the *central ray*.

With regard to distance, it has been common practice to use 40 inches as the distance between the beam source and the film in most skeletal radiographs. The other critical distance, that between the beam source and the particular structure in the patient being examined, varies. A calculation between these two distances gives the *magnification factor* of the image. Magnification is equal to the beam source–film distance divided by the beam source–patient distance. This means *the closer a structure is to the film plate,*

the less magnification distortion occurs and the better the detail. In viewing a radiograph and attempting to perceptually reconstruct the third dimension of depth, one must realize that subtle blurring and magnification indicate that this portion of the structure is brought forward out of the plane of the film, closer to the viewer, and sharp clarity indicates the portion of the structure farthest away from the viewer (Fig. 1–22).

Shape distortion results from unequal magnification of the structure being examined. The projected structure may appear *elongated*, of greater length and larger than the actual structure, or *foreshortened*, shorter than the actual structure and reduced in size (Fig. 1–23). Although adjustments are made to minimize distortion, the irregular planes of the skeleton, the distance between the skeleton and the film, and the divergence of the beam always permit some degree of shape distortion to occur. The concept of beam divergence is basic to understanding how this distortion is created. Like projected light, x-rays emitted from the narrow focal spot diverge outward in straight lines to the patient and the film. *Only at the central ray, the portion of the beam striking the structure and film perpendicularly, is the image accurate*. The farther from the central ray, the greater the distortion, because of increases in the angles of divergence. Additionally, the more inclined the structure, the greater the distortion. To diminish distortion, the radiographer centers the central ray over the area of interest and positions the body as parallel to the film as possible. Correct body alignment results in less distortion and more "open" joint spaces. That is, the joint space itself is visualized and not superimposed by overlapping bone ends.

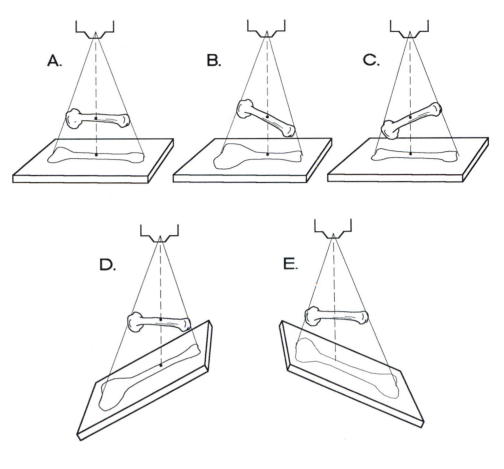

FIGURE 1–21. Foreshortening and magnification caused by anatomic part and image receptor alignment. (*A*) Normal relationship between part and image receptor. (*B,C*) Foreshortening and magnification caused by changes in anatomic part alignment. (*D,E*) Elongation and magnification caused by changes in part/image receptor and central ray/image receptor alignment. (From Carlton and Adler,[5] p 422, with permission.)

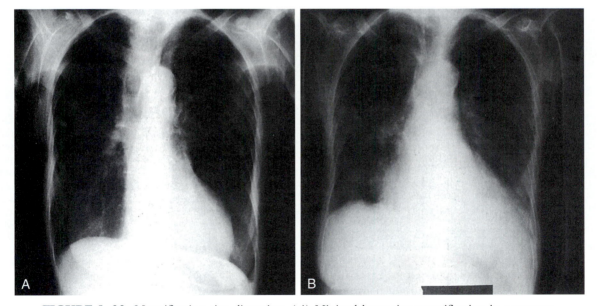

FIGURE 1–22. Magnification size distortion. (*A*) Minimal heart size magnification in a posteroanterior chest radiograph. (*B*) An anteroposterior projection of the same patient demonstrating greater heart size magnification. (From Carlton and Adler,[5] p 424, with permission.)

60 kVp	15 mAs	72″ SID
No grid	100 RS	11.9 mR

60 kVp	15 mAs	72″ SID
No grid	100 RS	11.9 mR

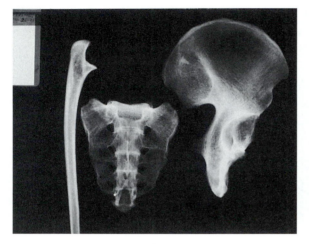

A

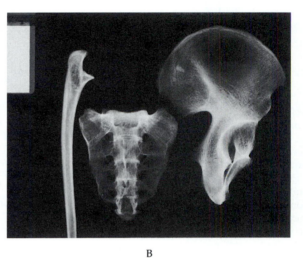

B

60 kVp	15 mAs	72″ SID
No grid	100 RS	11.9 mR

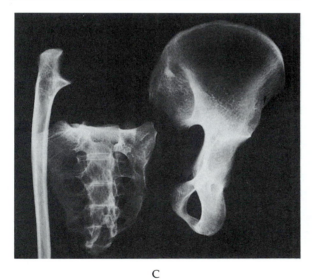

C

FIGURE 1–23. Shape distortion. (*A*), This radiograph was taken with a central ray perpendicular and centered to the center of the film. (*B*), This radiograph was taken with a central ray perpendicular to but off-centered to the left (away from the pelvis). The effect on distortion is not significant; however, changes in the image appearance are evident, particularly when studying the pelvis, which was farthest from the central ray. (*C*), This radiograph was taken with a central ray angle of 25 degrees and centered to the center of the film. Notice the significant distortion created by angling the central ray. (From Carlton and Adler,[5] p 425, with permission.)

OTHER COMMON IMAGING STUDIES IN ORTHOPEDIC RADIOLOGY

The develpment of new imaging modalities in recent years has expanded the armamentarium of the radiologist. The sometimes difficult process of diagnosis has been greatly facilitated by these advances in technology. This rapid progress, however, has made the determination of the *best* diagnostic protocol for an individual patient increasingly complex. Each imaging study differs in tissue specific sensitivity, structural clarity, radiation exposure, invasiveness, risk, and cost (Table 1–3). Thus, the *choice* of modality and the *sequence* in which additional imaging studies are performed are important to efficiently obtain a comprehensive diagnosis, without redundant or extraneous studies being performed (Fig. 1–24).[36,37]

The orthopedic radiologist first attempts to diagnose an *unknown* musculoskeletal disorder with plain-film routine projections and other special projections and techniques of *conventional radiography*, before employing costlier, more invasive, or riskier modalities. It is important to re-emphasize that plain-film radiography remains the most effective means of demonstrating bone and joint abnormalities.[38] Additional modalities are subsequently employed if conventional radiography is inconclusive. Once the diagnosis is *known*, additional modalities may also be used to dem-

TABLE 1–3 Common Imaging Examinations, Their Cost, and Their Radiation Dosage

Examination	Costs: Professional and Technician Time	Radiation Dose, Average
Plain film series lumbar spine	$250	2000–3000 MR
PF knee	$161	50–100 MR
Contrast arthrogram knee	$716	50–100 MR
Myelography lumbar spine	$1100	2500 MR
Conventional tomography		
knee	$438	2000 MR
Lumbar spine	$438	8000–10,000 MR
Computed tomography		
knee	$923	2000–4000 MR
Lumbar spine	$970	200–400 MR
MRI		
knee (avg)	$1000	No radiation
Lumbar spine	$1000	No radiation
Bone scan (Technetium) Whole skeleton	$581	20–25 millicuries

*Average 1996 hospital costs for technical & professional charges. From correspondence—North Hills Passavant Hospital, Pittsburgh, PA. MR = millirads

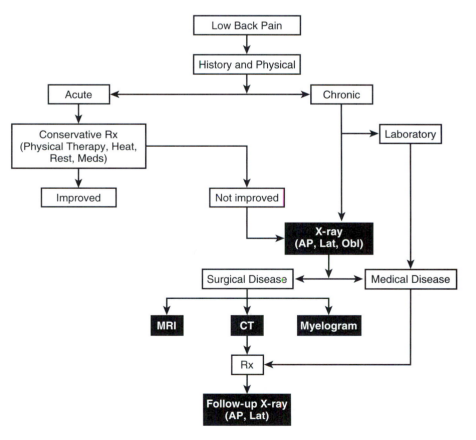

FIGURE 1–24. Algorithm for evaluation of low back pain. The clinical, laboratory, and/or imaging findings will determine the next step. Imaging studies are highlighted. (Adapted from Daffner, 1993, p 28.)

onstrate the exact location of the lesion, to identify the distribution of the lesion in the skeleton, to gain pertinent information for the surgeon, or to monitor the response of the lesion to medical intervention.[39]

The role of the radiologist and the other clinicians involved in the patient's care is not minimized by the sophistication of modern imaging modalities. Technology is not infallible; false-negative and false-positive results will occur. *It is the clinician's responsibility to recognize that if the results of any imaging study do not fit the physical findings, further clinical evaluation and diagnostic investigation are warranted.*

Common imaging modalities in orthopedic radiology other than plain-film radiography are *contrast-enhanced radiography* and *conventional tomography*, which are modifications of conventional radiography, *computed tomography (CT)*, *nuclear imaging*, and *magnetic resonance imaging (MRI)*. A brief description and an ex-

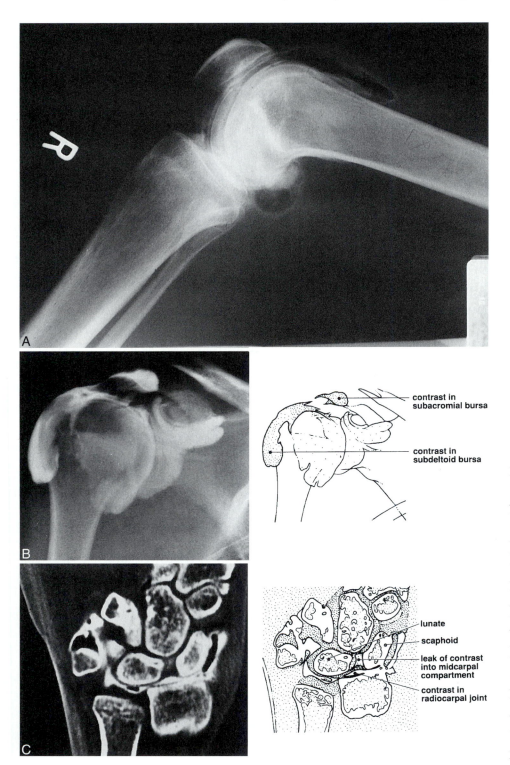

FIGURE 1–25. Examples of *contrast media* studies of synovial joints. (*A*) Negative contrast study of the knee. Note that the full extent of the capsule is illustrated as it is distended with contrast. (*B*) Shoulder arthrogram. After injection of contrast into the glenohumeral joint, there is filling of the subacromial-subdeltoid bursae complex, indicating rotator cuff tear. (From Greenspan,[2] p 2.5, with permission.) (*C*) Coronal computer tomography (CT) arthrogram of the wrist demonstrates a subtle leak of contrast from the radiocarpal joint through a tear in the scapholunate ligament, a finding not detected on routine arthrographic examination of the wrist. (From Greenspan,[2] p 2.6, with permission.)

planation of the capabilities and limitations of these modalities specific to the area of orthopedic radiology follow.

Contrast-Enhanced Radiographs[40,41]

In contrast-enhanced radiography, a *contrast medium* is injected into the body prior to taking a radiograph. The purpose of contrast-enhanced studies is to improve visualization by increasing radiographic contrast in areas with minimal inherent contrast. Contrast media may be radiolucent (negative contrast), radiopaque (positive contrast), or a combination of the two (dual contrast). The process may be monitored by fluoroscopy, which allows dynamic radiographic imaging of the contrast medium in the body and is recorded either on conventional radiographic film or similar fluoroscopic spot film. Two types of contrast studies are *arthrography* and *myelography*.

ARTHROGRAPHY

Arthrography[42,43] is a contrast-media study of the synovial joints and related soft tissue structures. Contrast material is injected into the joint space, distending the capsule and outlining internal tissues. Arthrography is frequently used in the evaluation of the shoulder, elbow, wrist, knee, and ankle joints (Fig. 1–25). Arthrography effectively demonstrates rotator cuff tears and adhesive capsulitis at the shoulder, osteochondritis dissecans and articular cartilage abnormalities at the elbow, and triangular fibrocartilage complex tears at the wrist. Arthrography at the knee can demonstrate meniscal tears, synovial abnormalities, ligamentous tears, osteochondral fractures, osteochondritis dissecans, and joint capsule abnormalities.

Arthrography is also used in conjunction with other advanced imaging modalities to provide more information than is possible on conventional radiographs. Examples of this include *arthrotomography*, *CT-arthrography*, and *digital subtraction arthrography*.

MYELOGRAPHY

Myelography[44–46] is a contrast-media study of the spinal cord, nerve root, and dura mater (Fig. 1–26). Contrast is injected into the subarachnoid space and mixes with the cerebrospinal fluid to produce a column of radiopaque fluid. The table on which the patient is positioned is tilted until the contrast flows under the influence of gravity to the specific spinal level being evaluated. Myelograms are imaged via radiographs; it is also common to perform a CT scan while the contrast is still localized in order to visualize greater anatomic detail in cross-section. This combination of modalities is referred to as a *CT myelogram*. Abnormal results of a myelogram may reveal a ruptured intervertebral disc, spinal cord compression, spi-

nal stenosis, intravertebral tumor, obstruction in the spinal canal, or nerve root injury.

Arthrography and myelography are valuable diagnostic tools, assisting in clinical decision making primarily when determining the need for surgical intervention. Some limitations in these modalities are that they are invasive and pose a certain amount of risk to the patient, anatomic detail may vary in clarity, and the recorded image does not visualize the third dimension of depth. For these reasons, contrast studies have been replaced in some areas of clinical practice by CT and MRI.

Conventional Tomography[47,48]

Conventional tomography is the radiographic evaluation of one predetermined plane of the body (Fig. 1–27). Structures above and below the plane of interest are blurred out. This is accomplished by accessory equipment that allows the x-ray tube and film to move about a fulcrum point during a film exposure. The plane of the body that is level with the fulcrum will be

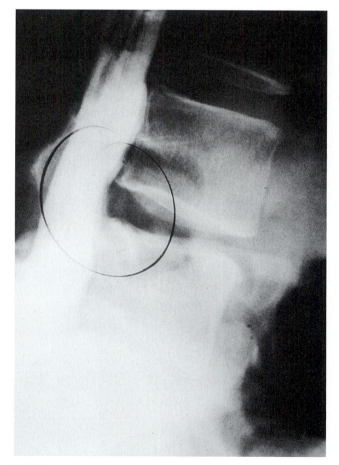

FIGURE 1–26. Myelogram of the lumbar spine. Contrast injected into the subarachnoid space mixes with cerebral spinal fluid to produce a column of radiopaque fluid. The *herniated disc at L4–5* protrudes posteriorly and causes an indentation of the column.

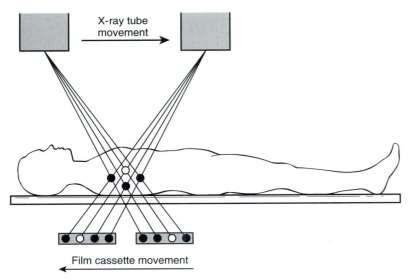

FIGURE 1–27. Principle of conventional tomography. The x-ray tube and the film move in opposite directions. The focal point (open circle) remains in sharp focus, whereas the other planes of the body (dark circles) are blurred by motion. (Adapted from Daffner,[8] p 25.)

in focus, with the rest of the body blurred by motion. Various *depths* of planes are imaged by preadjusting the fulcrum.

A major clinical application of tomography is in the evaluation of fractures (Fig. 1–28). Fractures of irregularly shaped bones such as the skull, the tibial plateau of the knee, or the cervical vertebrae may be difficult to visualize on plain films because of the depth of the structure or the amount of superimposition of adjacent structures. By imaging different depths of the bone, the extent of the fracture line can be determined. Additionally, tomography is used to assess healing of fractures. Whereas signs of healing may be obliterated on plain films by metallic fixation devices or callus formation, tomography can image *under* these obstructions. Other clinical applications include evaluating the extent of tumors within bone (Fig. 1–29).

A limitation of conventional tomography is that it cannot enhance detail; it is a process of controlled blur-

ring. Patient and equipment motion variables can easily alter the image quality. Other disadvantages are insufficient soft tissue detail and difficulty positioning a traumatized patient for various angles of projection. For these reasons, conventional tomography has, in some areas of clinical practice, been replaced by CT.

Computed Tomography[49,50]

Computed tomography merges x-ray technology with that of the computer. In CT the x-ray beam and detector system is housed in a circular scanner and moves through an arc of 360 degrees about the patient. The tissues absorb various levels of radiation according to their densities, and the detector system measures and transmits this information to the computer. The computer mathematically reconstructs an image based on the geometric plots where the measurements were taken. Each image represents an axial cross-sectional slice of the body measuring 0.3 to 1.5 cm thick (Fig. 1–30). By viewing a consecutive series of axial slices, the clinician can evaluate the dimensions of a structure. Additionally, the latest advances in computer software make it possible for the computer itself to reconstruct multiplanar and 3-D images of a structure (Fig. 1–31). CT images are displayed on television screens, are recorded on magnetic tape on discs, and may further be photographed or recorded on x-ray film.

CT can be described as an anatomic technique; it provides geography of body structures with much greater sensitivity than plain films. This is achieved by computer enhancement and magnification of subtle chemical and density differences that are present in similar tissues. The shades of gray (or color) on a CT image are assigned by the computer specific to each tissue's exact radiation absorption properties. In comparison, a plain-film radiograph images all soft tissues cartilage, organs, and vessels in the approximately same water-density shade of gray.

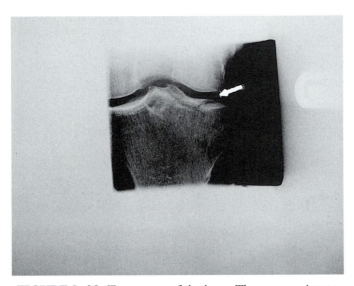

FIGURE 1–28. Tomogram of the knee. The arrow points to a tibial plateau fracture.

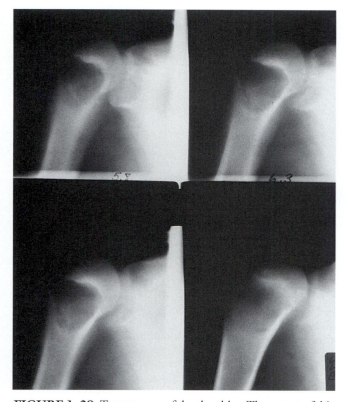

FIGURE 1–29. Tomograms of the shoulder. The extent of this chondroblastoma of the proximal humerus of a 15-year-old girl is evaluated by imaging successive depths through the bone. Numbers marked on the films (e.g., 5.8, 6.3) refer to millimeters of depth.

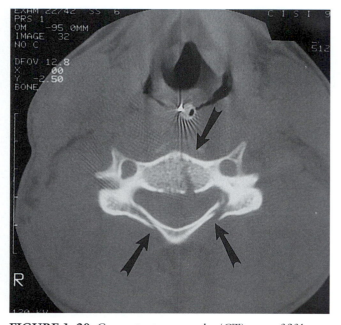

FIGURE 1–30. Computer tomography (CT) scan of fifth cervical vertebrae. This axial view of C5 demonstrates a burst fracture of the vertebral body and both lamina.

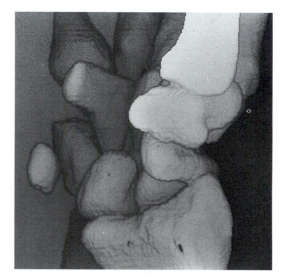

FIGURE 1–31. Three-dimensional CT reformation of the wrist. This oblique view of the wrist demonstrates a fracture through the waist of the scaphoid bone, complicated by avascular necrosis of the proximal fragment. (From Greenspan,[2] p 2.4, with permission.)

CT is valuable in the evaluation of various bone and soft tissue tumors, subtle or complex fractures, intra-articular abnormalities, the detection of small bone fragments, and quantitative bone mineral analysis important in the management of osteoporosis and other metabolic bone disorders. Some disadvantages of CT include the so-called average volume effect, which refers to the computer applying average values to a small volume of homogeneous tissue, and thus displaying it in one shade of gray. This becomes important when normal and pathologic processes interface within a tissue (Fig. 1–32). Despite the ability of CT to discriminate among subtle density differences, precise histologic differences are not visualized. So, for example, a tumor within soft tissue may not be visualized. Furthermore, patient movement or metal implants will produce significant artifacts, and some examinations incur high radiation doses.

Nuclear Imaging

RADIONUCLIDE BONE SCAN[51,52]

Nuclear imaging involves the diagnostic use of radioactive isotopes. A *radionuclide bone scan* is a nuclear imaging test of the skeletal system. Radiopharmaceuticals that are tissue-specific to bone are injected intravenously. The patient is placed under a *scintillation camera*, which detects the distribution of radioactivity in the body and records the image on x-ray film. Thus, this modality is also referred to as *scintigraphy*.

Radiopharmaceuticals concentrate differently in normal versus pathologic bone. Information is gained by viewing where and how much the radiopharma-

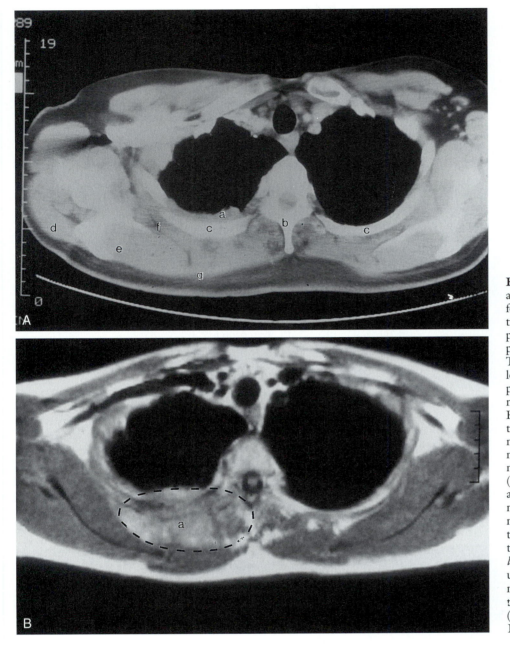

FIGURE 1–32. (*A*) Transverse axial CT image at the level of fourth thoracic vertebra. The patient was a retired coal miner. Note pleural thickening caused by occupational hazards in the left lung (a). The patient's chief complaint was left scapular and radiating left upper extremity pain. This image is negative for pathologic disease. See Figure 1–32*B* for further evaluation results. Note (b) vertebral spinous process, (c) rib, (d) infraspinatus muscle, (e) supraspinatus muscle, (f) subscapularis muscle, (g) trapezius. (From Richardson and Iglarsh, 1994, p 685, with permission.) (*B*) Transverse axial magnetic resonance image (MRI) at the level of the fourth thoracic vertebra. Note the large expanse of *lung tumor* invading the subscapularis muscle (a). This tumor was not detectable on the CT scan of the same patient in Figure 1–32*A*. (From Richardson and Iglarsh, 1994, p 685, with permission.)

ceuticals have concentrated in the body. Abnormal conditions generally show an *increased* uptake of the radiopharmaceuticals and image as *black areas* or *"hot spots"* on the scan. Normal bone appears transparent and gray, with the exception of some structures that under normal conditions do show increased uptake (e.g., the growth plates in children or the sacroiliac joints. In general, a bone scan designates areas of *hyperfunction*, or *increased mineral turnover* (Fig. 1–33).

A bone scan is best described as a sensitivity test, an early indicator of bone activity. Bone scans are most valuable in confirming the presence of disease and demonstrating the distribution of disease in the skeleton much earlier than possible on plain films or tomography. Indications for bone scans include the evaluation of subtle fractures, primary and metastatic

tumors, various arthritides, infections, avascular necrosis, metabolic bone disease, or any *unexplained bone pain*.

The major limitation of bone scans is the lack of specificity in the differential diagnosis of disease. It is not possible to distinguish among the various processes that can cause increased uptake. Thus, a bone scan is not useful as an independent study; rather, the results of other clinical evaluations are correlated with the bone scan to determine a diagnosis.

Magnetic Resonance Imaging[53,54]

Magnetic resonance imaging does not involve ionizing radiation; it produces information via the inter-

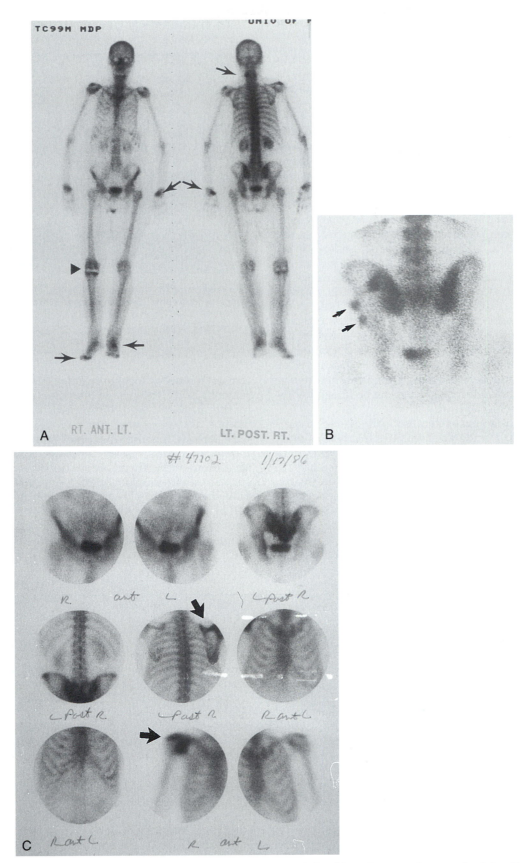

FIGURE 1–33. (A) Whole skeleton bone scan. Diagnosis for this patient was degenerative joint disease in multiple sites (see arrows indicating increased uptake in the cervical spine, wrist, ankle, and toes). The arrowhead indicates a total joint prosthesis at the knee. (B) Bone scan of the pelvis. This patient suffered a contusion to the gluteus medius muscle during injury in a football game. In this case the increased uptake was an early indication of myositis ossificans developing in the muscle. (From Richardson and Iglarsh, 1994, p 684, with permission.) (C) This bone scan shows increased uptake at the right scapula and right shoulder area. In this case these findings demonstrated the increased bone activity associated with Paget's disease. (From Richardson and Iglarsh, 1994, p 646, with permission.)

action of tissue with radiofrequencies in a magnetic field. The image obtained is based on a patient's re-emission of absorbed radiofrequencies while in the magnetic field.

The process begins with the patient positioned in a scanner containing magnetic field coils, radiowave transmitters, and radiowave receivers. In the magnetic field, previously random atomic nuclei align themselves with the field. These nuclei are not static but spin around parallel axes at frequencies specific to their tissue type. Radiowaves are pulsed to the patient at this frequency and are absorbed by the nuclei; this transfer of energy induces *resonance* among the nuclei. Different tissues resonate at different frequencies, and this is the basis for how tissues are identified on the final image. When the radiowaves are turned off, all the nuclei relax into their random patterns and release the resonant energy they had absorbed. Radio receivers pick up the energy the tissues emit in the form of radiowaves and transmit them to the computer. Through complex calculations an image is constructed and displayed on screen, then photographed and recorded on x-ray film. The images obtained from MRI are not limited to one plane of the body. Multiple views can be imaged without moving the patient.

The musculoskeletal system is ideally suited to evaluation by MRI. The signal intensities from bone, muscle, articular cartilage, fibrocartilage, ligaments, tendons, vessels, nerves, and fat differ sufficiently to create high-quality images of anatomy. Additionally, pathologic changes in different tissues can be highlighted through contrast manipulation. Thus, major uses of MRI in orthopedic radiology are in the evaluation of soft tissue trauma and tumors (Fig. 1–34).

Contraindications to MRI include the presence of

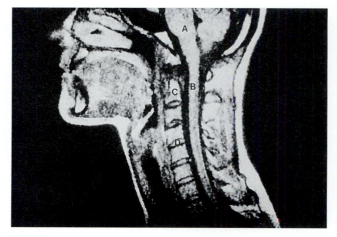

FIGURE 1–34. Magnetic resonance image of the cervical spine, sagittal view. No pathology is evident. Note cerebellum (a), spinal cord (b), marrow of C2 vertebral body and dense (c), intervertebral disc of C4–5 (d).

ferrous metals or mechanical devices implanted in the patient's body; these have the potential to be disrupted by the magnetic field. Orthopedic appliances such as fixation devices or total joint components are not made with ferrous metal and are not contraindications, although they may distort the image if near the area of investigation. Furthermore, various patient conditions such as claustrophobia, obesity, or severe pain can prohibit the use of MRI, which requires the patient to lie still in a small space for an average of 1 hour per study. Recent modifications in scanners addressed these problems, and open-type designs are now coming into use.

SUMMARY OF KEY POINTS

1. A radiograph is an x-ray film containing an image of an anatomic part. A plain-film or conventional radiograph designates a radiograph made without contrast enhancement or other modifications.

2. Plain-film radiography is the first-order diagnostic study to be done following the clinical examination. Plain films are the most effective means of demonstrating a bone or joint abnormality. The results of plain-film studies direct treatment or nontreatment of the patient, or serve as a departure point for additional studies that may be necessary to complete the diagnosis.

3. The gray images on the radiograph represent the sum of the radiodensities of the structures that the x-ray beam has passed through. Radiodensity is determined by a structure's material composition and its thickness.

4. The human body has four inherent radiodensities: air, fat, water, and bone. When radiographed, four distinct radiographic densities, or shades of gray, are apparent. Identification of structures is based on the analysis of the contrast between these different densities.

5. An inverse relationship exists between the amount of radiodensity of an object and the amount of blackening on film. Air images the blackest. Fat, water, and bone image in progressively lighter shades of gray. Contrast media such as barium image in bright white outline, heavy metals in prosthetic devices image solidly white.

6. At least two images, as close to 90 degrees to each other as possible, are required to view all three dimensions of a structure. Remember the old adage "one view is no view."
7. Routine projections or the basic series of films made to evaluate a body segment consist of a standardized selection of positions and projections chosen to provide the greatest visualization with minimal radiation exposure. AP, lateral, and oblique projections comprise most routine series.
8. The quality of a radiograph is evaluated by four image quality factors: density, contrast, detail, and distortion.
9. Diagnosis of unknown musculoskeletal disorders is first attempted with plain films and techniques of conventional radiography. When further investigation is needed, the selection of modalities and order in which they are performed is chosen to most efficiently obtain a comprehensive diagnosis without extraneous or redundant studies being done. The radiologist considers tissue specific sensitivity, structural clarity, radiation exposure, invasiveness, risk, and cost when planning the diagnostic investigation.
10. It is wise for all clinicians to remember that no matter how sophisticated medical imaging becomes, technology is not infallible. The clinician's responsibility is to recognize that if the results of any imaging study do not fit the physical findings, further clinical evaluation and diagnostic investigation is warranted.

REFERENCES

1. Clayton, CL (ed): Taber's Cyclopedic Medical Dictionary, ed 17. FA Davis, Philadelphia, 1993.
2. Greenspan, A: Orthopedic Radiology: A Practical Approach, ed 2. Raven Press, New York, 1992, p 2.1.
3. Bontrager, KL: Textbook of Radiographic Positioning and Related Anatomy, ed 3. Mosby, St Louis, 1993, p 14.
4. Weissman, B and Sledge, CB: Orthopedic Radiology. WB Saunders, Philadelphia, 1986, p 1.
5. Carlton, R and Adler, A: Principles of Radiographic Imaging. Delmar Publishers, Albany, NY, 1992, p 140.
6. Ibid, p 236.
7. Squire, LF and Novelline, RA: Fundamentals of Radiology, ed 4. Harvard University Press, Cambridge, MA, 1988, p 10.
8. Daffner, RH: Clinical Radiology: The Essentials. Williams & Wilkins, Baltimore, 1993, p 4.
9. Ibid.
10. Carlton, p 237.
11. Squire, p 7.
12. Ibid, p 10.
13. Carlton, p 222.
14. Squire, p 12.
15. Carlton, p 222.
16. Squire, p 10.
17. Swain, JH: An Introduction to Radiology of the Lumbar Spine: Orthopedic Physical Therapy Home Study Course 94-1. © 1994 Orthopaedic Section, APTA, Inc, p 2.
18. Bontrager, p xi.
19. Ibid, pp 15.
20. Ibid, p 15.
21. Ibid, p 18.
22. Ibid, p 17.
23. Swain, p 2.
24. Squire, p 13.
25. Bontrager, p 31.
26. Ibid.
27. Ibid, pp 32–37.
28. Carlton, p 398.
29. Bontrager, p 32.
30. Ibid, p 33.
31. Ibid.
32. Ibid, p 34.
33. Carlton, p 398.
34. Bontrager, p 35.
35. Carlton, p 413.
36. Daffner, p 27.
37. Greenspan, p 2.1.
38. Ibid.
39. Ibid, p 1.1.

40. Daffner, p 10.
41. Bontrager, p 668.
42. Greenspan, p 25.
43. Bontrager, p 668.
44. Ibid, p 674.
45. Greenspan, p 2.6.
46. Ibid, p. 2.8.
47. Daffner, p 16.
48. Bontrager, p 670.
49. Greenspan, p 2.3.
50. Daffner, p 14.
51. Ibid, p 17.
52. Greenspan, p 27.
53. Daffner, p 21.
54. Greenspan, p 2.11.

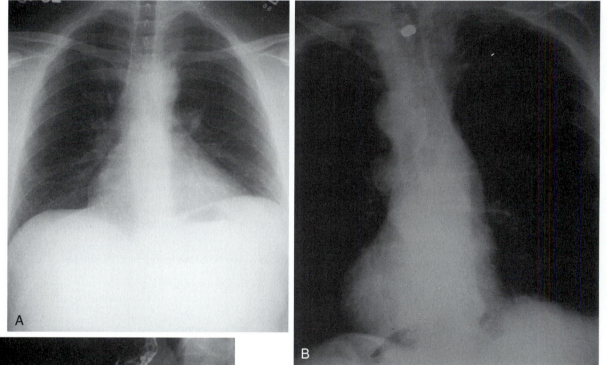

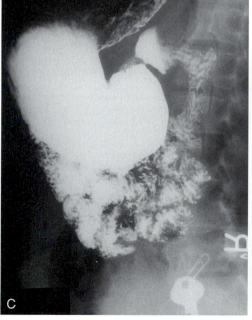

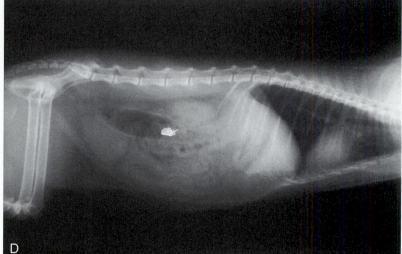

SELF-TEST

Chapter 1

REGARDING FILM A:

1. Is <u>high</u> or <u>low radiographic contrast</u> evident between the soft tissues and bones?
2. Based on the type of radiographic contrast that was produced, do you think this film is intended to be a <u>chest film</u> or an <u>AP thoracic spine film</u>?
3. Is the film <u>positioned correctly</u> for viewing? What anatomic structure verifies this?

REGARDING FILM B:

4. Is this film <u>positioned correctly</u> for viewing? Why or why not?

5. Note the <u>foreign object</u>. What is its likely <u>material composition</u>?
6. Can you determine <u>where</u> in the patient's anatomy this object is located? Why or why not?

REGARDING FILM C:

7. Identify this <u>imaging study</u>.
8. What <u>mistake</u> was made during the radiographic examination?

REGARDING FILM D:

9. Use your knowledge of <u>form</u> to identify this common domestic pet. Hint—This lateral projection demonstrates a long flexible spine, tail, and small pelvis.
10. Use your knowledge of <u>radiographic densities</u> to infer why the pet's owner is distraught.

CHAPTER 2

Radiographic Evaluation of Normal Versus Pathologic Bone

Prerequisite to comprehending the radiographic appearance of abnormal skeletal conditions is a foundation in the growth and development of normal bone. Once the architecture of normal bone and its relative radiographic image are known, the destructive and reparative processes resulting from disease states can be identified. Each pathologic process has characteristic radiologic hallmarks, and evaluation of these variations from normal leads to diagnosis.

The goals of this chapter are to (1) review the growth and development of bone, (2) present a systematic approach to the radiographic evaluation of bones and joints, (3) identify the six pathologic categories of skeletal disease, (4) allow the clinician to become familiar with the 11 radiographic predictor variables that lead to specific diagnosis of a bone or joint lesion, and (5) help the clinician to recognize the radiographic characteristics of some common pathologic processes.

GENERAL ANATOMY[1,2]

Bone can be considered from two different perspectives. As an *anatomic structure*, bone provides the architectural framework that protects vital organs, serves as a leverage system for muscles, and allows for func-

tional movement. As a *physiologic organ*, bone stores reserves of calcium, phosphorus, magnesium, and sodium and contains the marrow that produces erythrocytes, granular leukocytes, and platelets.

The 206 bones of the skeleton are varied in shape and are designated as long bones, short bones, flat bones, irregular bones, sesamoid bones, and accessory

TABLE 2–1 General Characteristics of Joints

Joints are classified into five types:

1. *Syndesmotic*—Two bones are bound by fibrous connective tissue. An example is the distal tibiofibular joint.
2. *Synchondrodial*—Two bones are bound together by cartilage. An example is the temporary epiphyseal plate.
3. *Synostotic*—The joint has been obliterated by bony union across the joint space. All synchondroses of growing bones eventually fuse, as do some syndesmoses.
4. *Symphyseal*—Two bones with articulating hyaline cartilage are bound tightly by dense fibrous connective tissue. The best example is the pubic symphysis.
5. *Synovial*—Two bones with articulating hyaline cartilage are nutritionally supported by synovial fluid and peripherally encased by the joint capsule. The inner layer of the capsule specializes into the synovial membrane, while the outer layer differentiates into fibrous tissue that blends with stabilizing ligaments and anchors to bone.

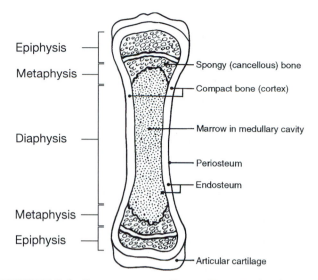

Epiphysis

Metaphysis

— Spongy (cancellous) bone

— Compact bone (cortex)

Diaphysis

— Marrow in medullary cavity

— Periosteum

— Endosteum

Metaphysis

Epiphysis

— Articular cartilage

FIGURE 2–1. Gross structure of bone. (From Richardson and Iglarsh,[9] p 638, with permission.

or supernumerary bones. The articulations or joints of the skeleton are classified as synovial, symphysis, synostosis, synchondrosis, and syndesmosis (Table 2–1).

The gross structure of bone exists in two forms: *compact bone* and *spongy bone*. Dense compact bone forms the outer shell of bone and is called the *cortex*. Spongy bone, also called *cancellous* bone, forms the inner aspect of bone, except for that tubular space that is the *medullary* or *marrow cavity* (Fig. 2–1).

The *periosteum* is a specialized dense fibrous tissue, containing blood vessels, nerves, and lymphatics, which envelops the cortex. The *endosteum* lines the inner aspect of the cortex and medullary cavity. Both

of these tissues have osteogenic properties in the maturing skeleton and also in response to fracture healing.

The *diaphysis, metaphysis,* and *epiphysis* are the shaft, flared expanse, and end of bone, respectively.

GROWTH AND DEVELOPMENT OF BONE[3,4]

Bone is a specialized type of connective tissue originating from the pluripotential cell mass of primitive mesoderm.[5] Beginning at the fifth week of embryonic life, mesenchymal cells become condensed in the form of short cylinders in each of the fetal limb buds. By the sixth week, cells have differentiated to form a cartilage model of future bone, and by the seventh week the process of ossification begins. Bone continues to grow and develop by two methods: endochondral and intramembranous ossification (Fig. 2–2).

Endochondral ossification is the replacement of the cartilage model by calcified bone. This transformation takes place at one or more ossific regions called *primary* and *secondary centers of ossification*. Primary centers of ossification are located in the center of newly developing bone, and ossification advances out toward each end of the cartilage model. The secondary centers of ossification are located at the cartilaginous ends or epiphyses of bone. The epiphysis is separated from the metaphysis by a cartilaginous *epiphyseal plate*, which provides growth in *length* of bone by *interstitial* growth of cartilage cells. At birth a secondary center of ossification is present in the large distal femoral epiphysis, but other secondary centers appear at varying ages after birth, from infancy through puberty.

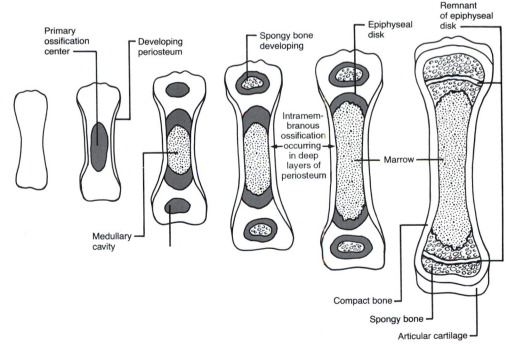

Primary ossification center

Developing periosteum

Spongy bone developing

Epiphyseal disk

Remnant of epiphyseal disk

Intramembranous ossification occurring in deep layers of periosteum

Marrow

Medullary cavity

Compact bone

Spongy bone

Articular cartilage

FIGURE 2–2. Schematic of the processes of endochondral and intramembranous bone growth and ossification. (From Richardson and Iglarsh,[9] p 638.)

In intramembranous ossification there is no intermediate cartilaginous phase; bone is formed directly from the deep layer of the periosteum. This direct appositional growth results in growth of bone *width*. Simultaneously, the endosteum acts to resorb bone, forming a larger medullary cavity in the growing bone.

REMODELING OF BONE[6]

Remodeling of bone occurs continuously during longitudinal growth. As the epiphysis moves progressively further away from the shaft, the metaphysis is remodeled by the simultaneous action of *osteoblastic cells* depositing bone on one surface and *osteoclastic cells* resorbing bone on another surface. In a growing child, bone deposition far exceeds bone resorption, and the body is in a state of *positive bone balance*. By contrast, in later life bone deposition cannot keep pace with bone resorption, and the elderly are thus in a state of *negative bone balance*.

Remodeling occurs constantly at different levels throughout life. Similar to other living tissues, bone maintains itself by undergoing the simultaneous processes of destruction and regeneration. Associated with this continual breakdown and rebuilding is an *adaptive* remodeling of bone in response to the *functional* demands placed on it.

Wolff's Law[7–9]

The phenomenon of remodeling related to function is generally referred to as *Wolff's law*. Put forth by Julius Wolff in 1892, this far-reaching principle states that "Every change in the form and the function of bones, or in their function alone, is followed by certain definite changes in their internal architecture, and equally definite changes in their external conformation, in accordance with mathematical laws."[10] To paraphrase, *bone is deposited in sites subjected to stress, and bone cells will align in such a way as to most efficiently withstand stress* (Fig. 2–3).

Increased physical stresses imposed on bone, either by the forces of weight-bearing or the forces of tension from muscles and other soft tissues, cause an acceleration of bone deposition resulting in *bone hypertrophy*. The thick, heavy bones of athletes and laborers contrasted with the lighter bones of sedentary individuals illustrate this point.[8] Of clinical importance is the *reverse* of this phenomenon, whereby *lack* of physical stress causes a predominance of bone resorption and results in *bone atrophy*. The best example of this is the generalized skeletal atrophy that develops during prolonged bedrest. A more extreme example is the bone atrophy sustained by astronauts subjected to long periods of weightlessness while in space.

The implications of Wolff's law on remodeling also affect bone at a local or segmental level. Consider the successful healing of a distal radius fracture, as seen in

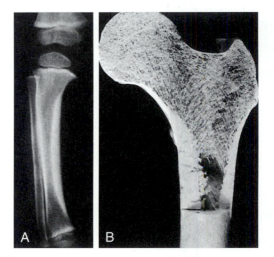

FIGURE 2–3. (*A*) An example of Wolff's law is seen in the tibia of a 2-year-old child with a bow-legged deformity. Note the marked thickening of the medial cortex, which is on the concave side of the deformity, which is subjected to the most stress on weight bearing. (*B*) An example of Wolff's law is seen in the internal architecture of this dried specimen of the upper end of a femur of an adult. Note the alignment of the trabecular systems of cancellous bone along the lines of weight-bearing stresses. (From Salter,[4] p 9, with permission.)

Figure 2–4. The phenomenon of Wolff's law and the reverse of it are both clearly demonstrated in the following events: (1) callus unites the fracture fragments and later remodels, restoring the normal internal and external architectures of the bone; (2) the imposed disuse of the limb while immobilized in a cast results in resorption of bone density in the entire hand and forearm, evidenced radiographically by osteopenia at 3 weeks postfracture; (3) complete resolution of the osteopenia is evidenced in follow-up films made 9 months postfracture, a direct result of active use of the limb. In this case the patient's cast had been removed 8 weeks postfracture, and the patient returned to full upper extremity function after 2 months of physical therapy.

A SYSTEMATIC APPROACH TO THE RADIOGRAPHIC EVALUATION OF BONES AND JOINTS

A popular method of introducing the novice to musculoskeletal radiographic analysis exists in the form of the acronym *ABCs*.[11,12] This approach concisely organizes the essentials of radiographic analysis into four divisions:

A: Alignment
B: Bone density
C: Cartilage spaces
S: Soft tissues

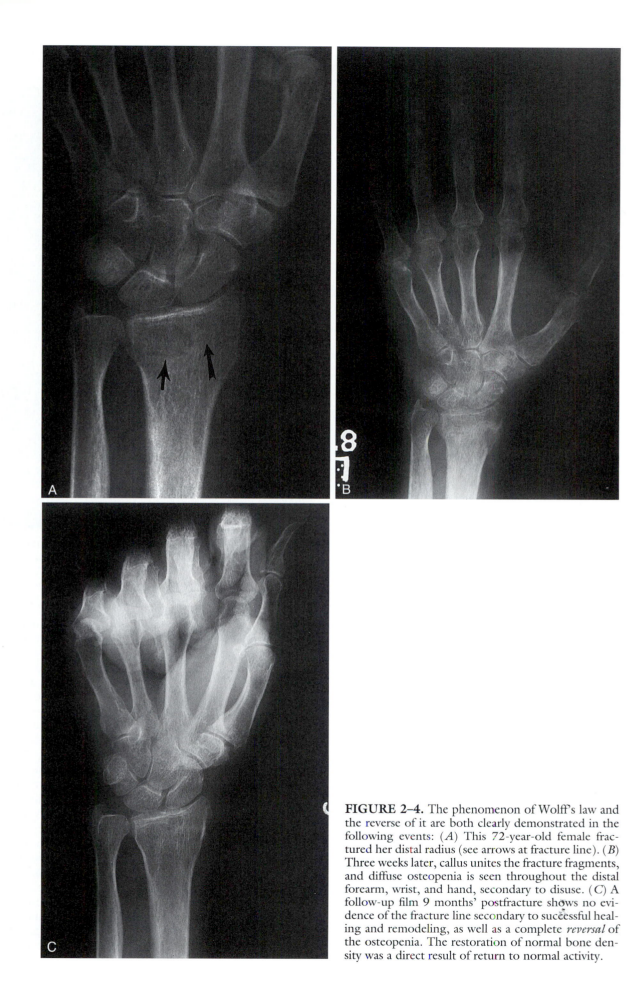

FIGURE 2–4. The phenomenon of Wolff's law and the reverse of it are both clearly demonstrated in the following events: (*A*) This 72-year-old female fractured her distal radius (see arrows at fracture line). (*B*) Three weeks later, callus unites the fracture fragments, and diffuse osteopenia is seen throughout the distal forearm, wrist, and hand, secondary to disuse. (*C*) A follow-up film 9 months' postfracture shows no evidence of the fracture line secondary to successful healing and remodeling, as well as a complete *reversal* of the osteopenia. The restoration of normal bone density was a direct result of return to normal activity.

These four divisions can be further subdivided into greater detail, as follows.

A: Alignment

Alignment analysis includes evaluation of:

General skeletal architecture: *Assess gross normal size and appearance of the anatomic form.* Routine films image anatomy approximately 30 percent larger than real life (although specific magnification can vary with the object-to-film distance). Note any *aberrant size* of bones. Gross enlargement of bone is seen in conditions such as gigantism, acromegaly, or Paget's disease (see Fig. 2–18); grossly undersized bone may similarly be related to congenital, metabolic, or endocrine abnormalities.[13] Note the presence of any *supernumerary bones,* such as an extra navicular among the tarsals or an extra digit in polydactyly (Figs. 2–5, 2–6). Note any congenital *anomalies,* such as a cervical rib or a transitional vertebra at the lumbosacral junction. Note the *absence of any bones* resulting from amputation or failure to develop (Fig. 2–7). Note any developmental or congenital *deformities* such as scoliosis or genu valgum.

General contour of bone: *Assess each bone for normal shape and contour.* Note any internal or external irregularities that may be related to pathologic, traumatic, developmental, or congenital factors. Trace the *cortical outline* of each bone, which should be *smooth and continuous.* Note any outgrowth of

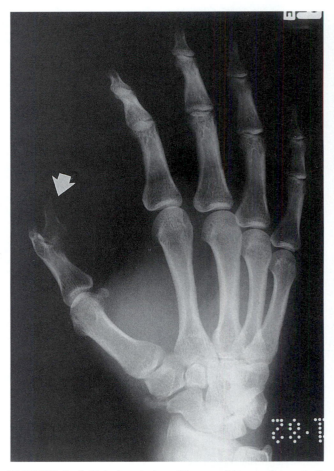

FIGURE 2–6. Polydactyly in a 31-year-old man. Arrow indicates an extra distal phalanx at the thumb.

spurs at joint margins indicative of degenerative joint changes, or spurs resulting from tension at areas of tissue attachment (Fig. 2–8).[14] Note any breaks in continuity of the cortex signifying *cortical fracture* (Fig. 2–9). Sharp angles in the cortex may be a sign of *impaction fracture* (Fig. 2–10). The sites of attachment of muscles, tendons, and ligaments are noted in trauma cases to evaluate for *avulsion fractures* (Fig. 2–11).[15] Note the markings of any past surgical sites, such as bone graft donation areas or drill holes for orthotic appliances (Fig. 2–12).

Alignment of bones relative to adjacent bones: Normal alignment of bones implies that the position of bones is not disrupted by fracture, or by joint subluxation or dislocation.[16] The most common cause of alignment abnormalities is trauma, whereby fracture and/or dislocation alters normal bone and joint relationships (Fig. 2–13). Other causes of abnormal alignment may be any of the inflammatory arthritides or degenerative joint diseases that erode articular cartilage and promote joint laxity (Fig. 2–14).[17] In evaluation of routine films in the coming chapters, mention is made where applicable of radiographic line images that serve as clues to assessment of nor-

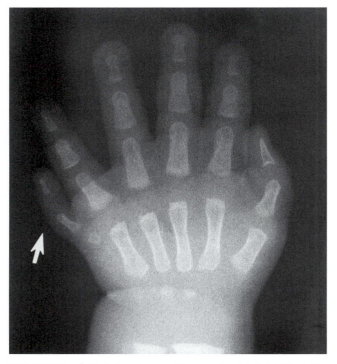

FIGURE 2–5. Polydactyly in a 10-month-old child. Note the extra sixth digit indicated by the arrow.

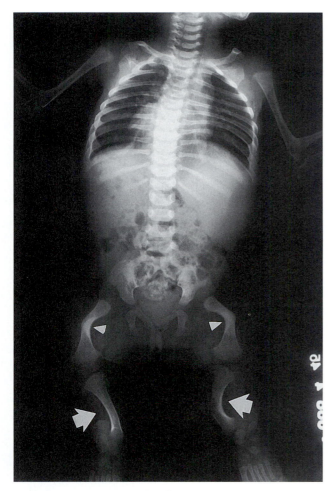

FIGURE 2–7. Congenital deformities in an 8-month-old female include bowing of the femurs (arrowheads) and bowing of the tibias with absence of the fibulas (large arrows).

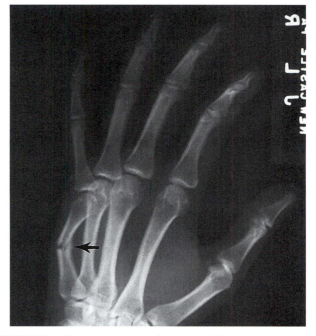

FIGURE 2–9. An example of a cortical fracture seen in the complete midshaft fracture of the fifth metacarpal (arrow). (From Richardson and Iglarsh,[9] p 681, with permission.)

mal spatial relationships. For example, in assessment of a lateral projection of the lumbar spine, normal positioning of the vertebrae is denoted by the parallel relationships of lines drawn connecting the anterior borders, the posterior borders, and the spinous process margins of each of the vertebrae. Disruptions in vertebral alignment would be evident in acute conditions such as traumatic spondylolisthesis, or in chronic conditions such as degenerative spondylolisthesis.[18]

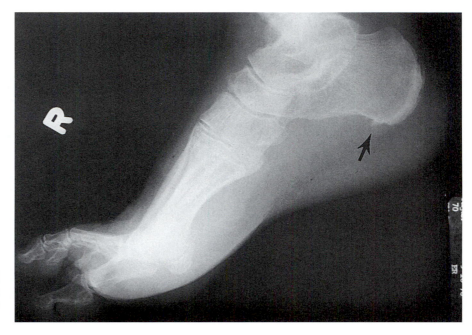

FIGURE 2–8. Heel spur is represented as a radiodense projection at the margin of the anterior-inferior surface of the calcaneus (arrow).

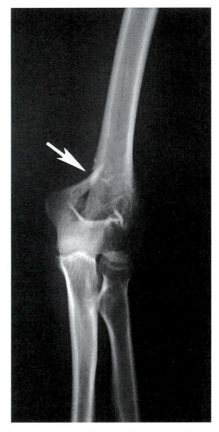

FIGURE 2–10. An example of an impaction fracture is seen in the *supracondylar* area of the distal humerus (arrow).

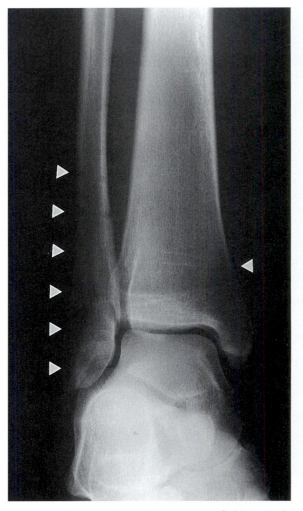

FIGURE 2–12. Note the odd appearance of old surgical sites as seen in the drill holes through the distal fibula and tibia of this patient who had fixation screws removed after successful healing (arrowheads).

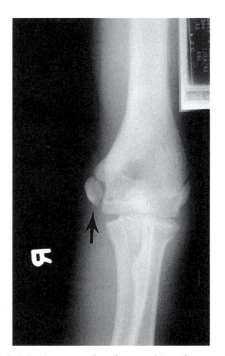

FIGURE 2–11. An example of an avulsion fracture is seen in this medial epicondyle avulsion of the distal humerus of the 10-year-old Little League pitcher. (From Richardson and Iglarsh,[9] p 663, with permission.)

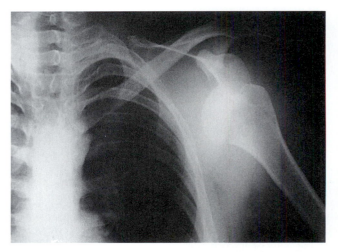

FIGURE 2–13. Anterior dislocation of the glenohumeral joint.

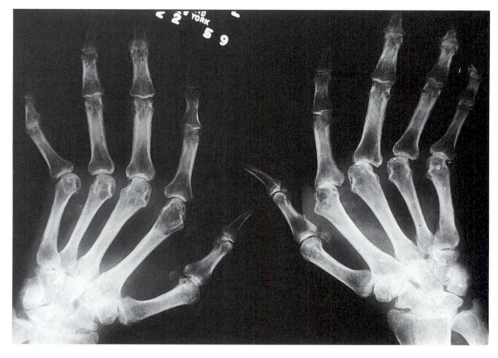

FIGURE 2–14. Advanced rheumatoid arthritis of the hands. Note the subluxation of the metacarpal joints, greater on the right hand, because of ligamentous laxity and joint erosion. The other classic hallmarks of rheumatoid arthritis include symmetric joint space narrowing and osteoporosis in the periarticular regions. A boutonnière deformity (hyperextension at the DIP joint with hyperflexion of the PIP joint) is present in the left fifth digit. Swan-neck deformities (hyperflexion of the DIP joints and hyperextension of the PIP are present in the third, fourth, and fifth right fingers. (From American College of Rheumatology Clinical Slide Collection on the Rheumatic Disease, 1991.)

B: Bone Density

Bone density analysis includes evaluation of:

General bone density: Normal bone density, or normal mineral content of bone, is evidenced by the presence of a sufficient amount of radiographic contrast between the skeleton and surrounding soft tissues. Additionally, sufficient contrast should exist within the skeleton itself, between the denser cortical shell of each bone and its relatively less dense cancellous bone center. Healthy cortex images with greater density than cancellous bone and thus appears as a white outline enveloping the form of bone (Fig. 2–15). *Loss of this distinct cortical image and loss of contrast between bone and soft tissues indicate loss of bone mass.*

   The degree of mineralization of bone is directly related to the patient's age, physiologic state, and the amount of activity or stress placed on the skeleton.[19] Certain diseases alter the mineral content of the skeleton. An overall increase in skeletal density is seen in some developmental bone disorders such as osteopetrosis or osteopoikilosis (Fig. 2–16). An overall decrease in skeletal density is seen in osteoporosis and in the hypocalcification characteristic of osteomalacia (Fig. 2–17).[20]

Texture abnormalities[21]: When the mineralization of bone is altered, the appearance of the trabeculae is also altered. The image of the trabeculae is often described in terms likened to texture, such as *thin, delicate, coarsened, smudged,* or *fluffy*. Altered trabecular appearance is often a radiologic hallmark in the di-

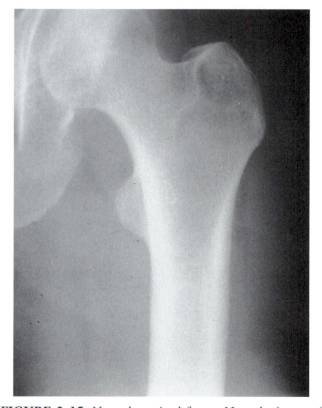

FIGURE 2–15. Normal proximal femur. Note the image of healthy cortex is evident in the increased radiodensity of the margins of the femur in contrast with the density of the medullar cavity.

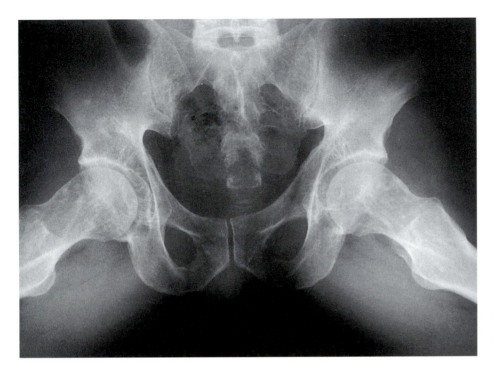

FIGURE 2–16. Osteopoikilosis is a benign bone disease characterized by spotty areas of calcification in bone as evidence in this pelvis of a 43-year-old man.

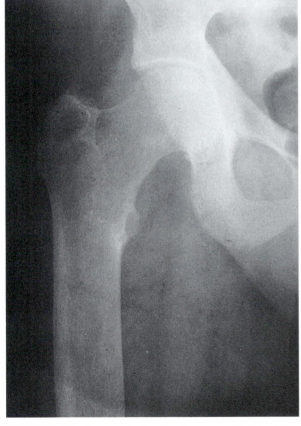

FIGURE 2–17. Osteomalacia, also known as "adult rickets," is a hypocalcification disorder. As seen in this proximal femur, the body is able to produce bone but is unable to calcify it. The result here is a very wide but porous femur. (From Richardson and Iglarsh,[9] p 642, with permission.)

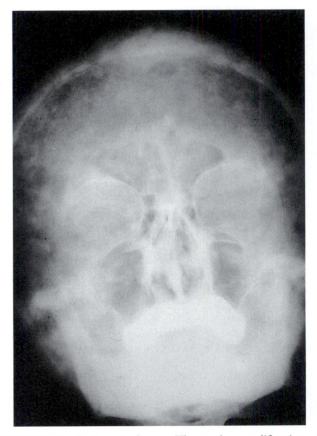

FIGURE 2–18. Paget's disease. The random proliferation of both osteoblastic and osteoclastic activity produces the curious fluffy sclerosis of the skull in this elderly male with Paget's disease. (From Richardson and Iglarsh,[9] p 644, with permission.)

agnosis of disease processes. For example, the random proliferation of both osteoblastic and osteoclastic activity produces the curious fluffy sclerosis of the skull in Paget's disease (Fig. 2–18) and in hyperparathyroidism (Fig. 2–19). Smudged and indistinct trabeculae are a characteristic of osteomalacia. Coarsening of trabeculae and osteoporosis are often seen in patients with chronic renal failure. The lacy, delicate appearance of trabeculae is secondary to thalassemia (Cooley's anemia), as seen in Figure 2–20.

Local bone density[22]:   Normal local increases in bone density are seen in areas subjected to increased physical stress, such as the weight-bearing areas of joints. These areas of localized increased density or *sclerosis* are actually signs of *repair*—extra bone is deposited here to fortify bony architecture to withstand weight-bearing. Bone also reacts to many other normal and abnormal conditions by increasing osteoblastic activity and forming new bone. This may be seen in the reparative attempts of bone to strengthen the subchondral bone of an osteoarthritic

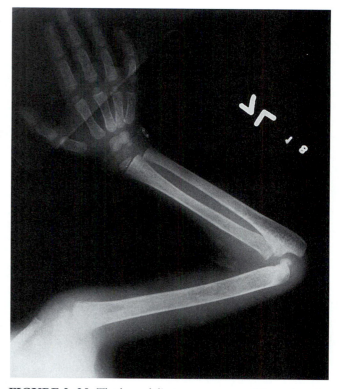

FIGURE 2–20. The lacy, delicate appearance of the trabeculae of the upper extremity of this child is secondary to thalassemia (Cooley's anemia).

joint (Fig. 2–21); at the site of a healing fracture as callus is formed and new bone is remodeled; and as *reactive sclerosis* as bone attempts to surround and wall off a diseased area, such as a tumor or infection (Fig. 2–22).[22]

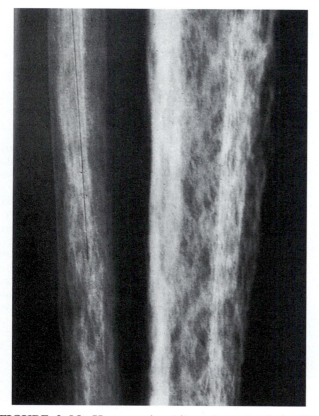

FIGURE 2–19. Hyperparathyroidism. A previously healthy 21-year-old man had been troubled for the past 18 months by increasing loss of strength in the lower extremities. Patient was found to have primary hyperparathyroidism secondary to a tumor of the parathyroid. Radiograph of his leg shows generalized skeletal changes with considerable decalcification of the bones and erosions of the cortex. (From Eiken, M: Roentgen Diagnosis of Bones: A Self-Teaching Manual. FADLs, Forlag, AS, Copenhagen, 1975, p 39, with permission.)

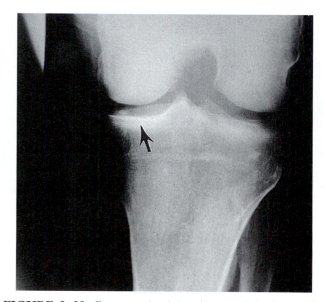

FIGURE 2–21. Degenerative joint disease of the knee. The arrow points to the sclerotic subchondral bone of the medial tibial plateau, which is a reparative response to the thinning of the articular cartilage.

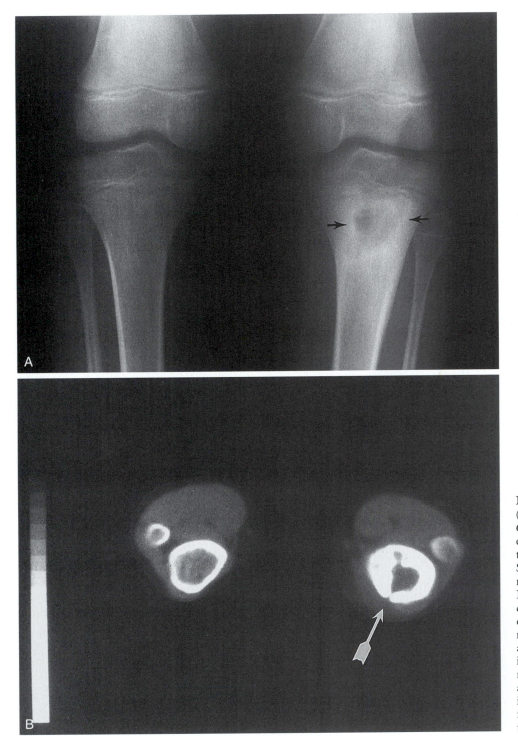

FIGURE 2–22. Osteomyelitis. (*A*) This 9-year-old female had a 6-month history of progressive, enlarging soft tissue swelling at the left anterior proximal tibia. She was diagnosed with osteomyelitis of the proximal tibia. Note how the lesion is well circumscribed by the active sclerosis of bone in an attempt to surround and wall-off the infected area (arrows). (*B*) The CT axial image further demonstrates the reactive sclerosis of the left tibia and also reveals a draining defect in the anterior tibia, which formed to relieve the pressure of the pus (white arrow).

C: Cartilage Space

Analysis includes evaluation of:[23–25]

Joint space width: The articular cartilage of joints or the cartilaginous intervertebral discs of the spine are not well demonstrated on plain films because of their water-like density. Cartilages and discs can be analyzed, however, by examining the space they oc-

cupy. A *well-preserved joint space* implies that the cartilage or disc is of normal thickness. A *decreased joint space* implies that the cartilage or disc is thinned down from degenerative processes (Fig. 2–23). Joint space is also referred to as the *potential space* and the *radiographic joint space*. Radiographic joint space is specific in that it encompasses both the cartilage and any actual space present in the joint. Evaluation of weight-bearing joints is best done *during weight-*

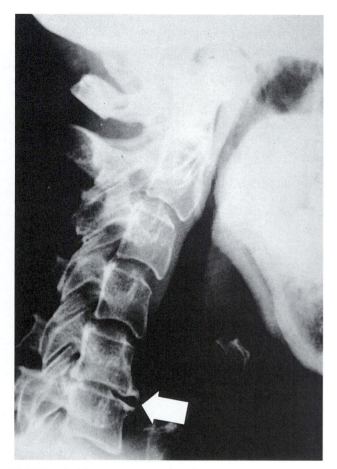

FIGURE 2–23. Degenerative disc disease of the cervical spine. This lateral view of the cervical spine shows the classic hallmarks of degenerative disc disease at C5–6 incuding a narrowed joint space and osteophyte formation at the joint margins (arrow).

bearing for accurate assessment of the articular cartilages, as this will effectively eliminate any actual space.

Subchondral bone:[26]   The appearance of the bone directly under the articular cartilage, the subchondral bone, is significant in the radiologic diagnosis of the various forms of arthritis. In osteoarthritis (degenerative joint disease) subchondral bone becomes sclerotic in appearance as new bone is formed to help withstand the increased stresses directed at it due to the thinning of articular cartilage (Fig. 2–24). In rheumatoid arthritis, there is no reparative sclerosis seen in the subchondral bone. Rather, erosions of the subchondral bone form radiolucent cysts and are hallmarks of rheumatoid arthritis, gout, and other inflammatory arthritides (Fig. 2–25).

Epiphyseal plates: Although the previous points were in regard to joints, epiphyseal plates in a growing child are cartilaginous, and thus fit into this category. The epiphyseal plates are evaluated by the presence of the epiphysis (Fig. 2–26). The epiphyses are evaluated for their size in relation to both skeletal maturity and chronologic age. The borders of the epiphyses are bounded by a smooth margin with a band of sclerosis indicating increased bone activity associated with linear growth. Disruptions in the epiphyseal plates can be difficult to diagnose, and contralateral films may be needed for comparison.

S: Soft Tissues

Soft tissue analysis includes evaluation of:[27,28]

Muscles: Plain films do not image muscles with distinction, but enough of an image is created to assess

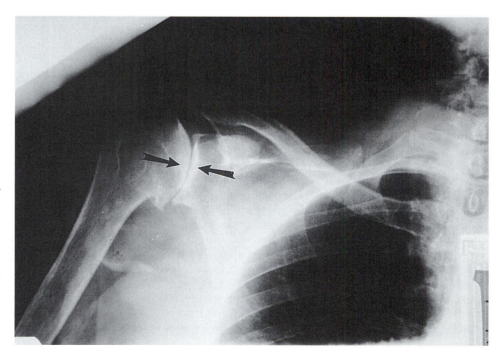

FIGURE 2–24. Osteoarthritis of the glenohumeral joint. Note the radiographic hallmarks of OA including decreased joint space, sclerotic subcondral bone (arrows), and osteophyte formation on the inferior joint margins. The severity of these degenerative changes is usually more common in weight-bearing joints. The arthritic changes here were probably accelerated by a prior trauma.

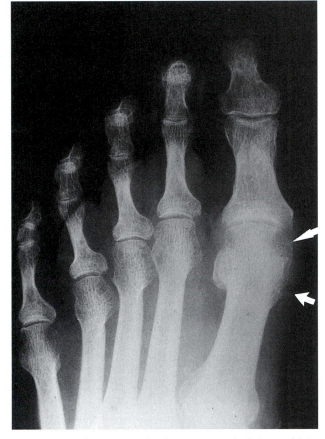

FIGURE 2–25. Gout at the first metatarsal phalangeal joint. Joint erosions in gout and other inflammatory arthritides show no reactive subchondral sclerosis as seen in osteoarthritic conditions. Rather, erosions of the subchondral bone in knee inflammatory conditions form radiolucent cysts in the articular and periarticular regions (arrows).

some generalities. Gross muscle wasting suggests a primary muscle disease, paralysis, inanition associated with severe illnesses, or disuse atrophy secondary to trauma (Fig. 2–27). Gross swelling of muscles and soft tissues may be indicative of inflammation, edema, hemorrhage, or tumor (Fig. 2–28).

Fat pads and fat lines: The loss or displacement of fat lines from their normal positions in the soft tissues is usually due to swelling and as such is an indicator of adjacent abnormality. For example, displacement of the pronator quadratus fat line at the wrist usually indicates a wrist fracture.[29] *Generally, displacement of fat pads out of their bony fossae is a result of increased joint volume from swelling and is a clue to adjacent trauma.* An example of this is the displacement of the fat pads out of the olecranon fossa posteriorly and out of the coronoid and radial fossae anteriorly at the elbow in the presence of elbow fracture[30] (Fig. 2–29).

Joint capsules: Normally rather indistinct, joint capsules will become visible under abnormal conditions when distended by effusion. This is seen in exacer-

bations of arthritic conditions and in acute joint trauma[31] (Fig. 2–30).

Periosteum: Normally rather indistinct, the periosteum becomes evident in its response to abnormal conditions. Periosteal reaction (Fig. 2–31) is generally described as being one of four types, named by the characteristic radiographic images.[32,33]

Solid: Indicates a benign process; seen in fracture healing and osteomyelitis (Fig. 2–32)

Laminated or onionskin: Indicates repetitive injury, as in the battered child syndrome; also associated with reticulum cell sarcomas such as Ewing's sarcoma

Spiculated or sunburst: Almost always associated with malignant bone lesions such as osteogenic

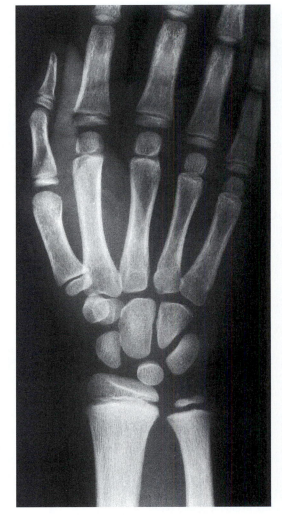

FIGURE 2–26. Normal radiographic appearance of hand of an 8-year-old child. The epiphyseal plates are evidenced by the radiolucent zones adjacent to the maturing epiphyses. The borders of epiphyses are normally bounded by a smooth margin with a band of sclerosis indicating increased bone activity. This is how they are distinguished from fracture fragments. Discriminating epiphyseal plate regions from fracture lines can at times be difficult, and contralateral films may be needed for comparison purposes.

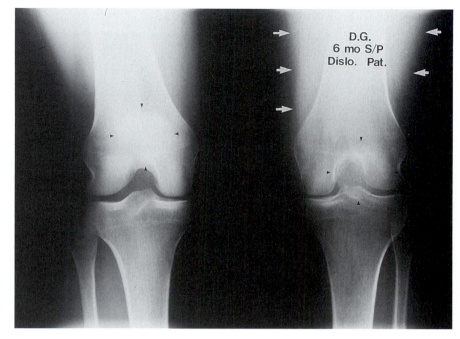

FIGURE 2–27. Disuse atrophy of the quadriceps secondary to traumatic patellar dislocation is evidenced by the shrunken appearance of the soft tissue outline of the thigh. Note the inferior position of the patella (patella baja) caused by quadriceps insufficiency.

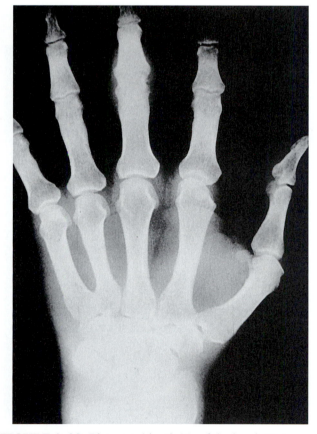

FIGURE 2–28. Rheumatoid arthritis of the hand. Note gross swelling of the hand and the proximal interphalangeal joint of the third digit, indicating an inflammatory phase. (From American College of Rheumatology Clinical Slide Collection on Rheumatic Disease, 1991.)

sarcomas and less frequently seen in metastatic squamous cell tumors. The distinct appearance of the periosteum is due to the repeated breakthrough of the neoplastic process followed by new periosteal response.

    Codman's triangle: A piece of periosteum elevated by abnormal conditions ossifies in a triangular shape. This may be present in a variety of conditions including tumor, subperiosteal hemorrhage, and battered child syndrome.

Miscellaneous soft tissue findings:[34] *Gas* in soft tissues is an indication of gas gangrene or trauma. *Calcifications* in soft tissues may be the result of old trauma whereby bloody hemorrhage has coagulated and calcified (Figs. 2–33, 2–34). Additionally, calcifications occur in vessels and organs, for example, renal calculi, gallstones, or calcifications in the abdominal aorta. *Foreign bodies* (e.g., metal shards) may also be evident in the soft tissues.

RADIOGRAPHIC EVALUATION OF SKELETAL PATHOLOGY

There are six basic categories of pathology in the classification of skeletal diseases: *congenital, inflammatory, metabolic, neoplastic, traumatic,* and *vascular.*[35] A seventh category, *miscellaneous or other,* is added to encompass any conditions that do not fall strictly into one category, such as *musculoskeletal infections* or *osteoarthritis.* A systematic method of evaluating and distinguishing the radiographic characteristics of these categories facilitates diagnosis.

    Daffner[36] describes a logical approach to musculoskeletal radiologic diagnosis as beginning with (1) *de-*

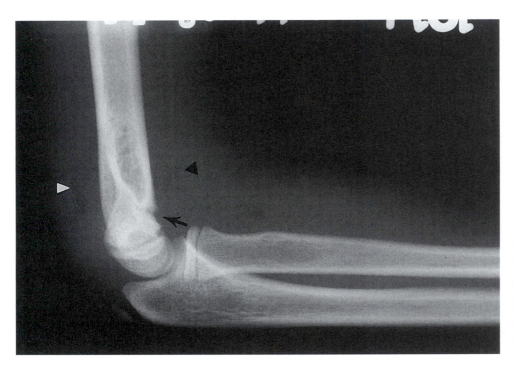

FIGURE 2–29. Fat pad sign at the elbow. This 12-year-old boy sustained a supracondylar fracture (arrow) of his distal humerus in a fall. Swelling of the joint has displaced the anterior and posterior fat pads out of their bony fossas, and they become evident as radiolucencies in the soft tissues (white and black arrowheads).

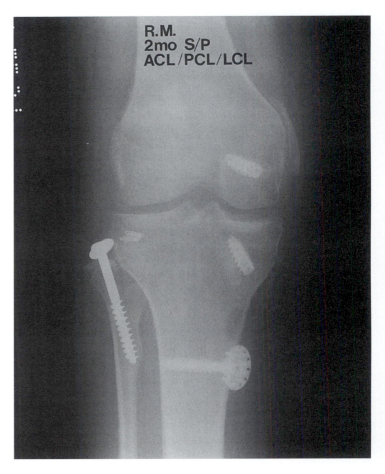

FIGURE 2–30. Soft tissue swelling. This film was made immediately after reduction of a traumatic knee dislocation in a 22-year-old male. Note the gross amount of soft tissue swelling present secondary to the recent trauma.

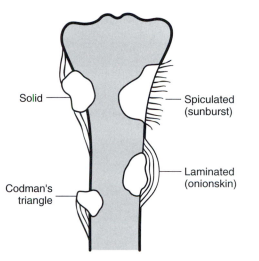

FIGURE 2–31. Periosteal reactions to abnormal conditions appear on radiograph in four characteristic images: solid, spiculated, laminated, or Codman's triangle. (Adapted from Greenspan,[2] p 15.17.)

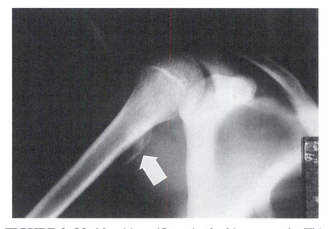

FIGURE 2–33. Myositis ossificans in the biceps muscle. This 28-year-old weight lifter felt a tear in his biceps while he was curling weights. Initial films were negative for fracture. Follow-up film 6 weeks later identified a calcified mass (arrow). Clinically, a palpable mass was evident in the bulk of the biceps muscle.

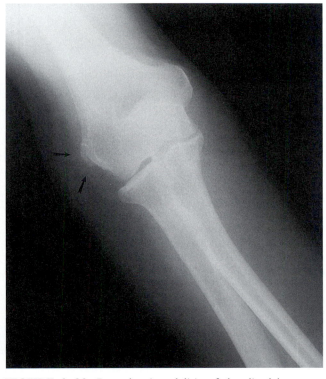

FIGURE 2–32. Lateral epicondylitis of the distal humerus. Note the solid periosteal reaction (arrows) indicating bone healing in response to the microtrauma of excessive, repetitive tension generated by the extensor muscles of the forearm.

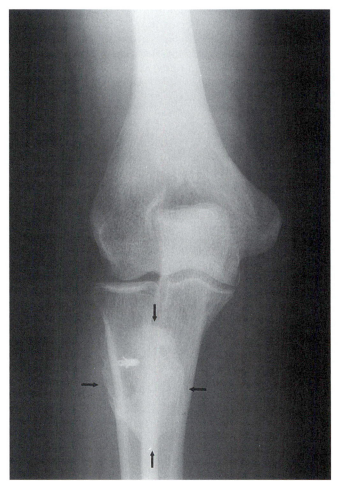

FIGURE 2–34. Heterotopic bone developed in the soft tissues of the forearm of this 53-year-old male after a biceps tendon repair with a mytex suture anchor. The boundaries of the abnormal bone tissue are indicated with arrows.

TABLE 2–2 Pathology Related to Skeletal Distribution

Category	Distribution		
	Monostotic	Polyostotic	Diffuse
Congenital	X	X	
Inflammatory	X	X	
Neoplastic	X	X	X
Metabolic	X	X	X
Traumatic	X	X	
Vascular	X	X	
Miscellaneous	(X)	(X)	

fining the distribution of the lesion and then (2) applying a number of factors that further limit the diagnostic choices. These factors are referred to as *predictor variables.*

Distribution of the Lesion

The distribution of a lesion refers to how many locations in the body the lesion involves and is a significant clue to the etiology of that lesion. A lesion may be *monostotic or monoarticular,* affecting only one bone or one joint; *polyostotic or polyarticular,* affecting multiple bones or multiple joints; or *diffuse,* affecting all bones or joints.

Only two disease categories occur diffusely, neoplastic and metabolic (Table 2–2). The other categories occur in either monostotic/monoarticular or polyostotic/polyarticular patterns. Occasionally, however, metabolic disease may manifest in monostotic or polyostotic forms. Examples of pathology as related to distribution appear in Table 2–3.

Predictor Variables

Daffner[37] cites 11 predictor variables that may be applied to any bone or joint lesion to assist in making a diagnosis. These are the behavior of the lesion; the bone or joint involved; the locus within a bone; the age, gender, and race of the patient; the margin of the lesion; the shape of the lesion; involvement or crossing of a joint space; bony reaction (if any); matrix produc-

TABLE 2–4 Predictor Variables for Bone and Joint Lesions

1. *Behavior of the Lesion*
   A. Osteolytic (or osteoclastic, bone destroying)
   B. Osteoblastic (reparative or reactive bone forms)
   C. Mixed
2. *Bone or Joint Involved*
3. *Locus within a Bone*
   A. Epiphysis (or apophysis)
   B. Metaphysis (or equivalent)
   C. Diaphysis
   D. Articular surface
4. *Age, Gender, and Race of Patient*
5. *Margin of Lesion*
   A. Sharply defined (slow-growing lesion)
   B. Poorly defined (aggressive lesion)
6. *Shape of Lesion*
   A. Longer than wide (generally slow-growing lesion)
   B. Wider than long (generally aggressive lesion)
      a. Cortical breakthrough
      b. No breakthrough
7. *Joint Space Crossed/Joint Space Preserved*
8. *Bony Reaction (If Any)*
   A. Periosteal
      a. Solid
      b. Laminated ("onionskin")
      c. Spiculated, sunburst, "hair-on-end"
      d. Codman's triangle
   B. Sclerosis
   C. Buttressing
9. *Matrix Production*
   A. Osteoid
   B. Chondroid
   C. Mixed
10. *Soft Tissue Changes*
11. *History of Trauma or Surgery*

tion by the lesion; soft tissue changes; and a history of trauma or surgery (Table 2–4).[38]

Many of these predictor variables apply directly to the diagnosis of bone tumors. Specific diagnoses can at times still be difficult even if all of the predictor variables are applied; the information gained by plain-film evaluation, however, is usually sufficient for the radiologist to determine whether a lesion is *nonaggressive* (benign) or *aggressive* (malignant) and in need of biopsy.

Daffner's description of the predictor variables follows:

TABLE 2–3 Examples of Pathology Related to Skeletal Distribution

Category	Monostotic/Monoarticular	Polyostotic/Polyarticular	Diffuse
Congenital	Cervical rib	Cleidocranial dysostosis	
Inflammatory	Osteomyelitis, gout	Congenital lues, rheumatoid arthritis	
Neoplastic	Any primary bone tumor	Myeloma	Metastasis
Metabolic	(Paget's disease)	(Paget's disease, fibrous dysplasia)	Osteopetrosis, hyperparathyroidism
Traumatic	Single fracture	Multiple fractures, battered child	
Vascular	Legg-Calvé-Perthes disease	Legg-Calvé-Perthes disease	
Miscellaneous (osteoarthritis)	OA at first carpometacarpal joint.	OA in all large weight-bearing joints	

BEHAVIOR OF THE LESION

Bone lesions are described as either **osteolytic**, meaning bone has been destroyed by osteoclastic activity, or **osteoblastic**, meaning new reparative or reactive bone is present. Occasionally, a mixture of the two processes may be present. Osteolytic lesions take on three forms of destruction: *geographic destruction*, whereby large areas of bone are destroyed and appear as radiolucent areas on film; *moth-eaten appearance*, whereby there are several small holes throughout the bone appearing on film similar to moth-eaten cloth; and *permeative destruction*, very fine destruction of bone through the haversian system, sometime requiring a magnifying lens to recognize on film (Fig. 2–35).

BONE OR JOINT INVOLVED

Some diseases manifest characteristically at specific bones or joints. Gout and rheumatoid arthritis, for example, appear primarily in the small joints of the hands and feet. Osteoarthritis commonly develops at the knees. Examples of other nonneoplastic and neoplastic diseases with predilection for certain areas are shown in Figure 2–36.

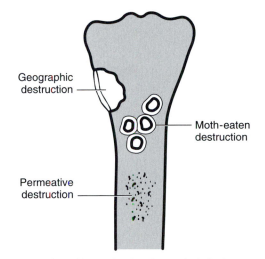

FIGURE 2–35. Different kinds of osteolytic lesions cause different types of bone destruction. The radiographic image that correlates with the pathologic process may be described as geographic, moth-eaten, or permeative. (Adapted from Greenspan,[2] p 5.20.)

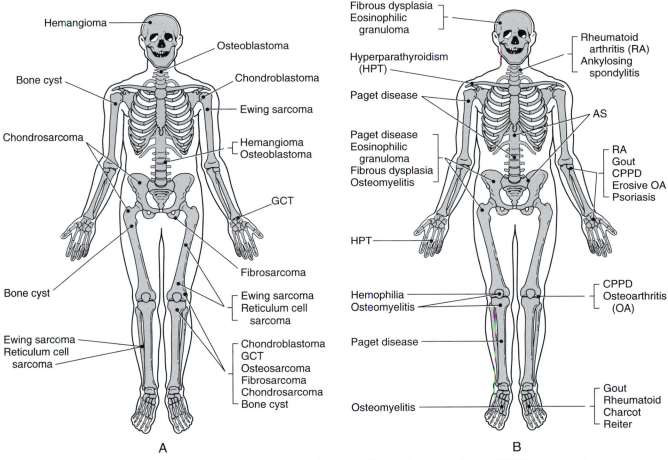

FIGURE 2–36. Preferred locations for bone lesions. (*A*) Neoplastic conditions. (*B*) Nonneoplastic conditions. (From Daffner,[8] p 288, with permission.)

LOCUS WITHIN A BONE

The site of the lesion within the bone itself is a significant clue to etiology. Certain tumors have a predilection for the bony shaft, whereas others favor the metaphyseal or epiphyseal regions. The arthritides have characteristic locations on the articular surfaces of bone. Osteoarthritis affects weight-bearing areas, whereas rheumatoid arthritis affects the entire joint surface.

AGE, GENDER, AND RACE

Age is a significant factor in predicting the type of malignant bone tumor as well as some benign tumors.

TABLE 2–5

PEAK AGE INCIDENCE OF BENIGN AND MALIGNANT TUMORS AND TUMOR-LIKE LESIONS

Age scale: 0, 10, 20, 30, 40, 50, 60, 70, 80, 90

Legend: Benign, Malignant

- Metastatic neuroblastoma
- Osteofibrous dysplasia
- Simple bone cyst
- Fibrous cortical defect
- Nonossifying fibroma
- Eosinophilic granuloma
- Aneurysmal bone cyst
- Fibrous dysplasia (polyostotic)
- Fibrous dysplasia (monostotic)
- Chondroblastoma
- Ewing's sarcoma
- Periosteal desmoid
- Conventional osteosarcoma
- Chondromyxoid fibroma
- Multiple enchondromatosis
- Multiple osteocartilaginous exostoses
- Osteoblastoma
- Osteochondroma
- Osteoid osteoma
- Enchondroma
- Benign fibrous histiocytoma
- Giant cell tumor
- Fibrosarcoma Malignant fibrous histiocytoma
- Parosteal osteosarcoma
- Adamantinoma
- Conventional chondrosarcoma
- Histiocytic lymphoma
- Metastatic lesions
- Myeloma
- Secondary osteosarcoma

Source: Greenspan, A: Orthopedic Radiology: A Practical Approach, ed 2. Raven Press, New York, 1992, with permission.

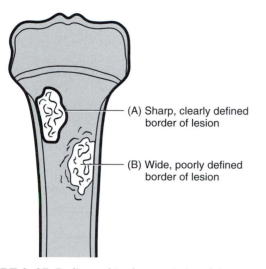

(A) Sharp, clearly defined border of lesion

(B) Wide, poorly defined border of lesion

FIGURE 2–37. Radiographic characteristics of the margins of (A) slow-growing, benign lesions versus (B) fast-growing, malignant lesions. (Adapted from Greenspan,[2] p 15.18.)

See Table 2–5 for peak ages of various tumors.[39] In addition to age predominance, there is gender predominance (rheumatoid arthritis—female, Paget's disease—male) and race predominance in some diseases (sickle cell disease, thalassemia).

MARGIN OF LESION

In general, margins are either *sharp and clearly defined*, indicative of a slow-growing benign lesion, or *wide and poorly defined*, characteristic of an aggressive lesion (Fig. 2–37). This relationship is logical: In the slow-growing process, bone has time to effectively wall off the abnormal bone with a border of new bone

growth. In contrast, a malignant lesion or aggressive process like osteomyelitis (bone infection) progresses so rapidly that bone is unable to respond adequately.

SHAPE OF LESION

Similar to margins, the shape of a lesion helps determine whether it is aggressive or nonaggressive. Lesions that are *longer than wide* are likely to be benign, as the lesion appears to be growing slowly along with bone. By contrast, lesions that are *wide and breaking out of bone* and extending into the soft tissues are aggressive.

JOINT SPACE CROSSED

As a rule, *tumors*, benign or malignant, do not cross joint spaces (Fig. 2–38) or epiphyseal growth plates. *Infections*, however, do cross joint spaces. *Inflammatory processes* are characteristic in that they cause destruction of bone on both sides of a joint (Fig. 2–39).

BONY REACTION

The response of bone to lesion, trauma, or degenerative processes can include *periosteal reaction, sclerosis*, and *buttressing*. Descriptions of various periosteal reactions to trauma and tumor were noted in the *ABCs* section. Sclerosis has been defined as new bone growth established to contain an area of abnormal bone (see *margin of lesion*), or new growth deposited to fortify an area subjected to increased stress, as in the sclerosis of subchondral bone in osteoarthritis. Buttressing is the formation of bony exostoses or osteophytes at a joint which serve to strengthen the architecture of the joint.

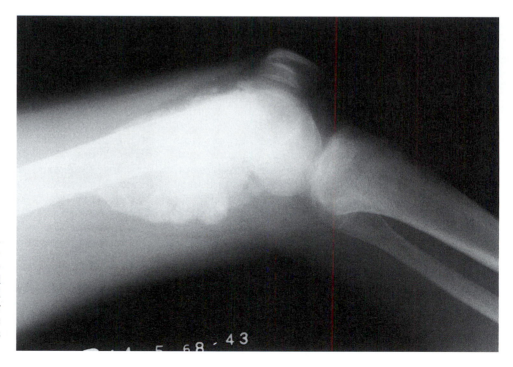

FIGURE 2–38. Osteosarcoma. This 16-year-old female with a 3-month history of pain and swelling in her knee was diagnosed with an osteosarcoma of the distal femur. Note that this large tumor extends to, *but does not cross*, the joint space of the knee. This is characteristic of all tumors.

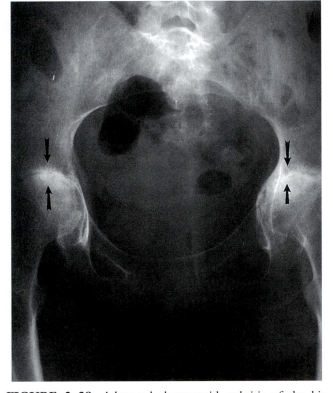

FIGURE 2–39. Advanced rheumatoid arthritis of the hip joints. Note that the destruction caused by rheumatoid arthritis involves the entire joint space and the bony regions on either side of the joint space.

MATRIX PRODUCTION

Matrix is the intercellular tissue produced by certain bone tumors. Matrix may be *chondroid* (cartilaginous), *osteoid* (bony), or *mixed*, a combination of the two. Chondroid matrix appears as stippled or popcorn-like calcifications seen in tumors invading soft tissues. Osteoid matrix appears as similar to bone density and occurs most often in osteogenic sarcoma.

SOFT TISSUE CHANGES

Examining soft tissue density changes may provide clues to the underlying abnormality. Fractures and other trauma will have associated soft tissue edema or hemorrhage, or joint effusion. All of these conditions alter the normal soft tissue outline and add density to the soft tissue image. Displacement of fat pads and fat lines is also associated with trauma (see section on ABCs). Tumor masses may develop in soft tissues or extend from adjacent bone or organs and become visible by the substance of their matrix or their disruption of normal soft tissue geography. Infections and inflammation also add density to the soft tissue image. Calcifications in soft tissues result from connective tissue disorders or old trauma.

HISTORY OF TRAUMA OR SURGERY

As trauma represents the most common disorder of bone, a clear clinical history including descriptions of any present or prior trauma is a significant factor in the radiologic examination. Some traumatic conditions may have similar radiographic appearances to pathological processes. As Daffner[34] elaborates, a stress fracture may be misdiagnosed as a malignant bone tumor unless a specific history of pain related to activity and relieved with rest is elicited from the patient. Additionally, a history of past injury or surgery to a bone is necessary to account for the odd appearance of old surgical sites or remodeling deformities.

RADIOGRAPHIC CHARACTERISTICS OF COMMON PATHOLOGIES

A brief review of the radiographic characteristics of some of the more frequently encountered pathologic conditions of the musculoskeletal system follows. Examples from each of the major pathologic categories are presented, with the exception of *trauma* conditions, which are covered in the following chapter on fractures and additionally in each anatomic chapter, and *congenital* conditions, which are covered by body segment in each of the anatomic chapters.

When reading the descriptions of the radiologic characteristics of the following pathologies, the clinician should recognize how each feature can be associated with a *predictor variable*. Furthermore, it should be noted how some radiographic features are unique to that diagnosis, and how others are pathognomonic for multiple conditions, necessitating differential diagnoses.

Adult Rheumatoid Arthritis[40–43]

Rheumatoid arthritis is a progressive, systemic, inflammatory connective tissue disease affecting primarily the synovial joints, although it may involve nonarticular tissues including blood vessels, muscle, heart, and lungs. This disease is estimated to affect 3 percent of the populations of countries with temperate climates. Women are afflicted with three times greater incidence than men, and peak age at onset is between 35 and 40 years old. The detection of specific antibodies or *rheumatoid factors* in the joint fluid or serum is significant in diagnosis. Although the course of the disease may vary in individual patients, it is generally characterized by spontaneous exacerbations and remissions of bilateral and symmetrical joint inflammation. Early stages exhibit involvement of the small joints of the wrists, hands, and feet. Later stages exhibit various degrees of joint deformities, contractures, and ankylosis, affecting both small and large weight-bearing and non-weight-bearing joints (Fig. 2–40).

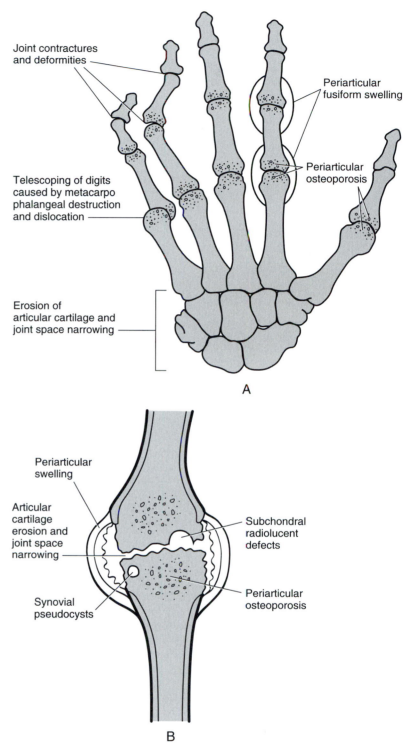

FIGURE 2–40. (*A*) Radiographic hallmarks of rheumatoid arthritis in small joints. (*B*) Radiographic hallmarks of rheumatoid arthritis in large joints. (Adapted from Greenspan, p 12.21)

Radiographic features characteristic of rheumatoid arthritis are:[44]

SOFT TISSUE CHANGES

The earliest sign of the disease is *periarticular swelling* of the small joints representing a combination of joint effusion, tenosynovitis, and edema (see Figs. 2-28 and 2–41). Swelling of both small and large joints continues to be evident throughout periods of exacerbations.

ARTICULAR EROSIONS

Central or peripheral joint surfaces may show articular erosion, evidenced by altered joint congruity and altered joint surface topography (Fig. 2–42). The sub-

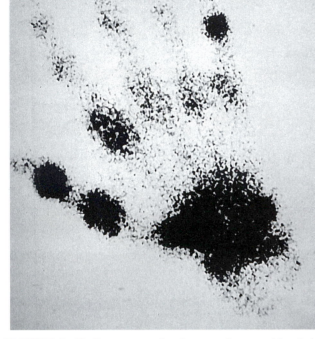

FIGURE 2–41. Bone scan of early-stage rheumatoid arthritis of the hand. There is abnormal uptake in the wrist, distal interphalangeal joint of the fifth digit, first and second metacarpal phalangeal joints, and the interphalangeal joint of the thumb. This represents an inflammatory phase of the disease.

chondral bone may show localized areas of resorption, appearing as *radiolucent defects*. Additionally *synovial cysts or pseudocysts*, formed by intrusion of synovial fluid into porous subchondral bone. Reparative processes such as sclerosis or osteophyte formation (hallmarks of osteoarthritis) are usually minimal or absent; these processes may be evident, however, if degenerative changes were preexisting or superimposed on the underlying inflammatory condition.

JOINT SPACE NARROWING

Erosion of articular cartilage results in *joint space narrowing*. Because the entire joint surface is affected in rheumatoid arthritis, narrowing is often *concentric*. At the hip, concentric narrowing results in axial or medial *migration* of the femoral head, leading to *acetabular protrusio* (see Fig. 7–27), an outpouching of the acetabular cup caused by upward pressure from the femoral head. At the shoulder, cephalad migration of the humeral head can occur as a result of articular erosion and associated rupture of the rotator cuff (Fig. 2–43).

OSTEOPOROSIS

Localized areas of decreased bone density or *rarefaction* appear in the early stages of rheumatoid arthritis at periarticular regions. In later stages, generalized osteoporosis is seen (Fig. 2–14).

JOINT DEFORMITIES

Joint *subluxations* and *dislocations* occur secondary to a combination of capsular and ligamentous laxity, destruction of joint surfaces, and tendon rupture. *Flexion contractures* are the result of maintaining the joints in a position of maximum capsular volume to gain pain relief from the pressure of joint swelling. Characteristic of but not solely pathognomonic for rheumatoid arthritis are these deformities of the hands (see Fig. 2–14): *swan-neck deformity*, which refers to hyper-extension of

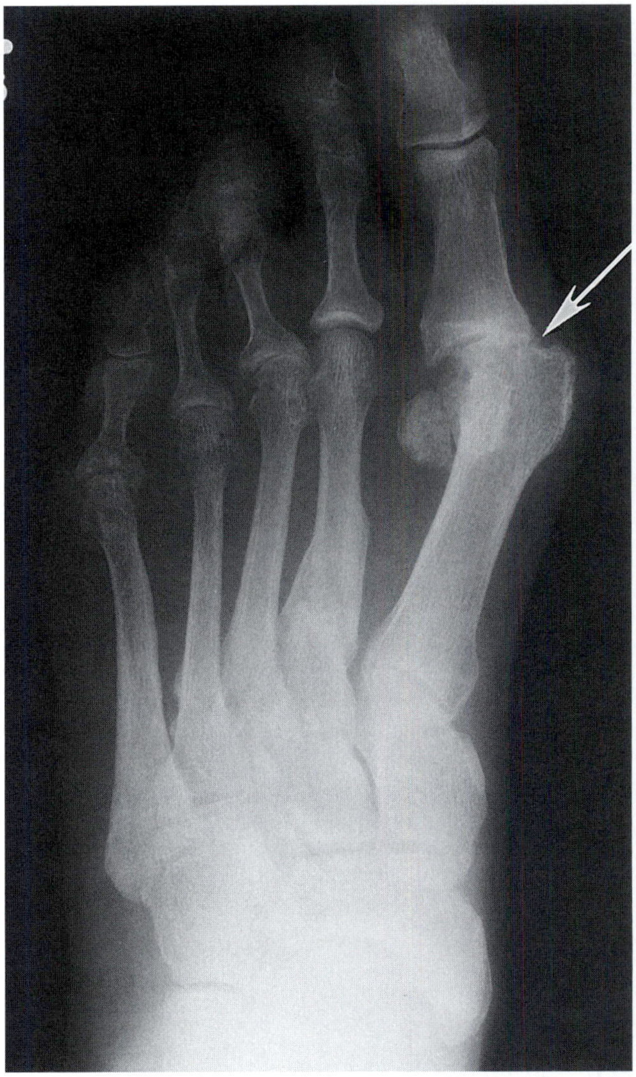

FIGURE 2–42. Rheumatoid arthritis of the foot. First MTP joint shows severe *erosion* of the joint surface with *subluxation* of the metatarsal (arrow).

from subluxations at the metatarsophalangeal joints of the great toe and remaining digits, respectively.

CHANGES IN THE CERVICAL SPINE

Although the thoracic and lumbar spines are infrequently affected, the cervical spine is involved in approximately 50 percent of patients with rheumatoid arthritis.[38] Erosion and narrowing of the apophyseal (facet) joints and intervertebral joints which may lead to slight subluxations are common findings. Life threatening, however, is the subluxation of the atlantoaxial joint (C1–C2), resulting from laxity in the transverse ligament of atlas combined with erosive changes in and superior migration of the odontoid process. This segmental instability requires surgical intervention, as even minor trauma may result in fatal spinal cord compression (Fig. 2–45).

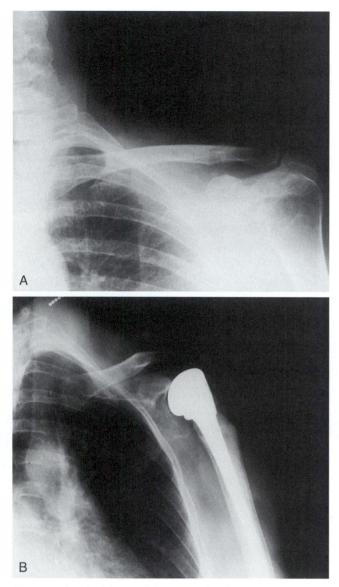

FIGURE 2–43. Advanced rheumatoid arthritis at the shoulder joint. (*A*) This anterior-posterior view shows migration of the humeral head occurring as a result of articular erosion and associated rupture of the rotator cuff. (*B*) Post-op film showing resection of humeral head and prosthetic replacement.

the proximal interphalangeal joints with flexion of the distal interphalangeal joints; *boutonnière deformity*, which refers to the opposite configuration, flexion of the proximal interphalangeal joints with extension of the distal interphalangeal joints; *telescoping* or *main en lorgnette deformity*, which describes the shortened appearance of the phalanges due to metacarpophalangeal joint destruction and dislocation; and joint *ankylosis*, or bony fixation across a joint space, which is a relatively rare finding in adult rheumatoid arthritis but when present is most frequently encountered at the midcarpal articulations (Fig. 2–44). Joint deformities are also at the feet: *hallux valgus* and *hammer-toe* result

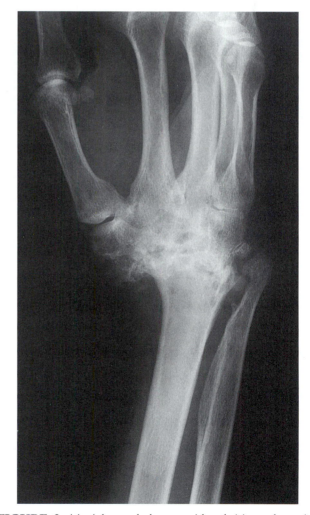

FIGURE 2–44. Advanced rheumatoid arthritis at the wrist. Note the diffuse ankylosis that has occurred throughout the carpals and radiocarpal joint. Note the marked erosion of the distal radius.

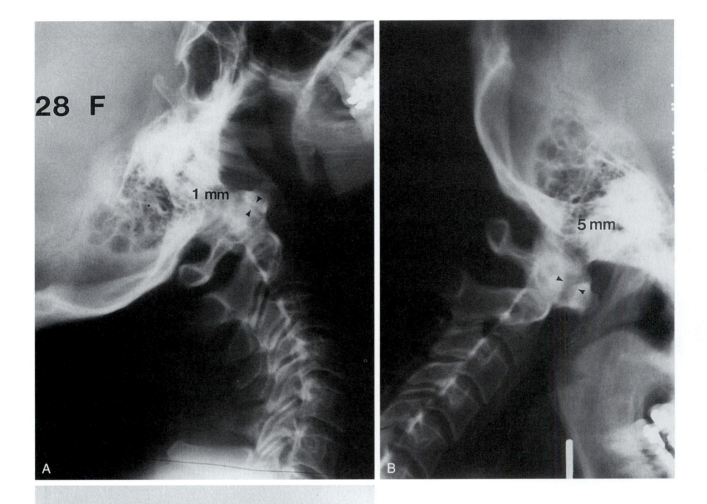

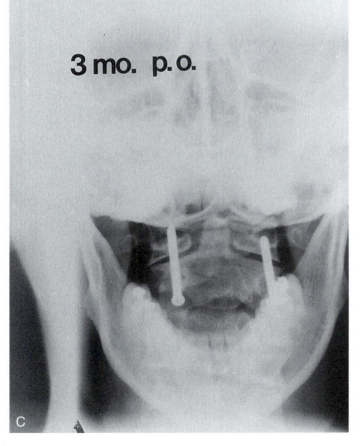

FIGURE 2–45. Instability of C1–2 as demonstrated in this 28-year-old female with rheumatoid arthritis. (*A, B*) On extension and flexion films the atlantodens interface is noted to gap from 1 to 5 mm. Normally this interface is to remain constant in any degree of flexion or extension. (*C*) Based on these findings, the patient underwent surgical fixation of the C1–2 segment.

Osteoarthritis (Degenerative Joint Disease)[45-48]

Osteoarthritis (degenerative joint disease, osteoarthrosis, degenerative arthritis) is by far the most common type of arthritis. Some degree of osteoarthritis is evidenced radiographically in the majority of the population over age 55 in the United States.[49] Osteoarthritis is characterized by changes in articular cartilage and bony overgrowth at joint margins (Fig. 2–46). Clinical symptomatology, including pain, deformity, and loss of joint function, may range from absent or minimal to severe and necessitating surgical intervention. Osteoarthritis fits into the miscellaneous category of the pathologic conditions as outlined earlier, as its etiology appears to be multifactorial and at times even obscure. Genetics, aging, gender, obesity, race, and mechanical trauma may all contribute to the condition.

Osteoarthritis is classified into two types—*primary* and *secondary*. Primary osteoarthritis is idiopathic, develops spontaneously in middle age, and progresses slowly as an exaggeration of the normal aging process of joints.[50] Women are affected with somewhat greater frequency than men. In the population over age 65, whites are more frequently affected than blacks.[51] Secondary osteoarthritis develops at any age and is the result of a clearly defined underlying condition. Any injury, disease, or deformity that damages the articular cartilage or promotes excessive friction in the joint by disrupting optimal joint congruity or altering joint kinematics may contribute to the development of secondary osteoarthritis.[52] Examples include inflammatory arthritides, joint infections, congenital defor-

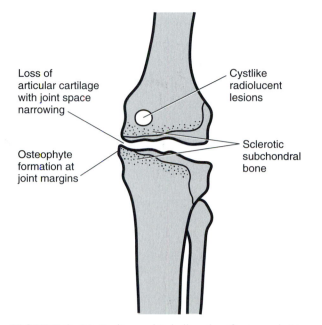

FIGURE 2–46. Radiographic hallmarks of osteoarthritis.

mities, major joint trauma such as torn menisci or torn ligaments, and microtrauma from repetitive occupational or athletic stresses. The secondary osteoarthritis that develops after *fracture*, caused by either an intra-articular extension of the fracture line or the altered surface kinematics from a malunion deformity, is often referred to as *posttraumatic arthritis*.

Radiographic features characteristic of osteoarthritis are:[53,54]

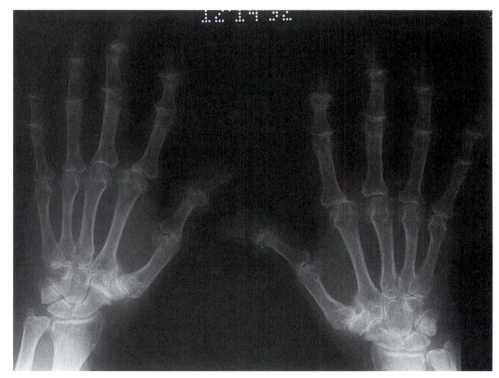

FIGURE 2–47. Osteoarthritis of the hands in a 75-year-old female. The radiographic hallmarks of osteoarthritis, including joint space narrowing, sclerosis of the subchondral bone, and osteophyte formation at joint margins, is evident throughout the distal and proximal interphalangeal joints of all the fingers, the interphalangeal joints of the thumb, and the radial side intercarpal joints, bilaterally.

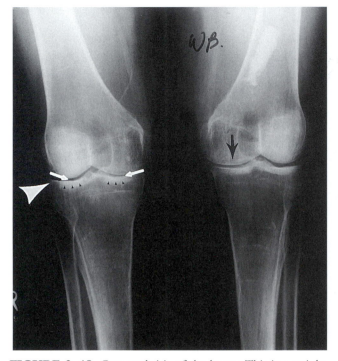

FIGURE 2–48. Osteoarthritis of the knees. This is a weight-bearing film of a 66-year-old female. At the patient's right knee, osteoarthritis is evidenced by narrowed joint space (white arrows), osteophyte formation at the joint margins (large white arrowhead), and sclerotic subchondral bone (small black arrowheads) of both the medial and lateral tibial plateaus. At the patient's left knee, it is interesting to note that in the area of minimal weight-bearing stress, the subchondral bone has lost density and rarefaction is present on the medial aspect of the joint.

JOINT SPACE NARROWING

The earliest biochemical change in osteoarthritis is loss of proteoglycan from the matrix of articular cartilage. The biomechanical consequences of this include loss of normal elastic resilience; loss of support for collagen fibrils, rendering them more susceptible to joint friction; and a resultant acceleration of shedding of the

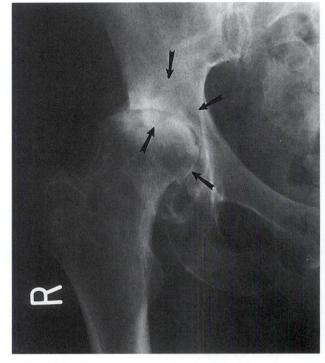

FIGURE 2–49. Severe osteoarthritis of the hip with pseudocysts. The radiolucent cystlike areas (arrows) are caused by intrusion of synovial fluid into areas of subchondral bone that has become weakened by microfractures.

cartilaginous surface layers with vertical splitting of deeper layers (fibrillation and fissuring). Repair efforts are insufficient, and degeneration of the cartilage progresses, evidenced radiographically by diminution of the joint space (Fig. 2–47).

SUBCHONDRAL SCLEROSIS

The reactive response of the subchondral bone to degeneration of the articular cartilage is a prominent feature of osteoarthritis (Fig. 2–48). Loss of the buffering effects of cartilage results in increased forces directed

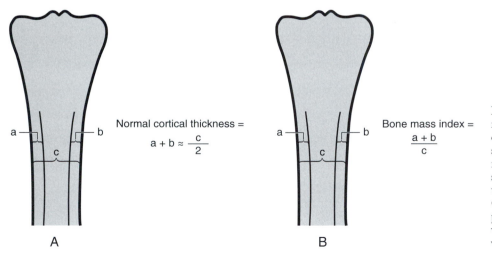

Normal cortical thickness =

$$a + b \approx \frac{c}{2}$$

Bone mass index =

$$\frac{a + b}{c}$$

A   B

FIGURE 2–50. (*A*) Cortical thickness measurements are usually based on the cortices at the midshaft of the second or third metacarpal. Normally, the sum of the two cortices should equal approximately one-half the overall diameter of the shaft. (*B*) Cortical thickness may also be expressed as an index of bone mass, which is the sum of the cortices divided by diameter.

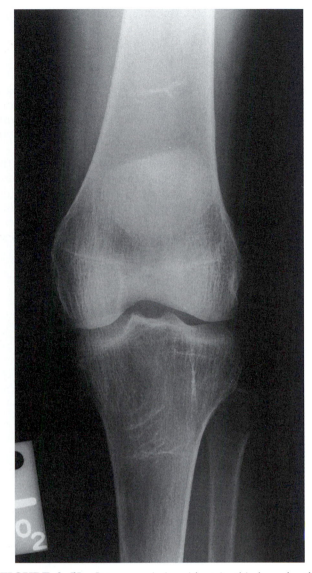

FIGURE 2–51. Osteoporosis is evident in this knee by the accentuation of the remaining trabeculae. The trabeculae have diminished in number and in thickness, and the remaining vertically oriented trabeculae stand out as thin, delicate line images.

TABLE 2–6 Examples of Conditions Associated with Osteoporosis

---

Generalized Osteoporosis (Most of Skeleton, Especially Axial Components, Involved)

Endocrine

- Estrogen deficiency
- Hyperparathyroidism
- Hyperthyroidism
- Diabetes mellitus
- Pregnancy

Neoplastic

- Malignant bone disease
- Leukemia
- Lymphoma
- Metastatic disease

Iatrogenic

- Drug-induced
  Heparin
  Phenytoin (Dilantin)
  Steroids

Genetic

- Osteogenesis imperfecta
- Hemophilia
- Gaucher's disease

Deficiency states

- Anorexia
- Alcoholism
- Weight loss
- Malnutrition

Miscellaneous

- Involutional
  Senile osteoporosis
  Postmenopausal osteoporosis
- Paraplegia
- Weightlessness

Regional Osteoporosis (a Limb, or Region of the Skeleton Involved)

- Migratory osteoporosis
- Transient osteoporosis
- Reflex sympathetic dystrophy syndrome
- Paget's disease
- Disuse/pain

Localized Osteoporosis (Focal Involvement)

- Neoplasm
- Inflammatory arthritis

---

to the subchondral bone, which gradually becomes the weight-bearing surface. *Eburnation* describes the polished ivory appearance of the exposed surface of subchondral bone. In central areas of maximal stress and friction, the subchondral bone hypertrophies to the extent that it becomes radiographically more dense or *sclerotic*. In areas of minimal stress, however, subchondral bone may atrophy, and loss of density or *rarefaction* may be evident (see Fig. 2–48).

OSTEOPHYTE FORMATION

A reparative response of articular cartilage results in hypertrophy and hyperplasia at the peripheral margins of the joint. This thickened rim of cartilage even-

tually ossifies and becomes radiographically evident (see Fig. 2–46). This formation of bony outgrowth is described as *osteophyte formation, bone spurs, osteoarthritic lipping,* or *osteophytosis.* Osteophytes may enlarge enough to impinge on adjacent tissues or restrict joint function.

CYSTS OR PSEUDOCYSTS

Excessive pressure, especially in weight-bearing joints, leads to microfractures of the trabeculae of subchondral bone. Intrusion of synovial fluid into the altered spongy bone forms cystlike lesions, evident on radiographs as radiolucent areas (Fig. 2–49).

ADDITIONAL FINDINGS—SOFT TISSUE SWELLING

Fragments of dead cartilage can dislodge into the joint, irritating the synovial membrane and causing acute inflammation and *synovial effusion*. The synovium may encapsulate this joint debris, thus enlarging and deforming the joint, as, for example, in Heberden's

nodes in the distal interphalangeal joints (see Fig. 12–51).

JOINT DEFORMITIES

Other joint deformities can result from contractures (related to maintaining joints in positions of maximum capsular volume for pain relief) or from altered joint surface congruity (due to loss of articular cartilage) (see Figs. 8–35, 8–36).

It is interesting to note that the *severity of osteoarthritic findings demonstrated radiographically does not always correlate with the clinical symptoms*. That is, a patient with marked osteoarthritic changes may experience relatively minor pain and loss of function, whereas one with minimal osteoarthritic changes may experience

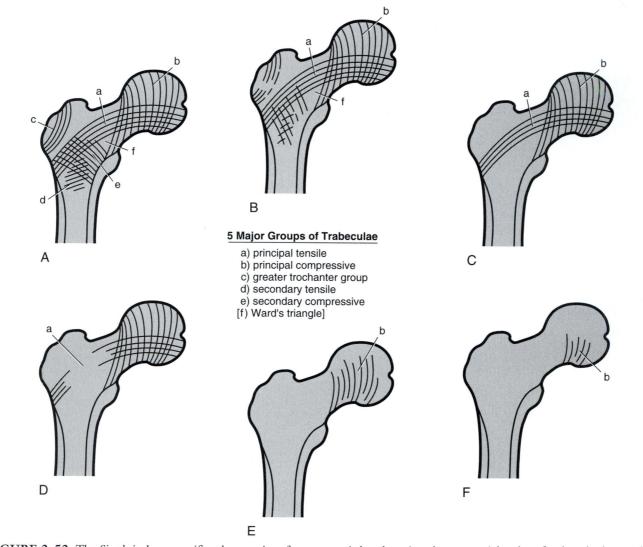

5 Major Groups of Trabeculae

a) principal tensile
b) principal compressive
c) greater trochanter group
d) secondary tensile
e) secondary compressive
[f) Ward's triangle]

FIGURE 2–52. The Singh index quantifies the severity of osteoporosis by observing the sequential order of trabecular loss at the proximal femur. Bone loss occurs in order of increasing importance of structural strength. There are five major groups of trabeculae: (a) principal tensile, (b) principal compressive, (c) greater trochanter, (d) secondary tensile, (e) secondary compressive and (f) Ward's triangle, a radiographic image formed by the borders of the principal tensile groups. (*A*) Grade 6: All normal trabecular groups visible. Femoral head and neck completely occupied by cancellous bone. (*B*) Grade 5: Principal tensile (a) and compressive (b) trabeculae are accentuated. Ward's triangle is prominent (f) as an area of increased radiolucency. (*C*) Grade 4: Principle tensile (a) trabeculae markedly reduced in number, but can still be traced from lateral cortex to femoral neck. (*D*) Grade 3: Break in continuity of principal tensile trabeculae (a) is seen opposite of greater trochanter. (*E*) Grade 2: Only principal compressive (b) trabeculae visible. (*F*) Grade 1: Principal compressive (b) trabeculae severely reduced in number. (Adapted from Greenspan, with permission.)

severe pain and impaired function. Thus it is important that intervention, especially surgical intervention, is predicated primarily on the severity of pain and loss of joint function, not on the severity of the radiographic findings.

Osteoporosis[55-57]

Osteoporosis is a metabolic bone disease characterized by decreased osteoblastic formation of matrix combined with increased osteoclastic resorption of bone. The result is a *decrease in total bone mass*. However, while the *amount* of bone is insufficient, the bone itself remains *normally mineralized*. The etiology of osteoporosis is widely varied, and consequently so is the manifestation of the disease. Possible causes of osteoporosis are divided into *congenital* and *acquired* categories. Manifestation of osteoporosis may be *generalized*, involving the entire skeleton, or *localized*, involving only a single bone or region (Table 2–6).[58]

The simplest and most widely used method of evaluating the severity of osteoporosis is plain-film radiography. Alterations in trabecular patterns, especially at the proximal femur, and diminishment of the thickness of cortical margins, are significant factors in the assessment of osteoporosis. Although diffuse radiolucency of bone is a striking feature in osteoporosis, it is a less reliable or objective measurement of bone density, as the image can easily be altered by technical errors such as overexposure or underexposure, and because at least a 30 percent reduction in bone mass is required before detection is evident on plain films.[59]

The characteristic radiolucency of osteoporosis often leads to the usage of the term as a radiologic *descriptor*. This is incorrect, as it is usually impossible to distinguish between the potential causes of increased bone radiolucency. Osteomalacia (see Fig. 2–17) (*normal matrix, deficient mineralization*) and hyperparathyroidism (see Fig. 2–19) (*normal matrix and mineralization, increased resorption*) are examples of distinct clinical entities other than osteoporosis (*deficient matrix, normal mineralization*) in which bone appears similarly radiolucent. Therefore, the term "osteoporosis" should not be used as a descriptor, but only when appropriate as a *clinical diagnosis*. The appropriate descriptor of bone that appears abnormally radiolucent is *osteopenia*, which means "poverty of bone."

Radiographic features characteristic to all forms of osteoporosis, regardless of their cause, are:[60]

CORTICAL THINNING

The first sites affected by osteoporosis, as well as the ones that are best demonstrated radiographically, are the periarticular regions where the cortex is normally thinner. Early bone density loss will be most obvious in these regions. Loss of the cortical outline indicates loss of density. Along the shafts of the long bones, loss of density is indicated by thinning of the cortices.

The normal amount of *cortical thickness* is an objective measurement and can be compared with normal standards or used as a baseline for subsequent studies in the same patient (Fig. 2–50A). Measured at the midpoint of a metacarpal shaft (usually the second or third), cortical thickness is simply the sum of the two cortices. This sum should equal approximately one-half the total diameter of the bone. Another measurement of density is the *index of bone mass*, which is simply the sum of the cortices divided by the total diameter (Fig. 2–50B).[61]

OSTEOPENIA

As just discussed, osteopenia is the radiographic description of increased bone radiolucency. Osteopenia, or, synonymously, rarefaction, is a hallmark of osteoporosis.

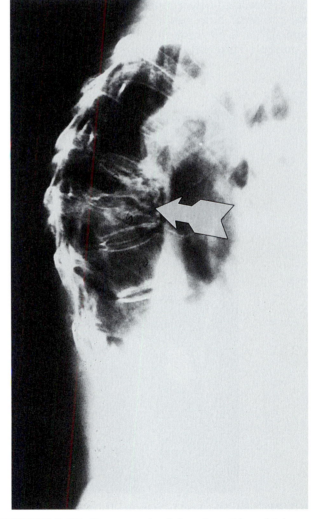

FIGURE 2–53. Osteoporosis of the spine with multiple compression fractures. The arrow points to the T8–9 disc space, which is deformed by the collapse of these two vertebrae from multiple compression fractures. This 94-year-old female has severe kyphosis of the thoracic spine (also known as a gibbous deformity) accentuated by vertebral collapse at multiple levels.

TRABECULAR CHANGES

In osteoporosis the trabeculae are diminished in number and thickness and so appear sparse, thin, and delicate (Fig. 2–51). This is best demonstrated at the proximal femur, where the trabecular architecture is easily recognized.

Because patterns of trabecular loss have been shown to correlate well with the increasing severity of osteoporosis, analysis of trabecular loss is used to evaluate the severity of osteoporosis. The *Singh index* defines six grades of osteoporosis, based on the fact that the five major trabecular groups of the proximal femur are resorbed in a predictable, sequential order as the disease progresses (Fig. 2–52).[62]

FRACTURES

Increased incidence of fractures is directly related to the loss of bone mass and thus the loss of structural integrity. The most common sites of fracture in patients with generalized osteoporosis are the vertebral bodies, ribs, proximal humerus, distal radius, and proximal femur (Figs. 2–53 through 2–56). A cumulative effect of multiple vertebral body compression fractures is a

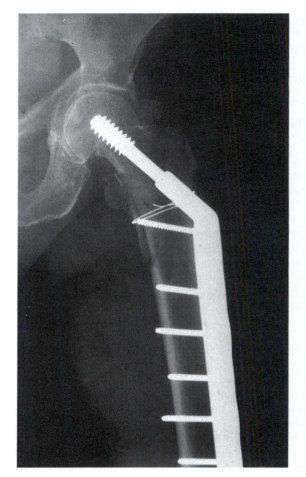

FIGURE 2–55. Intertrochanteric fracture of the left femur, fixated with compression plate and screws.

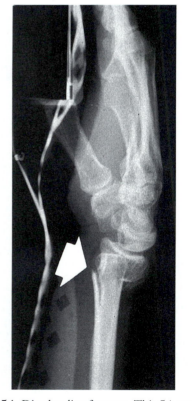

FIGURE 2–54. Distal radius fracture. This 54-year-old female fell on an outstretched arm and sustained a fracture of the distal radius, commonly known as a Colles' fracture. There is a volar apex of the fracture site with dorsal angulation. The osteoporotic changes present are difficult to visualize through the splint material.

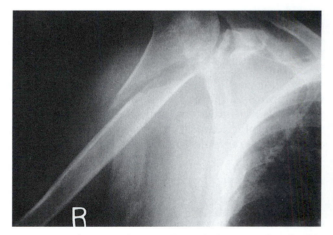

FIGURE 2–56. Spiral fracture through the surgical neck of the proximal humerus in a 62-year-old female. Osteoporosis is evidenced by the thinning of the cortices along the shaft of the humerus.

characteristic *kyphotic deformity* of the spine, commonly seen in elderly females.

Musculoskeletal Infections[63-65]

Infections of the musculoskeletal system can be divided into three categories: (1) infections of bone (*osteomyelitis*), (2) infections of joints (*septic or infectious arthritis*), and (3) infections of soft tissues (*cellulitis*). The three basic mechanisms or routes that permit an infectious organism to gain entry are (1) *hematogenous*, via the bloodstream from a distant site of infection in the body, (2) *contiguous*, from infection in adjacent soft tissues, and (3) *direct implantation*, from a puncture wound, open fracture, or operative procedure (Fig. 2–57).

Bone and joint infections may present in acute, subacute, or chronic forms, defined by the intensity of the infectious process and the associated symptoms. Furthermore, bone and joint infections may be distin-guished as either *pyogenic* (pus producing) or *nonpyogenic*. The most common organism of pyogenic infection is *Staphylococcus aureus*. Nonpyogenic infections may be caused by tuberculosis, syphilis, and fungus.

OSTEOMYELITIS[66]

Acute osteomyelitis is often pyogenic, resulting from hematogenous spread of the *S. aureus* organism. It most commonly presents in the long bones of children, with higher incidence seen in boys (see Fig. 2–22). The metaphyseal region is the primary site of involvement owing to the unique blood supply of this region during growth. The radiologic features characteristic of acute pyogenic osteomyelitis are:

Soft Tissue Swelling
The earliest signs of bone infection are soft tissue edema and loss of fascial planes, usually present within 24 to 48 hours after the onset of infection.

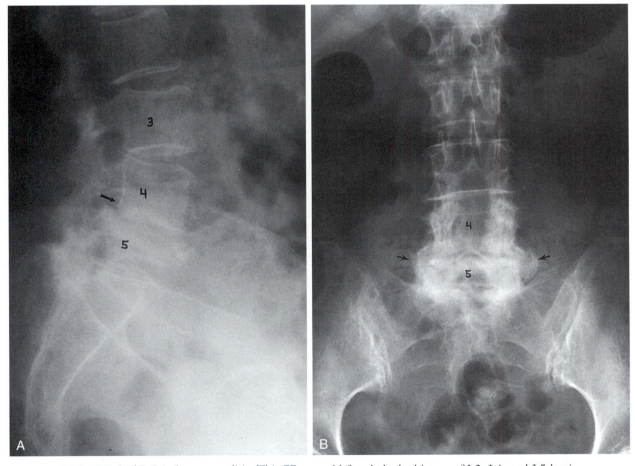

FIGURE 2–57. L4–5 osteomyelitis. This 77-year-old female had a history of L3, L4, and L5 lami-nectomies and an L4–5 diskectomy secondary to radiculopathy and decreased bowel and bladder function. An infection developed postoperatively. (*A*) On the lateral film, an anterolisthesis of L4 on the eroded body of L5 is seen (arrow). (*B*) On the anterior posterior view, the sequestra is noted (arrows).

Lytic Lesion

A destructive lytic lesion, represented by an area of increased bone radiolucency, is visible within 7 to 10 days after the onset of infection. Progressive cortical and cancellous destruction occurs over the next 2 to 6 weeks.

Sequestra and Involucra

In 6 to 8 weeks after onset, *sequestra*, isolated segments of dead bone usually surrounded by pus, become apparent. Sequestra are surrounded by the *involucrum*, an envelope of immature periosteal bone that also becomes infected. Draining *sinus tracts* (see Fig. 2–22B) often are formed through the involucrum, and pus and small bits of sequestra may be discharged. At this stage, the condition is designated as *chronic osteomyelitis* (Figs. 2–58, 2–59).

INFECTIOUS ARTHRITIS[67]

Infectious arthritis of the pyogenic type is seen in all age groups, but it is frequently seen in children, often paralleling the incidence of acute osteomyelitis. In children, the joints in which the metaphysis is entirely encapsulated—namely, the hip, elbow, and knee—are commonly affected (Figs. 2–60, 2–61). Destruction of epiphyseal plates with resultant growth arrest is a dreaded complication. In adults, infectious arthritis may develop in any joint, as it is unrelated to osteomyelitis (Fig. 2–62). Conditions that lower resistance, such as prolonged adrenocorticosteroid therapy, may influence development. The radiographic features characteristic of pyogenic infectious arthritis are as follows:

Soft Tissue Swelling

Early stages of joint infection are demonstrated by joint effusion and adjacent soft tissue swelling.

Periarticular Rarefaction

Radiolucency of bone at the periarticular regions is also demonstrated early.

Joint Space Narrowing

In later stages, destruction of articular cartilage on both sides of the joint will significantly narrow the joint space.

Subchondral Bone Erosion

As infectious arthritis involves all articular surfaces within the joint, erosion of subchondral bone may be evident on all joint surfaces in later stages.

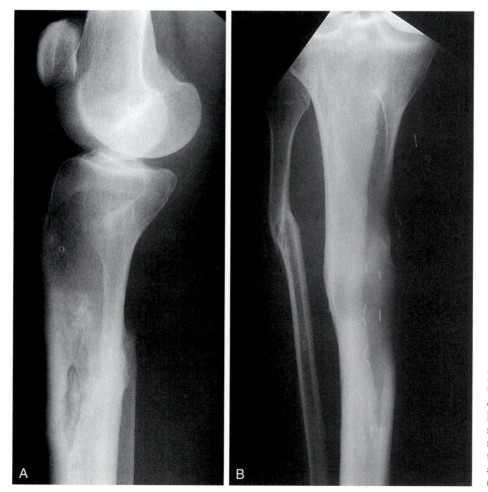

A   B

FIGURE 2–58. Chronic osteomyelitis of the tibia and fibula. This 44-year-old man developed osteomyelitis following a fracture. Involucrum (*A*) surrounds both the tibia and fibula, seen on a lateral view of the leg. Patient received an extensive course of antibiotics and surgical debridement. (*B*) Resection of dead bone.

CELLULITIS[68]

Cellulitis usually results from direct skin puncture but can also result from systemic disorders such as diabetes. The most common infectious organisms are the gas-producing *Clostridium novyi* and *C. perfringens*. The radiographic features characteristic of cellulitis are:

Soft Tissue Swelling
Cellulitis presents with soft tissue edema and obliteration of fat and fascial planes.

Radiolucent Streaks or Bubbles
The gas-forming organisms may cause an accumulation of gas within the soft tissues, which is demonstrated on film as radiolucent bubbles or streaks. This is usually an indication of gas gangrene (Fig. 2–63).

Bone Tumors[69]

Tumor refers to a *mass* of autonomous growth, an equivalent term being *neoplasm*. Tumors are generally divided into two categories, *benign* and *malignant*. Benign tumors usually are not recurrent or progressive. Malignant tumors, in contrast, are progressive and may produce local or remote *metastases*. Malignant tumors are thus further classified as *primary*, *secondary* (the result of a malignant transformation of a benign process), or *metastatic*. Specific histopathologic criteria additionally are applied in determining whether a tumor is malignant or benign.

Tumors are also classified by their tissue of origin. *Osteogenic benign tumors* are tumors originating

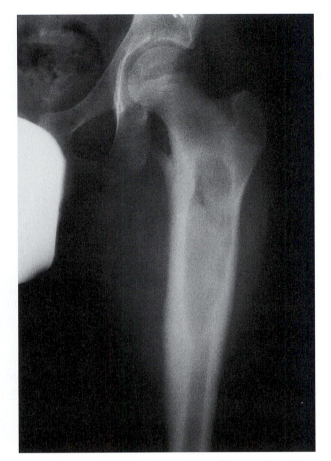

FIGURE 2–59. Chronic osteomyelitis of the proximal femur. This 13-year-old boy presented with complaints of left thigh pain and a 6-month history of fever and chills. Soft tissue swelling and a large lytic lesion are present along the entire upper half of the femur.

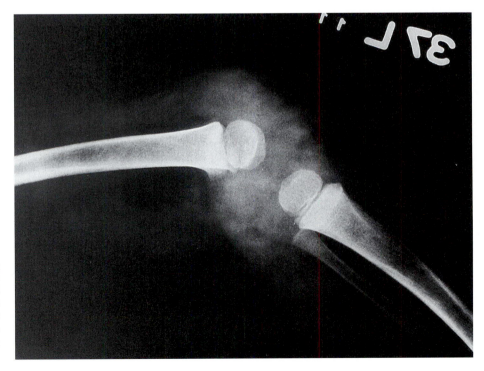

FIGURE 2–60. Infectious arthritis. This 3½-year-old toddler presented with a 3-month history of pain and swelling and with a visible lump on the knee. There was a history of frequent upper respiratory infections and pneumonia. Distension of the knee joint capsule with pus is evident.

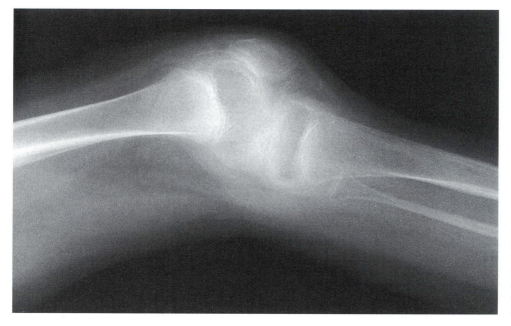

FIGURE 2–61. Infectious arthritis, differential diagnosis. This x-ray of an 8-year-old boy was made in 1921. Although some of the characteristic hallmarks of infectious arthritis were present, including soft tissue swelling, periarticular rarefaction, and joint space narrowing, the diagnosis was later correctly changed to hemophilia.

from bone tissue (e.g., *osteoma, osteoid osteoma,* and *osteoblastoma*). Examples of malignant osteogenic tumors are the variants of *osteosarcoma.* Tumors arising from tissues other than bone can still manifest in bone, such as two of the most common primary malignancies of bone, *multiple myeloma* and *Ewing's sarcoma* (Fig. 2–64) (both arising from cells of the bone marrow), or the most common benign tumor of bone, *osteochondroma* (arising from cartilage).

Some radiographic features generally characteristic of tumors that assist the radiologist in making a diagnosis are as follows:

SITE OF THE LESION

Some tumors have a predilection for specific bones or specific sites on individual bones, and diagnosis can sometimes be suggested on this basis alone. For example, multiple myeloma characteristically affects the vertebral bodies, pelvis, and calvaria of the skull. Parosteal osteosarcoma presents at the posterior aspect of the distal femur.

TYPE OF LESION BORDER

Slow-growing tumors, which are usually benign, have well-defined sclerotic margins, also referred to as a *narrow zone of transition* (Fig. 2–65). Fast-growing or malignant tumors typically show a *wide zone of transition,* with minimal or absent reactive sclerosis.

TYPE OF MATRIX

The tumor matrix can be identified radiographically as *osteoid* (bone-forming) or *chondroid* (cartilage-forming). Cloudlike, fluffy density within the medul-

lary cavity and in adjacent soft tissue suggests tumorous bone and a diagnosis of osteosarcoma. Cartilage growth typically appears as popcorn-like, punctate, annular, or comma-shaped calcifications.

TYPE OF BONE DESTRUCTION

The type of bone destruction is related to the growth rate of the tumor, thus providing a clue as to whether a lesion is benign or malignant (see Fig. 2–35). *Geographic destruction* with sharp borders suggests a benign process. *Moth-eaten* appearance with ragged borders suggests a likely malignant process. *Permeative* destruction with poorly defined borders suggests an aggressive or malignant process (Fig. 2–66).

TYPE OF PERIOSTEAL RESPONSE

Periosteal reaction to a neoplasm is usually characterized as *interrupted or uninterrupted.* Interrupted periosteal response suggests malignant or nonmalignant but highly aggressive lesions. It may present in a sunburst or spiculated pattern, laminated or onionskin pattern, or a Codman's triangle, as commonly seen in the osteosarcomas (see Fig. 2–31). Uninterrupted periosteal response suggests benign processes and presents as a solid density, either longitudinal, undulated, or buttressing in pattern.

SOFT TISSUE EXTENSION

Generally, benign tumors do not exhibit extension into the soft tissues. Extension of the mass through the cortex and into the soft tissues is typical of aggressive and often malignant tumors.

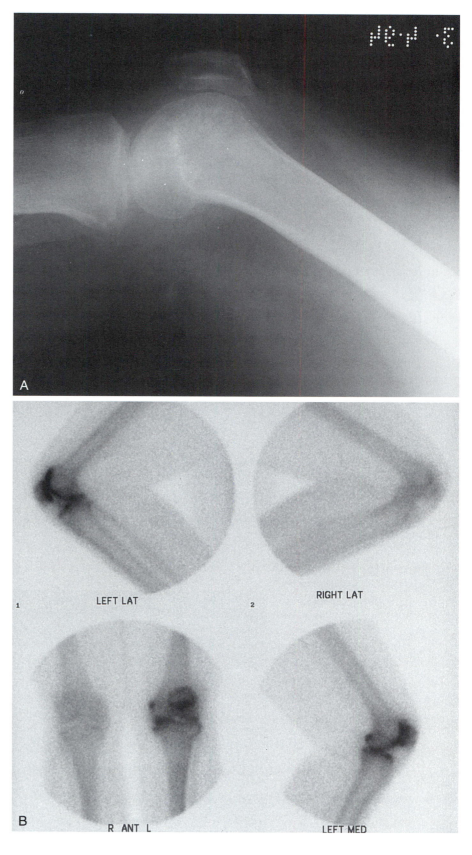

FIGURE 2–62. Infectious arthritis, bone scan. This 34-year-old male had a history of surgical debridement at the knee 1 year ago. He was re-evaluated for recurrent pain. (*A*) Plain film findings were suggestive of either mild osteoarthritis or infectious arthritis. (*B*) Bone scan showed increased uptake in the medial lateral compartment and patella of the knee. When these findings were correlated with the laboratory findings, a diagnosis of infectious arthritis was confirmed.

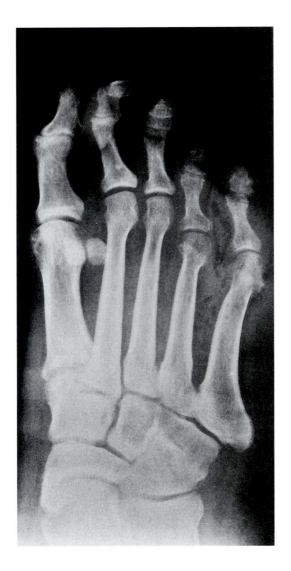

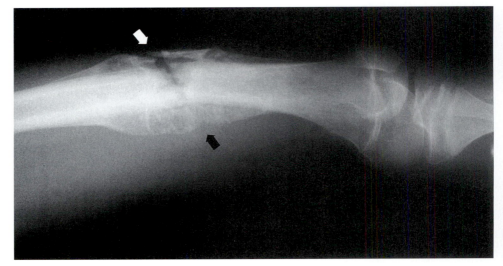

FIGURE 2–63. Gas gangrene. Anteroposterior plain film of the foot of a 59-year-old man with long-standing diabetes mellitus shows marked soft tissue swelling and edema, particularly in the region of the fourth and fifth digits. Radiolucent streaks of gas are typical of gangrenous infection. (From Greenspan,[2] p 20.17, with permission.)

FIGURE 2–64. Ewing's sarcoma of the femoral shaft with a pathologic fracture through the midshaft (arrows) in a 16-year-old boy.

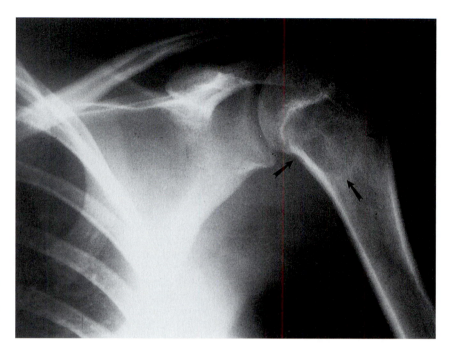

FIGURE 2–65. Chondroblastoma of the proximal humerus in a 15-year-old female. Note the narrow zone of transition, a well-defined sclerotic margin, associated with slow growing or benign tumors.

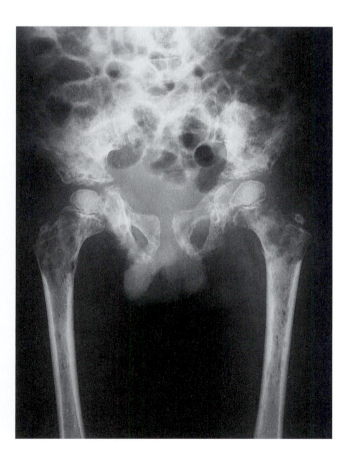

FIGURE 2–66. Diffuse lytic metastasis to bone secondary to rhabdomyosarcoma. Note the permeative destruction with poorly defined borders of the lesions which is characteristic of an aggressive or malignant process.

SUMMARY OF KEY POINTS

1. *Remodeling* of bone, which occurs continuously throughout life, is directly related to *function*. To paraphrase Wolff's Law, bone is deposited in the sites subjected to stress and resorbed in sites deprived of stress.
2. The essentials of radiographic analysis can be remembered with the acronym *ABCs*: Alignment, Bone density, Cartilage spaces, soft tissues.
3. There are six basic categories of pathology in the classification of skeletal diseases: congenital, inflammatory, metabolic, neoplastic, traumatic, and vascular. A seventh category, miscellaneous, encompasses those conditions that do not fall strictly into one category, such as osteoarthritis.
4. Radiographic diagnosis of skeletal pathology begins with 1) *defining the distribution of the lesion*, and 2) *applying predictor variables to the lesion*.
5. *Predictor variables* are factors that further limit diagnostic choices. Daffner described eleven: behavior of the lesion; the bone or joint involved; the locus within a bone; the age, gender, or race of the patient; the margin of the lesion; the shape of the lesion; involvement of the joint space; bony reaction; matrix production by the lesion; soft tissue changes; and history of trauma or surgery.
6. Radiographic characteristics of *adult rheumatoid arthritis* are: periatricular soft tissue swelling, articular erosions, minimal or absent reparative processes, concentric joint space narrowing, rarefaction of periatricular regions in early stages, generalized osteoporosis in later stages, and joint deformities.
7. Radiographic characteristics of *osteoarthritis (DJD)* are: joint space narrowing, sclerosis of subchondral bone, and ostephyte formation at joint margins.
8. Radiographic characteristics of *osteoporosis* are: rarefaction of bone at periatricular regions, loss of cortical thickness, generalized osteopenia, and associated fractures. The most common sites for fracture are the vertebrae, proximal humerus, distal radius, and proximal femur.
9. *Infections of the musculoskeletal system* can be divided into: infections of bone—*osteomyelitis*; infections of joints—*septic or infectious arthritis*; and infections of soft tissues—*cellulitis*. The earliest radiographic feature of any infection is soft tissue swelling.
10. The radiographic features that assist the radiologist in differentiating types of *bone tumors* include: site of the lesion; a narrow or wide zone of transition of the lesion; whether the matrix is osteoid or chondroid; the type of destruction—geographic, moth-eaten, permeative; an interrupted or uninterrupted periosteal response; and presence of soft tissue extension of the lesion.

REFERENCES

1. Schultz, RJ: The Language of Fractures, ed 2. Williams & Wilkins, Baltimore, 1990, p 2.
2. Greenspan, A: Orthopedic Radiology: A Practical Approach, ed 2. Raven Press, New York, 1992, p 3.1.
3. Ibid, p 3.1.
4. Salter, RB: Textbook of Disorders and Injuries of the Musculoskeletal System, ed 2. Williams & Wilkins, Baltimore, 1983.
5. Schultz, p 2.
6. Salter, p 9.
7. Ibid, pp 9, 361, 430, 479.
8. Brashear, HR and Raney, RB: Shand's Handbook of Orthopedic Surgery, Mosby, St. Louis, 1978, p 54.
9. Richardson, JK and Iglarsh, ZA: Clinical Orthopaedic Physical Therapy. WB Saunders, Philadelphia, 1994, p 653.
10. Salter, p 9.
11. Daffner, RH: Clinical Radiology: The Essentials. Williams & Wilkins, Baltimore, 1993, p 283.
12. Swain, JH: An Introduction to Radiology of the Lumbar Spine: Orthopaedic Study Course 94-1. © 1994, Orthopaedic Section, APTA, Inc, p 2.
13. Greenspan, pp 24.1, 25.1.
14. Ibid, p 12.1.
15. Ibid, p 4.7.

16. Richardson, p 636.
17. Greenspan, p 12.1.
18. Ibid, p 10.43.
19. Daffner, p 307.
20. Ibid.
21. Ibid.
22. Salter, p 27.
23. Ibid, p 65.
24. Daffner, p 309.
25. Greenspan, p 12.1.
26. Daffner, p 310.
27. Ibid, p 303.
28. Greenspan, p 4.9–4.13.
29. Daffner, p 303.
30. Greenspan, p 4.14.
31. Ibid.
32. Daffner, p 297.
33. Greenspan, p 15.20.
34. Daffner, p 303.
35. Ibid, p 283.
36. Ibid.
37. Ibid, pp 283–306.
38. Ibid, p 285.
39. Greenspan, p 15.14.
40. Ibid, p 13.4.
41. Richardson, p 649.
42. Daffner, p 310.
43. Salter, p 190.
44. Greenspan, p 13.14.
45. Richardson, pp 430, 645.
46. Daffner, p 310.
47. Salter, p 214.
48. Greenspan, pp 12.1–12.11.
49. Richardson, p 430.
50. Salter, p 214.
51. Greenspan, p 12.1.
52. Richardson, p 430.
53. Greenspan, pp 12.2–12.10.
54. Richardson, pp 430, 645.
55. Greenspan, pp 21.1–21.8, 22.1–22.5.
56. Richardson, p 639.
57. Daffner, p 307.
58. Greenspan, p 22.1.
59. Ibid, p 21.2.
60. Ibid, pp 22.1–22.5.
61. Ibid, p 21.2.
62. Ibid, p 22.4.
63. Ibid, pp 19-1–20.16.
64. Brashear, pp 105–135.
65. Salter, p 168.
66. Greenspan, pp 20.1–20.6.
67. Ibid, pp 20.7–20.9.
68. Ibid, p 20.16.
69. Ibid, pp 15.1–15.30.

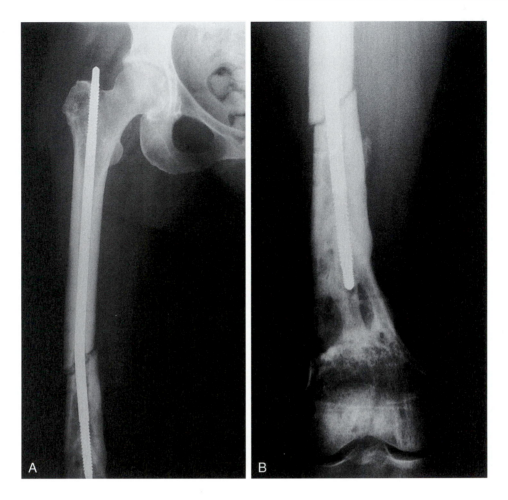

SELF-TEST

Chapter 2

REGARDING FILM A:

1. Identify this <u>projection</u>.
2. A fracture has occurred through the shaft of the femur. What radiographic evidence leads you to believe that this is a <u>pathologic fracture</u>?
3. Does this entire femur exhibit this radiographic evidence? Does the pelvis?
4. An intermedullary rod is present to unite the frac-

ture gap. Does this appear to be the <u>first</u> internal fixation device used at this site?
5. Does the <u>hip joint</u> appear normal?

REGARDING FILM B (SAME PATIENT):

6. Identify this <u>projection</u>.
7. The fracture is noted. Identify two other abnormal features of the distal femur.
8. Would you categorize this pathology as probably being related to an <u>infection</u>, an <u>inflammatory process</u>, or a <u>neoplasm</u>? What radiographic evidence suggests a likely category?

CHAPTER 3

Radiographic Evaluation of Fracture

Trauma is the most common disorder of the musculoskeletal system evaluated by radiology. The fractures and dislocations that comprise the majority of traumatic conditions are most effectively evaluated by plain-film radiography.[1] In dealing with trauma, the task of the radiologist is twofold: (1) to diagnose and evaluate the characteristics of the fracture or dislocation and (2) to assess the results of treatment and to monitor the healing process and potential complications.[2]

The words used to describe fractures as seen on plain films are based on anatomic and standardized terms. This is important because the information is then accessible to all clinicians involved in patient treatment.[3] *Eponyms* (e.g., *Colles' fracture*) are generally avoided in radiographic description because of their general reference characteristics, lack of descriptive detail, and ease of misinterpretation. Rather, the more precise and objective language of anatomy, which serves as the common ground between all medical and rehabilitative clinicians, is used.

The goals of the chapter are to define the elements that make up the radiographic evaluation of fractures; note the special characteristics of fractures in children; identify basic features of fracture treatment, healing, and possible complications of healing; and present a glossary of eponyms of orthopedic conditions, which although uncommon in radiographic description, do remain common in medical vocabulary.

DEFINITION OF FRACTURE

A fracture is a break in the continuity of bone or cartilage.[4] Fractures may be caused by *direct trauma* or *indirect trauma*, according to whether a force was applied directly to the bone or at a distance from the bone and then transmitted to it. The patterns in which fractures occur are somewhat predictable based on the *viscoelastic properties* of bone combined with the biomechanics of *load*. See Table 3–1 for a summary of long bone fracture patterns and their precipitating forces.[5]

A basic distinction in defining fractures is whether or not the fracture site is exposed to the external environment. A *closed or simple fracture* is one in which the skin and soft tissues overlying the fracture are intact (Fig. 3–1). An *open or compound fracture* exists any time the skin is perforated, regardless of the size of the wound. The older terms, simple and compound, do not offer any useful information and are thus fading from use.

Evaluation of fractures on plain films requires *at least two views of the bone involved, with each view including the joints adjacent to that bone.* This is significant because many injury patterns involve associated fractures, subluxations, or dislocations at sites remote from the apparent primary injury.[6]

71

TABLE 3–1 Summary of Long Bone Fracture Biomechanics

Fracture Pattern	Appearance	Mechanism of Injury	Location Soft Tissue Hinge	Energy
Transverse		Bending	Concavity	Low
Spiral		Torsion	Vertical segment	Low
Oblique-transverse or butterfly		Compression + Bending	Concavity or side of butterfly	Mod
Oblique		Compression + Bending + Torsion	Concavity (often destroyed)	Mod
Comminuted		Variable	Destroyed	High
Metaphyseal compression		Compression	Variable	Variable

From Gozna and Harrington,[5] with permission.

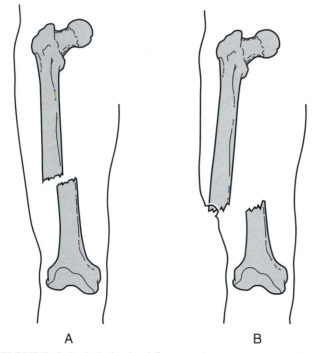

FIGURE 3–1. (*A*) A *closed* fracture does not communicate with the external environment. (*B*) An *open* fracture denotes an opening in the skin, and the fracture site is susceptible to infection from the external environment.

ELEMENTS OF FRACTURE DESCRIPTION

Greenspan[7] identifies seven elements that should be included in a complete radiographic evaluation of fractures:

1. The anatomic *site* and *extent* of the fracture.
2. The *type* of fracture, whether *complete* or *incomplete*.
3. The *alignment* of the fracture fragments.
4. The *direction* of the fracture line.
5. The presence of *special features* of the fracture, such as *impaction* or *avulsion*.
6. The presence of *associated abnormalities*, such as joint dislocations.
7. The *special types* of fractures that may occur as a result of *abnormal stresses* or secondary to *pathologic processes* in the bone, such as *stress fractures* or *pathologic fractures*.

Explanations of these seven points follow.

Anatomic Site and Extent of the Fracture[8,9]

Establishing the location of a fracture requires points of reference (Fig. 3–2). The *shafts* of long bones are divided into thirds: fractures may be present at the *proximal, middle, or distal thirds* of the shaft, or at the *junction* of these regions, for example, at the junction of the

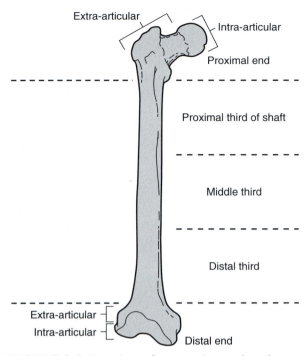

FIGURE 3–2. Location reference points on long bones.

middle and proximal thirds. The ends of long bones are designated as the *distal* or *proximal* end, and each end is divided into *extra-articular* and *intra-articular* portions (Fig. 3–3). The intra-articular portions are comprised of the joint surface areas. Fractures may *extend intra-articularly* from an extra-articular region (Fig. 3–4).

Reference points for flat or irregularly shaped bones may be noted as either the *intra-articular* or *extra-articular* regions. Additionally, all bones may be referenced by standard anatomic landmarks or parts, such as the *surgical neck of the humerus, the intertrochanteric region of the hip, the supracondylar area of the distal femur, or the medial malleoli at the ankle.*

Type of Fracture—Complete or Incomplete[10,11]

A *complete fracture* is a fracture in which all cortices of the bone have been broken (Fig. 3–5). In a complete fracture, what was once one bone is now *two frag-*

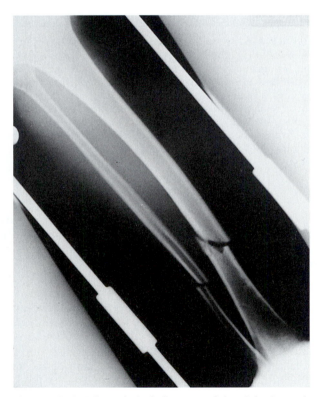

FIGURE 3–3. Bilateral shaft fracture of the right lower leg. These fractures are described as complete fractures occurring at the junction of the middle and distal thirds of the shafts. The fracture line is oblique in the fibula and is oblique in the tibia with comminution. In both fracture sites, some degree of apposition remains between the fragments, so they are described as minimally displaced, with slight lateral angulation of the distal fragments.

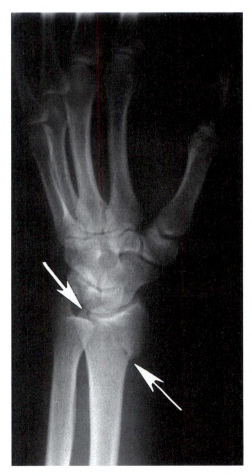

FIGURE 3–4. Intra-articular fracture of the distal radius. The arrows mark the extent of the fracture line. The fracture line is described as oblique, extending from the metaphysis on the radial side of the bone to the intra-articular surface. The fracture is complete, with minimal displacement and minimal angulation.

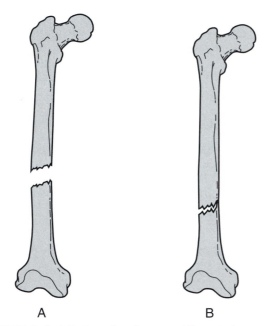

FIGURE 3–5. (*A*) Complete fracture. All cortical margins are broken and now there are two fracture *fragments*. (*B*) Incomplete fracture. One cortical margin remains intact.

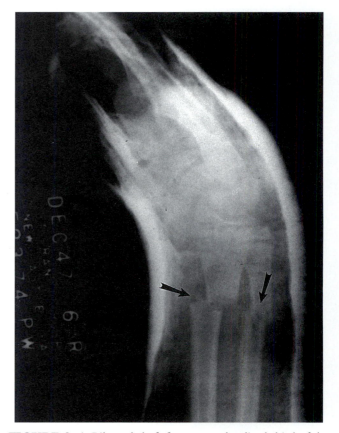

FIGURE 3–6. Bilateral shaft fracture at the distal third of the radius and ulna. This film was made through plaster to determine if fragment position was satisfactory after reduction. Both fractures are described as complete fractures with transverse fracture lines. The distal fragments are dorsally displaced, but good contact remains between the fracture fragments and good alignment is preserved. (From Richardson, JK, and Iglarsh, ZA: Clinical Orthopaedic Physical Therapy. WB Saunders, Philadelphia, 1994, p 679, with permission.)

ments (Fig. 3–6). If a fracture has more than two fragments, it is classified as a *comminuted* fracture.

An *incomplete fracture*, by contrast, has only one portion of the cortex disrupted (Fig. 3–7). Generally, incomplete fractures are relatively stable and will maintain their position indefinitely if no subsequent stresses are placed on them. Incomplete fractures are seen predominantly in short bones, irregularly shaped bones, and flat bones. There are some types of incomplete fractures that occur exclusively in children, and these are discussed under the section on fractures in children.

Alignment of Fracture Fragments[12]

Further description of a fracture includes identifying the position of one fracture fragment in relationship to the other fracture fragment. Common practice is to describe the position of the *distal fragment* in relation to the *proximal fragment*. Many terms are needed to accurately express this relationship.

Position refers to the relationship of the fragments to their normal anatomic structure. Loss of position is *displacement*. Fractures are *displaced* if there is no *apposition* or contact between the broken surfaces of the fragments. The direction of displacement (of the distal fragment) may be *medial, lateral, anterior, posterior, superior,* or *inferior* (Fig. 3–8). Additionally, displacement may result from *distraction, overriding,* or *rotation* of the fracture fragments. *Nondisplaced* fractures, by contrast, have some degree of contact remaining between the fracture fragments.

Alignment is the relationship of the longitudinal axis of one fragment to the other. Fracture fragments are said *to be in alignment* when the longitudinal axes of both fragments line up in tandem or in parallel (Fig. 3–9). Deviations from alignment are the result of *angulation* of the fracture fragments. Some confusion arises in describing the direction of angulation because two methods are in common usage. Angulation may be described by either (1) the direction of angular displacement of the distal fragment in relationship to the proximal fragment or (2) by the direction of the *apex* of the angle formed by the fracture fragments. To clarify angulation, both methods are often employed. Some examples are *volar apex with dorsal angulation of the distal fragment* and *medial angulation of the fracture site (medial apex) with lateral angular displacement of the distal fragment* (see Fig. 3–9).

Accurate description of a fracture site must address *both* position and alignment. Good position does not

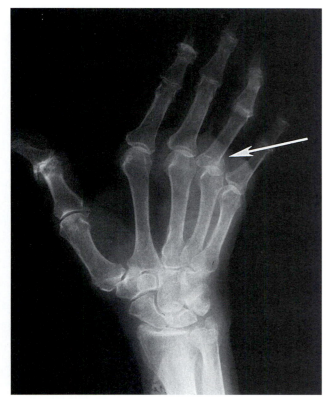

FIGURE 3–7. Incomplete fracture at the base of the proximal phalanx of the fourth digit, or ring finger. Note the abnormal position of the metacarpophalangeal joint, indicating possible subluxation or dislocation. Note also the great amount of soft tissue swelling and edema.

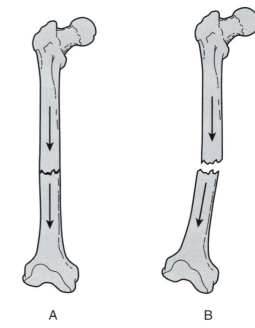

A   B

FIGURE 3–9. Alignment is the relationship of the longitudinal axes of the fracture fragments. (*A*) Fracture is in good alignment. (*B*) Fracture is poorly aligned, as the distal fragment is angulated.

imply good alignment, and vice versa; rather, the possible combinations are as follows (Fig. 3–10):

1. Good position with good alignment: In this fracture site, there is no displacement of the bone from its normal anatomic position and no angulation of the fragments.
2. Good position with deviated alignment: In this fracture site, some apposition remains between the frag-

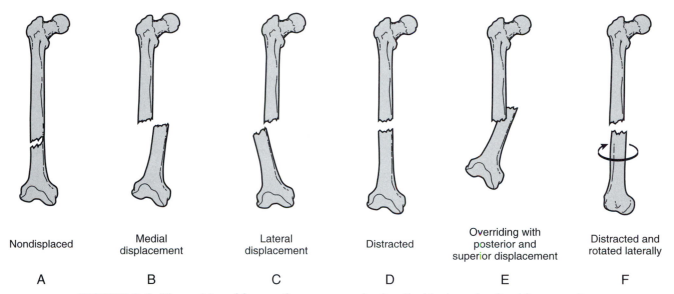

Nondisplaced	Medial displacement	Lateral displacement	Distracted	Overriding with posterior and superior displacement	Distracted and rotated laterally
A	B	C	D	E	F

FIGURE 3–8. The *position* of fracture fragments may be described by how the *distal* fragment displaces in relationship to the *proximal* fragment.

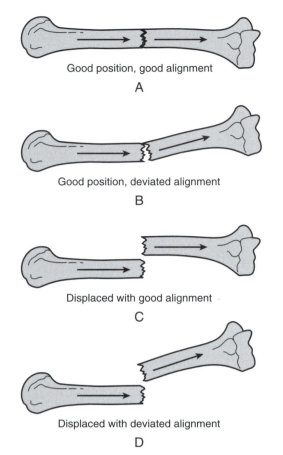

Good position, good alignment

A

Good position, deviated alignment

B

Displaced with good alignment

C

Displaced with deviated alignment

D

FIGURE 3–10. (*A–D*) Possible combinations of fracture position and alignment. (Adapted from Schultz,[4] p 24.)

ments (relatively nondisplaced) and the distal fragment is angulated.
3. Displaced with good alignment: In this fracture site, the fragment ends are no longer in contact, but the longitudinal axes are parallel. This side-by-side or

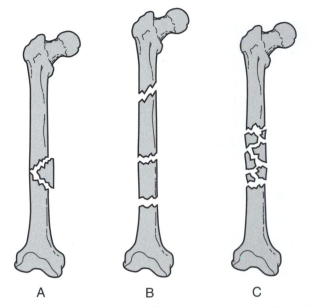

A   B   C

FIGURE 3–12. *Comminuted* fractures are fractures with more than two fragments. Some frequently occurring comminuted fracture patterns are (*A*) the wedge-shaped or butterfly pattern, (*B*) a two- or three-segmented level fracture. (*C*) Other fractures with multiple fragments, be it several or several hundred, are still described as comminuted.

overriding arrangement is commonly known as "bayonet apposition."
4. Displaced with deviated alignment: In this fracture site, the fragments are both displaced and angulated.

Direction of Fracture Lines[13,14]

The *direction* of the fracture line is described in reference to the longitudinal axis of a long bone and in

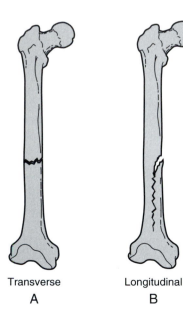

Transverse
A

Longitudinal
B

Oblique
C

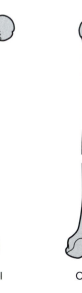

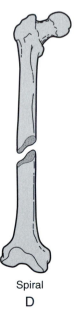

Spiral
D

FIGURE 3–11. (*A–D*) Directions of fracture lines are described in reference to the longitudinal axis of the bone.

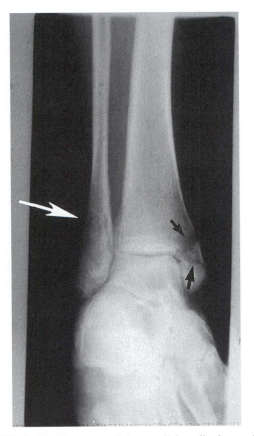

reference to the cortices of irregularly shaped bones. Fracture lines are *transverse, oblique, spiral, or longitudinal* (Fig. 3–11).

A transverse fracture line occurs at right angles to the longitudinal axis or cortices of a bone. An oblique line runs obliquely to the axis. A spiral line, usually resulting from torsional forces, is similar to an oblique line but spans a greater area of the shaft, encircling the shaft and thus forming a spiral in relationship to the long axis. Longitudinal fracture lines are approximately parallel to the shaft.

A *comminuted* fracture does not always have a clear direction, as it refers to any fracture with more than two fragments. Some frequently occurring comminuted fracture patterns are the *butterfly fragment*, a wedge-shaped fragment split from the main fragments, and the *segmental fracture*, where the bone is segmented by more than one fracture line (Figs. 3–12, 3–13).

Presence of Special Features[15,16]

Some special features of fractures are *impaction* and *avulsion* (Fig. 3–14).

Impaction fractures are the result of one fracture fragment being forcibly driven into the other fragment.

FIGURE 3–13. Fracture of the medial malleolus and distal fibula. The black arrows mark two distinct fracture lines at the medial malleolus. A wedge-shaped fragment is apparent. This fracture is described as complete, as both cortices are broken, and intra-articular, as it extends into the talocrural joint. The white arrow points to a fracture of the distal third of the fibula. Further description of this fracture is not possible without additional views. (From Richardson, JK, and Iglarsh ZA: Clinical Orthopaedic Physical Therapy. WB Saunders, Philadelphia, 1994, p 662, with permission.)

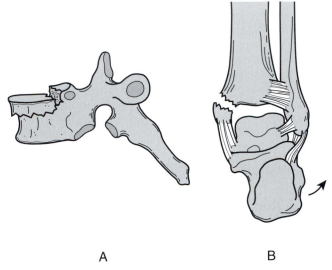

A   B

FIGURE 3–14. Special features of fractures include (*A*) impaction, seen, for example, in a compression fracture of a vertebral body, or (*B*) avulsion, as seen in a medial malleolar avulsion during an eversion force trauma at the ankle.

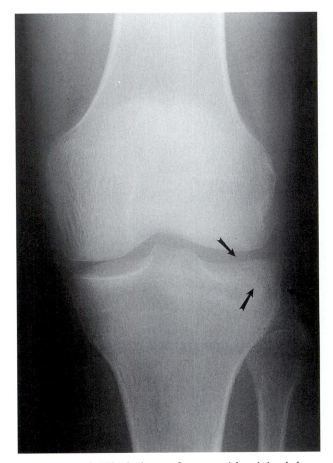

FIGURE 3–15. Tibial plateau fracture with minimal depression. Arrows mark the extent of the fracture line.

The trabeculae will telescope or enmesh into each other. This occurs predominantly in areas of cancellous bone, as its spongy nature permits the compression necessary to effect impaction. There is some degree of natural stability produced with impaction fractures, and this, combined with the close contact of the fragments, is advantageous for fracture healing. Two forms of impaction are *depression fractures*, in which the hard surface of one bone is driven into the softer surface of another, and *compression fractures*, in which both surfaces of a bone are forced together. By example, *a depression fracture of the tibial plateau* results from the impacting force of the hard distal femoral condyle into the relatively softer tibial plateau (Fig. 3–15). *A compression fracture of a vertebral body* results from forceful flexion of the spine, which compresses the vertebral body between superior and inferior adjacent vertebrae (Fig. 3–16).

Avulsion fractures are the result of fragments of bone being pulled away from their original position by active contraction of a muscle or by the passive resis-

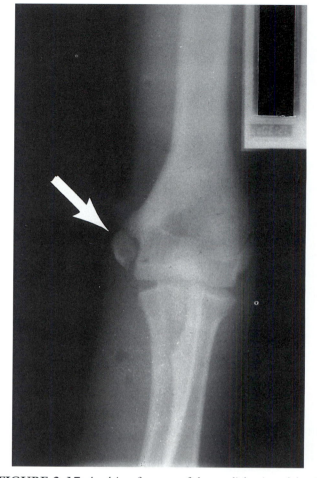

FIGURE 3–17. Avulsion fracture of the medial epicondyle of the distal humerus secondary to forceful contraction of the flexors of the forearm. (From Richardson, JK, and Iglarsh, ZA: Clinical Orthopaedic Physical Therapy. WB Saunders, Philadelphia, 1994, p 663, with permission.)

tance of a ligament against an opposing force (Fig. 3–17). Avulsion fractures occur at bony prominences, which serve as attachment sites for muscles, tendons, and ligaments. Avulsion fractures, similar to other fractures, are described by location and fracture line. For example, an eversion injury at the ankle may result in a *transverse avulsion fracture of the medial malleolus*.

Fractures of the epiphysis and *epiphyseal plates* are special features of fractures in children and will be discussed in that section.

Associated Abnormalities[17]

Abnormalities associated with fractures are varied. *Subluxations* and *dislocations* of related joints are probably the most common injuries associated with fracture (Fig. 3–18). Involvement in nearby soft tissues is also common (e.g., disruptions of the joint capsules, of the ligaments, or of the interosseous membrane be-

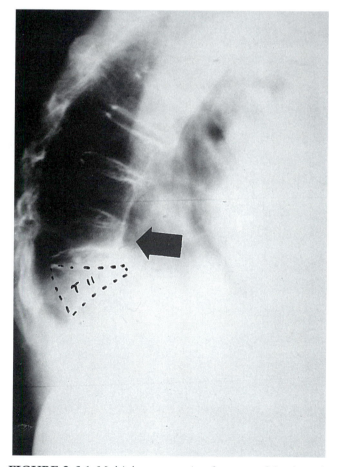

FIGURE 3–16. Multiple compression fractures of the thoracic spine. Severe osteoporosis is a striking feature. Much of the cortical outline of the vertebral bodies is no longer apparent because of bony demineralization, so the shape of the bodies is deduced primarily from the remaining fibrous disc spaces. The large arrow marks T10, which has collapsed from multiple compression fractures and is deformed into a wedge shape. T11 is similarly deformed but is largely obscured by the soft tissues.

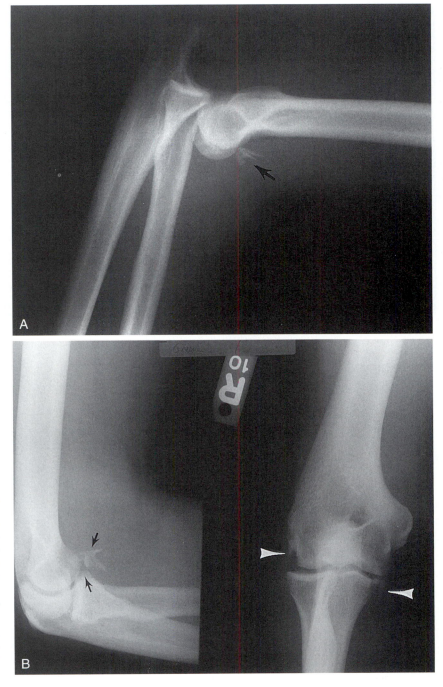

FIGURE 3–18. Posterior dislocation of the elbow with associated fractures. This 39-year-old man injured his elbow in a fall from a skateboard. (*A*) Lateral view of the elbow before reduction demonstrates the posterior position of the radius and ulna in relationship to the distal humerus. The black arrow marks a fracture fragment in the anterior soft tissues. (*B*) Lateral and (*C*) anteroposterior films made after reduction show good positioning of the joints and multiple fracture fragments in the soft tissue (arrows). Note the gross soft tissue swelling of the arm visible on the lateral view.

tween the long bones of the forearm or the tibiofibular syndesmosis).

Fractures due to Abnormal Stresses or Pathologic Processes[18,19]

Stress or fatigue fractures occur as a result of repetitive minor trauma to otherwise normal bone. Stress fractures are not acute breaks in bone like other types of fractures, but are alterations in the architecture of

bone secondary to gradual, local, resorptive activity of bone in response to repetitive trauma. Stress fractures are found most frequently in the lower extremities, and the predominant example is found in the stress fractures of the metatarsals associated with prolonged walking, marching, or running. Stress fractures appear on radiographs as linear areas of increased radiodensity (Figs. 3–19, 3–20).

Pathologic fractures are fractures that occur in bone that has been structurally weakened by a pathologic process (Fig. 3–21). The pathology that induces the susceptibility of bone to fracture may be systemic or lo-

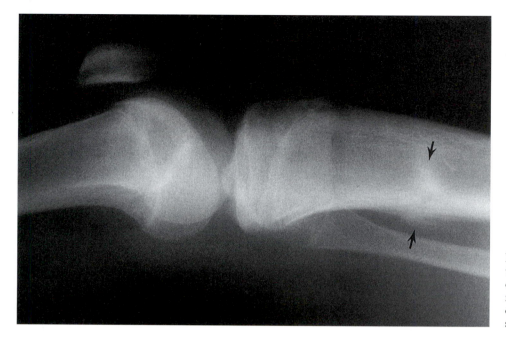

FIGURE 3–19. Stress fracture in the proximal third of the tibial shaft of a 15-year-old male runner. Arrows mark the zone of increased radiodensity representing bony response to repetitive trauma.

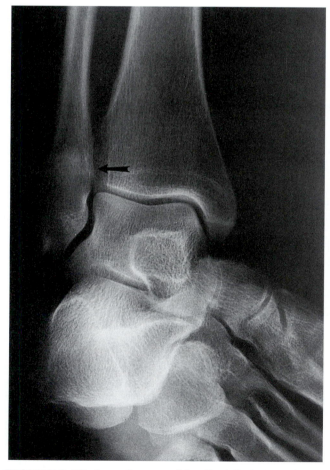

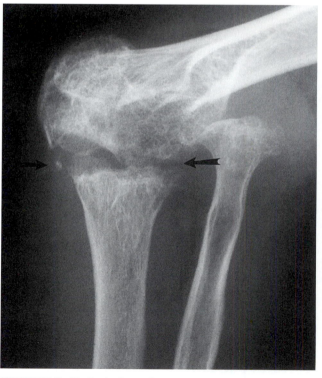

FIGURE 3–20. Stress fracture of the distal fibula in a 35-year-old female city police officer. Arrow marks the zone of increased radiodensity representing the reparative attempts of bone in response to repetitive trauma, in this case, walking on city sidewalks.

FIGURE 3–21. Pathologic fracture through the distal third of the olecranon in a 26-year-old male. The underlying pathology is *osteogenesis imperfecta*, a disease characterized by abnormal maturation of collagen affecting both intramembranous and enchondral bone formation. Note the diffuse decrease in bone density, pencil-thin cortices, flared metaphyses, and cysticlike appearance of the proximal ends of the radius and ulna.

calized in origin (Fig. 3–22). Systemic processes may be congenital (osteogenesis imperfecta, osteopetrosis) or acquired (osteoporosis, Paget's disease). Local processes may be tumors, infections, or disuse.

FRACTURES IN CHILDREN

Fractures occurring in growing bone have unique patterns of injury and present special problems in diagnosis, treatment, and healing. Although the primary advantage of fracture occurring in immature bone is rapid healing and great ability to remodel, the primary concern is the potential for disruption of growth.

The location of fractures in the long bones of children is generally described by the region of development (Fig. 3–23). *Diaphyseal* fractures involve the central shaft, *metaphyseal* fractures involve the expanding end, *physeal* fractures involve the epiphyseal growth plate, and *epiphyseal* fractures involve the epiphysis.[20]

The radiographic diagnosis of children's fractures can be complicated by the presence of epiphyseal growth plates, dense growth lines, secondary centers of ossification, and large nutrient foramina, all of

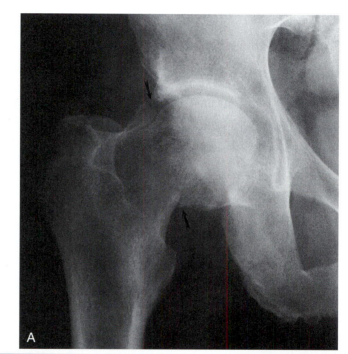

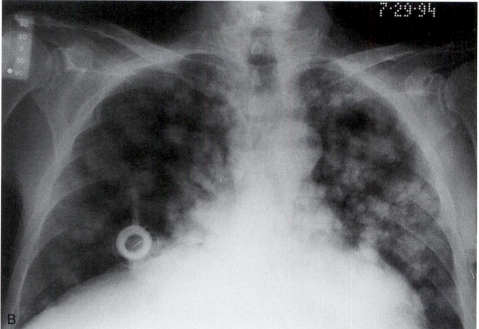

FIGURE 3–22. Pathologic fracture of the femoral neck. (*A*) Arrows mark the extent of the fracture line. Demineralization of the femur is evident by the thinning of the cortices. (*B*) The underlying pathology is lung cancer, revealed in the abnormal densities of the chest film.

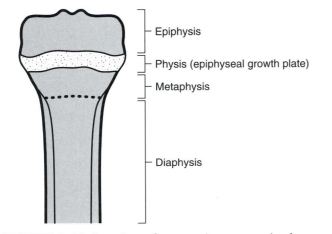

FIGURE 3–23. Location reference points on growing bone.

which may be confused with fracture lines.[21] For this reason, *comparison films* of the uninvolved extremity are often obtained to assist in diagnosis. An additional difficulty in radiographically examining immature bone is that only the ossified portions of bone have sufficient radiographic density to be imaged. The preformed cartilage model is not imaged.

The elements of radiographic description of fractures, as listed earlier, are the same for children as for adults. Additions within this list include describing (1) the patterns of incomplete shaft fractures seen predominantly in children and (2) the special features of fractures of the epiphysis and ephiphyseal plate. Descriptions of these points follow.

Incomplete Fractures

Incomplete fractures of the shafts of long bones in children are classified as (Fig. 3–24):

Greenstick fracture: This eponym has become almost standardized in usage as it accurately depicts the ap-

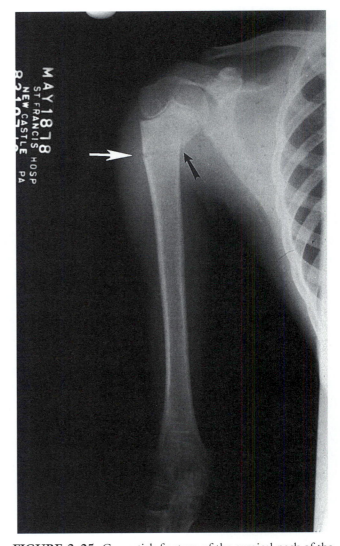

FIGURE 3–25. Greenstick fracture of the surgical neck of the humerus in a 13-year-old boy. The white arrow points to the incomplete transverse fracture line on the lateral aspect of the humerus. The black arrow points to an associated fracture on the medial aspect of the humerus, proximal to the greenstick fracture.

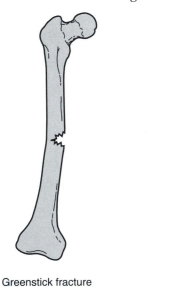
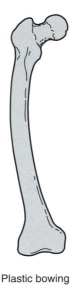
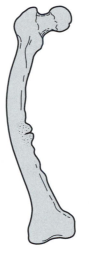

Greenstick fracture

A

Plastic bowing

B

Torus (buckle) fracture

C

FIGURE 3–24. *Incomplete* fractures in children exhibit characteristics unique to the structural architecture of growing bone.

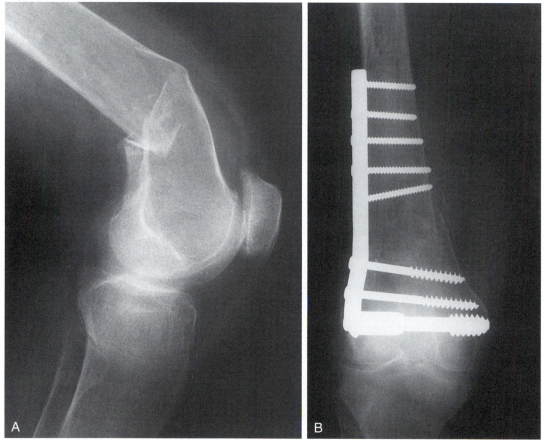

FIGURE 3–26. Buckle fracture of the distal femur. (*A*) The unusual buckle configuration of this fracture in a 56-year-old woman is secondary to decalcification of the skeleton as related to osteomalacia. (*B*) Postoperative film demonstrating open reduction and internal fixation of the fracture site.

pearance of this incomplete fracture: *one side of the shaft is fractured, whereas a portion of the cortex and periosteum remains intact on the compression side* (Fig. 3–25). Since this intact cortical bone is often *plastically deformed or bowed*, an angular deformity is common, sometimes necessitating conversion to a complete fracture by reversal of the deformity.[22]

Torus fracture: This eponym is also common, and describes an *impaction fracture that results in buckling of the cortex.* This pattern occurs predominantly at the metaphyseal regions, which are predisposed to a compressive response due to the amount of spongy bone and newly remodeled trabecular bone present.[23] Occasionally, this type of fracture is seen in adults if an underlying pathology exists (Fig. 3–26).

Plastic bowing: This is a result of the unique biomechanical nature of developing bone. When longitudinal compression forces imposed on a naturally curved, tubular growing bone exceed the point in which *elastic recoil* returns the bone to its prior position, that bone will become *plastically deformed or bowed.* Plastic bowing means that even when the force is removed, the bone remains bowed. Plastic bowing is a type of incomplete fracture, as microscopic fatigue lines, or *microfractures,* are evident in

plastically deformed bone. Note that with additional increased force, bone would continue to weaken and eventually fail, or fracture. It is reasonable to assume, then, that plastic bowing is a component of all fractures of childhood.[24]

The younger the child, the more likely plastic bowing is to occur. It is particularly common in the fibula and the ulna. Additionally, a common injury pattern is *bowing in one bone combined with greenstick type of fracture in the paired bone,* e.g., bowing of the fibula with fracture of the tibia, or bowing of the ulna with fracture of the radius. In some cases the bowed bone must be fractured in order to reverse the deformity and allow healing of both bones to proceed in good alignment.

Epiphyseal Fractures

Fractures involving the epiphyseal plate (also referred to as the *physis* or *physeal* region) have been estimated to account for 15 to 20 percent of all fractures in children.[25] An increased incidence of physeal fractures occurs at the onset of puberty, hypothesized to be related to biomechanical and structural weakness of

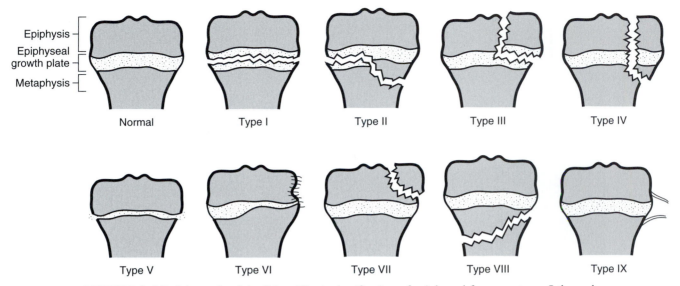

FIGURE 3–27. Schematic of the Salter-Harris classification of epiphyseal fractures, types I through V, with later additions made by Rang and Ogden, types VI through IX. Type II is the most common injury pattern.

the physeal cartilage during this stage of growth. Additionally, boys seem to be affected with greater frequency, possibly related to their higher propensity for injury and because their growth plates remain open longer than do those in girls.[26] Accurate diagnosis is critical, as the chosen treatment must strike the delicate balance of assisting healing without disrupting subsequent growth. The most commonly used method of radiographically identifying the varieties of epiphyseal fractures is the *Salter-Harris* classification system of types I through V (Fig. 3–27), with later additions made to this system by Rang and Ogden, types VI through IX[27,28]:

Type I: The fracture line extends through the physis, separating and displacing the epiphysis from the normal position. This type is common in younger children and is associated with birth injuries. Prognosis is good for normal growth.

Type II: The fracture line extends through the physis and exits through the metaphysis, creating a triangular wedge of metaphysis that displaces with the epiphysis. This is the most common type and occurs most frequently in children over 10 years of age (Fig. 3–28). Prognosis is good for normal growth.

Type III: The fracture line extends from the joint surface through the epiphysis and across the physis, resulting in a portion of the epiphysis becoming displaced. Partial growth arrest is a possibility, and surgical fixation may be warranted.

Type IV: The fracture line extends from the joint surface through the epiphysis, physis, and metaphysis, resulting in one fracture fragment. Partial growth arrest is possible, and surgical fixation may be necessary.

Type V: The fracture is a crush type of injury that

damages the physis by compression forces. It is difficult to diagnose this injury in acute stages. Eventual growth arrest may be the only clue that this injury occurred. Two nontraumatic causes of this type of injury are infection and epiphyseal avascular necrosis, which may cause dissolution of cartilage cells with resultant growth arrest.

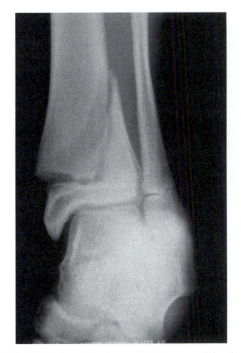

FIGURE 3–28. Salter-Harris type II fracture of the distal tibia. The fracture line extends through the physis and exits through the metaphysis, creating a triangular-shaped wedge of metaphysis that is displaced with the epiphysis.

Rang's type VI: This injury involves the *perichondrial ring* or the associated periosteum of the physis. While little or no damage occurs directly to the physes, the reparative process at the periosteum may cause an osseous bridge to develop between the metaphysis and the epiphysis, arresting growth and leading to angular deformity.

Ogden's types VII, VIII, and IX: These fractures do not directly involve the physis but may subsequently disrupt growth. Type VII is an osteochondral fracture of the articular portion of the epiphysis, type VIII is a fracture of the metaphysis, and type IX is an avulsion fracture of the periosteum.

REDUCTION AND FIXATION OF FRACTURES[29,30]

Although the fundamental principles of fracture reduction and fixation are beyond the scope of this text, a brief discussion of them introduces terms that may appear in the radiographic report.

Reduction

Once a fracture has occurred and the fracture fragments are *displaced*, restoration of the fragments to their normal anatomic positions or *reduction* is attempted. Reduction may be accomplished in two ways:

Closed reduction: During closed reductions of fractures, no surgical incisions are made. Rather, fragments are physically guided back into position via manipulation, traction, or a combination of both.

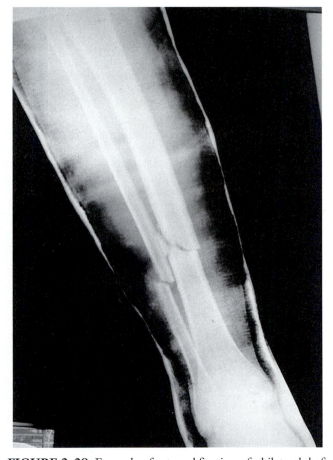

FIGURE 3–29. Example of external fixation of a bilateral shaft fracture of the lower leg. Much bony detail is lost when viewing through plaster; however, the visual information is sufficient to determine if good positioning of the fracture fragments exist. The tibial fracture is described as being located at the junction of the middle and proximal thirds of the shaft. The fracture line is oblique, and there is comminution with a large wedge-shaped fragment. The fragments are in good position and good alignment. The fibular fracture is located 1 inch distal to the tibial fracture. The fracture line is oblique, and the distal fragment is minimally displaced laterally and is in good alignment. (From Richardson, JK, and Iglarsh, ZA: Clinical Orthopaedic Physical Therapy. WB Saunders, Philadelphia, 1994, p 675, with permission.)

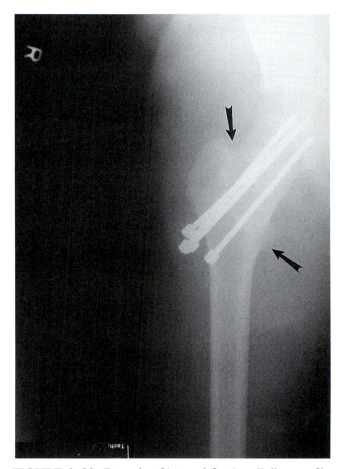

FIGURE 3–30. Example of internal fixation. Follow-up film for an intertrochanteric fracture of the right hip shows good healing. The arrows mark the extent of the fracture line. Note the four pins that were used to surgically compress the fracture site.

Open reduction: Open reductions of fractures surgically expose the fracture site. Although most open reductions involve the use of internal fixation devices, some do not.

Fixation

Fixation is the method of maintaining fracture fragments in position after reduction in order to achieve healing. The goals of fixation include (1) avoiding further compromise of the injured soft tissues, (2) maintaining the length of the bone, especially in the lower extremities, and (3) producing alignment of the fragments and particularly of the joints.[31] Fixation is of two types: *external fixation*, such as plaster cast immobilization or splints, and *internal fixation*, which employs orthopedic appliances such as pins, wires, plates, screws, and rods (Figs. 3–29, 3–30). Bone grafts could

also be thought of as a form of internal fixation. Additionally, methods of internal and external fixation and their devices may be combined.

FRACTURE HEALING AND COMPLICATIONS IN HEALING[32]

Fracture healing begins shortly after the fracture occurs. The mechanism of healing is not uniform and differs somewhat among cortical bone, cancellous bone, and bone that has been surgically compressed and fixated.

Briefly, cortical bone fractures heal by the formation of new bone or *callus* bridging the fracture gap (Fig. 3–31). This is achieved by a reaction of the periosteum and endosteum with organization and ossification of the acute fracture hematoma. New bone is initially deposited on either side of the fracture site, several millimeters away from the actual fracture line, and then proceeds toward the gap, eventually linking together and forming a collar of external *primary callus*. This randomly organized immature bone is gradually replaced by *secondary callus* via the resorptive activity of the osteoclasts combined with osteoblastic deposition of new bone. The secondary callus now becomes organized in response to the stresses of normal function in accordance with Wolff's law. Excessive bone is resorbed and remodeling continues, eventually restoring the natural contour of bone.

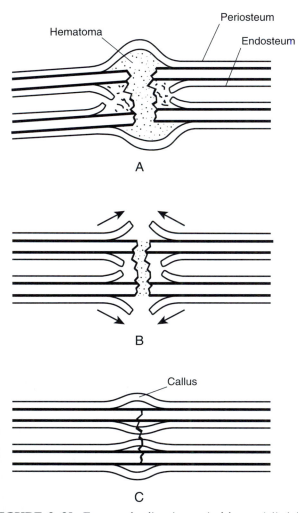

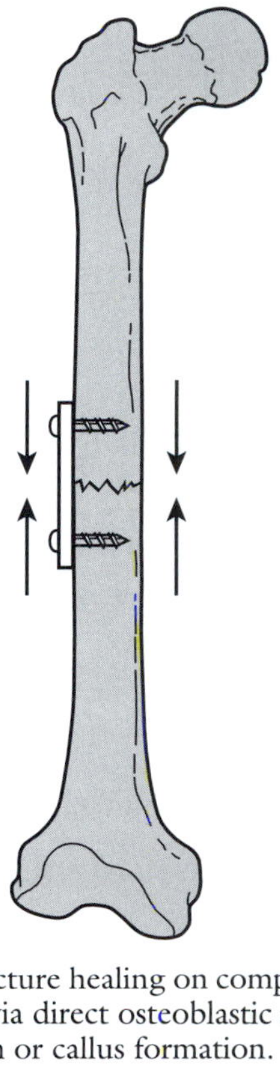

FIGURE 3–31. Fracture healing in cortical bone. (*A*) A hematoma fills in the fracture site after the periosteum and endosteum rupture. (*B*) Periosteal and endosteal response results in bone deposition that proceeds toward the fracture. (*C*) A collar of callus surrounds the fracture site and will progressively remodel over time. (Adapted from Schultz,[4] p 25.)

FIGURE 3–32. Fracture healing on compressed and surgically fixated bone occurs via direct osteoblastic activity, with little or no periosteal reaction or callus formation.

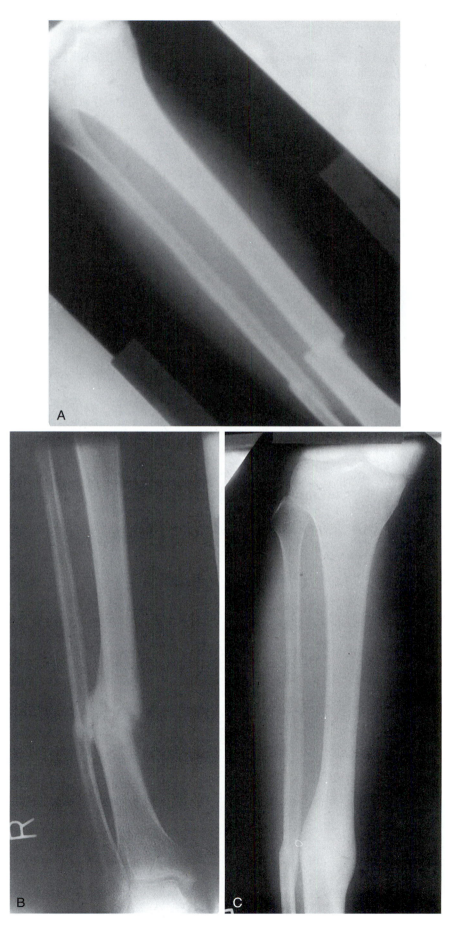

FIGURE 3–33. Successful healing of a bilateral shaft fracture of the lower leg in a 17-year-old female. (*A*) Emergency room film made after a sled-riding accident. The fracture is located at the junction of the distal and middle thirds of the shafts of the tibia and fibula. In both bones, the fracture fragments are overriding and displaced laterally. Good alignment exists. (*B*) Follow-up films 3 weeks later through plaster show formation of callus bridging the fracture gap. (*C*) Follow-up films 1 year later show no evidence of the fracture lines remaining, and good progression of remodeling.

Cancellous bone fractures unite with little or no callus formation. Healing occurs via direct osteoblastic activity at the fracture site, also referred to as *creeping substitution*. This method of healing requires that the fracture fragments be in close contact with each other. If approximation cannot be achieved, hematoma fills in the gap and healing proceeds by callus formation. Surgically compressed and fixated bone heals via direct osteoblastic activity with little or no periosteal reaction or callus formation (Fig. 3–32). Additionally, immediate remodeling occurs as bone deposition and resorption continue simultaneously as a result of osteoblastic and osteoclastic cell activity.

Some terms that describe the radiographic evidence of fracture healing are[33,34]:

Formation of callus: radiodense periosteal and endosteal lines bridge the fracture gap (Fig. 3–33A)

Primary bone union: healing of a fracture by trabecular new bone, without callus formation (due to perfect apposition)

Early union: appearance of a trabecular pattern across the fracture line

Clinical union: callus is seen uniting the fracture site, yet a radiolucent band remains between the fracture fragments, suggesting that the repair lacks normal strength (Fig. 3–33B)

Radiographic union: a dense bridge of periosteal and endosteal callus unites the fracture site

Established union: cortical structure and remodeling beginning to appear

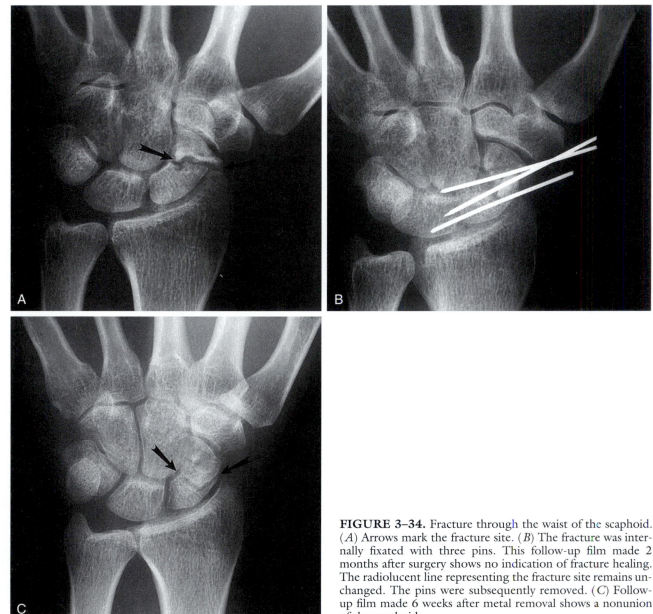

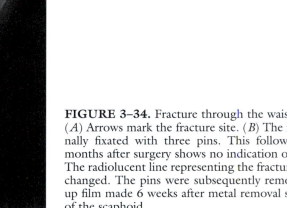

FIGURE 3–34. Fracture through the waist of the scaphoid. (*A*) Arrows mark the fracture site. (*B*) The fracture was internally fixated with three pins. This follow-up film made 2 months after surgery shows no indication of fracture healing. The radiolucent line representing the fracture site remains unchanged. The pins were subsequently removed. (*C*) Follow-up film made 6 weeks after metal removal shows a nonunion of the scaphoid.

Remodeling: trabeculae become reorganized along lines of weight-bearing stress

Fibrous union: a clinically stable, pain-free fracture site, without evidence of the fracture line repair remaining (Fig. 3–33C).

Some terms that describe complications of fracture healing, as described by Schultz,[35] are:

Delayed union: Delayed union exists any time a fracture fails to unite in the time frame usually required for union. Yet although fracture healing is delayed, the process of cellular repair is present and will continue on to complete union, provided the adverse factors are removed and/or no additional stresses are imposed. Causes of delayed union may be disrupted vascularity, infection, inadequate or interrupted immobilization, unsatisfactory reduction, severe local trauma, loss of bone substance, or wide distraction of fragments.

Slow union: Slow union is known to exist in many fractures, even when ideal conditions are present. The rate of union, although slow, may be average or normal for the significant factors involved, such as patient age and fracture site. Thus, slow union is distinct from delayed union, which is a pathologic state.

Nonunion: Nonunion exists when there is a failure of the fracture fragments to unite and the processes of bone repair have ceased completely (Fig. 3–34). The factors contributing to delayed union, if left un-

checked, will cause nonunion. The radiographic appearance of nonunion shows persistence of the fracture line, sclerosis and rounding-off of the fragment ends, and occlusion of the medullary canal. Callus and bony bridging are absent.

Malunion: This occurs when the fracture has successfully united, but a degree of angular or rotary deformity exists. If the deformity causes significant functional problems, surgery may be warranted for correction.

Pseudoarthrosis: This condition, also known as "false joint," refers to an abnormal condition at the fracture site associated with nonunion (Figs. 3–35, 3–36). In nonunion the fragment bone ends are usually connected by dense fibrous or fibrocartilaginous tissue. Sometimes, however, a false joint may form between the ends and be surrounded by a bursal sac containing synovial fluid.

Avascular necrosis: Avascular necrosis (aseptic necrosis, ischemic necrosis) exists when the blood supply to a bone or segment of a bone is compromised, leading to localized bone death. The initial stages of avascular necrosis are not evident on plain films, but in later stages increased density is present (Fig. 3–37).

Time Frame for Fracture Healing

Rockwood[36] illustrates the entire time frame for complete fracture healing as divisible into three phases, each of which overlaps somewhat. The *inflammation* phase occupies approximately 10 percent of total healing time, the *reparative* phase approximately 40 percent, and the *remodeling* phase approximately 70 percent.

The actual number of weeks or months that these three phases can extend over is influenced by innumerable factors. Because healing is carried out by living cells, the process of healing can be affected by almost any endogenous or exogenous factor that influences the metabolic function of cells. In clinical practice, however, fracture healing appears to proceed with a certain degree of predictability and is modified by relatively few influences. These are outlined by Rockwood[37]:

Age of the patient: Generally, the younger a patient, the more rapidly fractures heal, as opposed to the average rate at which adults heal. The positive bone balance state of growing children contributes to rapid healing and excellent remodeling capabilities. Additionally, the periosteum in children is thick and loosely attached to the shafts of bones, and thus is less likely to tear during fracture. Its presence acts as an aid in maintaining reduction and readily supplies critical vascular support to the repair process. In contrast, the periosteum of adult bone is relatively thin and firmly attached to the shaft, usually tearing during fracture.

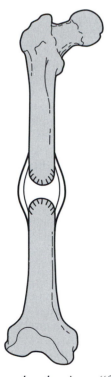

FIGURE 3–35. A pseudoarthrosis, or "false joint," is an abnormal condition at a nonunion fracture site, whereby a bursal sac surrounds the fracture site.

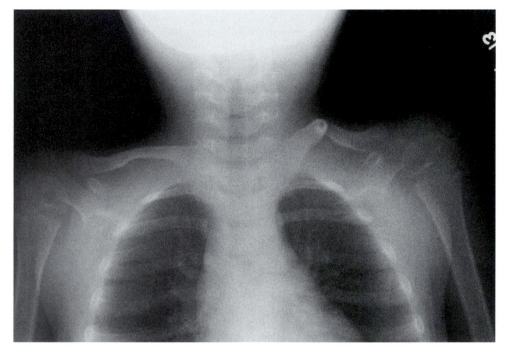

FIGURE 3–36. Pseudoarthrosis of the left clavicle, 1½ years after fracture, in a 5-year-old girl. The nonunion of the fracture site has resulted in the formation of a "false joint."

Degree of local trauma: Greater local trauma at the fracture site and in adjacent soft tissues delays fracture healing. More tissues involved in the injury diffuse the cellular repair effort to many different fronts. Greater displacement of the fracture fragments also is known to delay fracture healing.

Degree of bone loss: Loss of bone substance or excessive distraction of the fragments compromises the

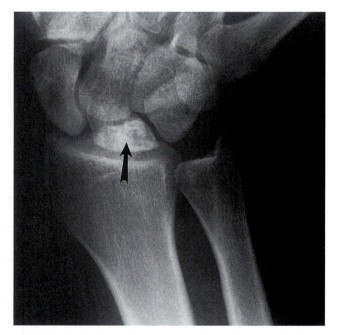

FIGURE 3–37. Avascular necrosis of the lunate in a 25-year-old male. The increased density of the lunate represents the body's attempt to revasculize and produce new bone.

ability of the cells to bridge the fracture site and contributes to delay in healing.

Type of bone involved: Cancellous bone unites rapidly but only at points of direct contact. Cortical bone unites by two mechanisms, depending on local conditions. A rigid immobilized site with contact of fragment ends will heal faster than a poorly immobilized site with displacement.

Degree of immobilization: The degree of immobilization, along with the amount of soft tissue trauma, is of paramount importance in fracture healing. Inadequate mobilization leads to delayed union or nonunion. If movement persists during the repair process, a cleft or false joint (pseudoarthrosis) can develop between the fragment ends.

Infection: When infection is imposed on a fracture, or results in a fracture, healing will be delayed or may not happen at all as the local cell response will be mobilized toward containing or eliminating the infection.

Presence of local malignancy: Unless the malignancy is treated, fractures through primary or secondary malignant tumor will not heal significantly, even though microscopic evidence of callus may be present.

Other local pathologic conditions: Fractures through nonmalignant but abnormal bone may heal, but in some instances (e.g. Paget's disease, fibous dysplasia) healing may be delayed or not happen at all.

Radiation necrosis: Bone that has been irradiated heals much more slowly and in some cases fails to unite because of local cell death, thrombosis of vessels, and fibrosis of the marrow, which all interfere with the ingrowth of capillaries necessary for repair.

Presence of avascular necrosis: Normally, healing occurs from both sides of a fracture site. If one fragment is rendered avascular, healing must proceed from only one side and thus is delayed. If both fragments have disrupted vascularity, the chances of healing are minimal.

Hormones: Corticosteroids are powerful inhibitors of the rate of fracture healing. Growth hormones are potent stimulators of fracture healing.

Exercise and local stress about the fracture: Bone formation is stimulated by forces acting across the fracture site, and weight-bearing techniques are used to take advantage of this fact. Appropriate stress, however, is not to be confused with imposing unwanted motion at a fracture site, which can result in delayed union.

SUMMARY OF KEY POINTS

1. The task of the radiologist who evaluates trauma is two-fold: 1) to diagnosis the physical characteristics of the fracture or dislocation and 2) to assess and monitor the results of treatment.
2. A fracture is a break in the continuity of bone or cartilage. A closed fracture denotes intact soft tissues over the fracture site. An open fracture communicates with the external environment through a tear or perforation in the skin over the fracture site.
3. Radiographic evaluation of fracture includes description of anatomic site and extent of the fracture, incomplete vs. complete fracture pattern, alignment of fragments, direction of fracture line, special features such as impaction or avulsion, associated abnormalities such as joint dislocation, and special types of fractures due to abnormal stresses or underlying pathology such as stress fractures or pathologic fractures.
4. Fractures in children have unique patterns of injury. Greenstick, torus, and plastic bowing describe fracture patterns predominant in immature long bones.
5. Fifteen to 20% of childhood fractures involve the epiphyseal region. Accurate diagnosis is critical to preventing growth arrest. Radiographic identification of the different types of epiphyseal injuries can be made by the Salter-Harris classification system. Type II is the most common injury pattern.
6. Fracture fragments are guided back to their best possible anatomic position by either closed reduction (manipulation, traction) or open reduction (surgical exposure of the fracture site).
7. Fractures are immobilized to facilitate the healing process by either external fixation methods (splints, casts) or internal fixation methods (pins, wires, compression plates, and screws). At times a combination of the two methods is used.
8. Fractures may heal by the formation of callus, or by direct osteoblastic activity referred to as creeping substitution. The time frame for healing is influenced by several factors including patient age; degree of tissue trauma; fracture site and configuration; type of bone; degree of immobilization; presence of infection, malignancy, avascular necrosis, pathologic process, or radiation necrosis; corticosteroids; exercise and local stress about the fracture.
9. Complications of fracture healing include delayed union; slow union; nonunion; malunion; pseudarthrosis; avascular necrosis.
10. The use of eponyms (e.g., Colles' fracture, hip pointer) to describe orthopedic trauma has historic roots and newer terms (e.g., keyboard wrist) continue to be generated today. Although eponyms serve as a type of orthopedic verbal shorthand, they should always be avoided in radiologic description due to anatomic inexactness.

APPENDIX: GLOSSARY OF ORTHOPEDIC EPONYMS

The use of eponyms to describe fracture anatomy and orthopedic trauma has historic roots and certainly predates the discovery of x-rays a century ago. Many current eponyms have survived for decades or longer, and newer eponyms continue to appear. As stated earlier, eponyms are usually avoided in radiographic description because of their sometimes general characteristics, anatomic inexactness, or ease of misinterpretation. Additionally, some terms have acquired new meanings over the years, and some have always been controversial. However, the use of eponyms survives because they serve as a convenient type of orthopedic shorthand. Kilcoyne and Farrar[38] have compiled an extensive list of common orthopedic eponyms, and it is reproduced here.

Anterior malleolus fracture: Uncommon fracture of the anterolateral margin of the distal tibia at the site of attachment of the anterior tibiofibular ligament. This fracture fragment is also known as the "tubercle of Chaput"

Aviator's astragalus: A variety of fractures of the talus that include compression fractures of the neck, fractures of the body or posterior process, or fractures with dislocations

Backfire: See Chauffeur fracture

Bado: A classification of Monteggia type fractures based on the direction of dislocation of the radial head

Bankart: A detached fragment from the anteroinferior margin of the glenoid rim; it is seen with anterior shoulder dislocations

Barton: Intra-articular fracture of the rim of the distal radius. It may involve either the dorsal or volar rim

Baseball finger: Hyperflexion injury to the distal interphalangeal joint, often associated with a dorsal avulsion fracture of the base of the distal phalanx; it is also called "dropped" or "mallet" finger

Basketball foot: Subtalar dislocation of the foot

Bennett: Intra-articular avulsion fracture subluxation of the base of the first metacarpal; the fracture produces a small volar lip fragment that remains attached to the trapezium and trapezoid by means of the strong volar oblique ligament while the shaft fragment is displaced by proximal muscle pull

Bennett "reverse": Intra-articular fracture subluxation of the base of the fifth and/or fourth metacarpal

Boot-top: Ski boot fracture of the midportion of the distal one-third of the tibia and fibula

Boutonnière deformity: Hyperflexion of a proximal interphalangeal joint of a finger due to disruption of the central slip of the extensor tendon

Boxer: Fracture of the neck of the fifth metacarpal with dorsal angulation, and often volar displacement of the metacarpal head

Boyd: A classification of intertrochanteric hip fractures

Buckle: See Torus fracture

Bumper: Compression fracture of the lateral tibial plateau often associated with avulsion of the medial collateral ligament of the knee; it is also called "Fender fracture"

Bunkbed: Intra-articular fracture of the base of the first metatarsal in a child

Burst: Severe comminution of a vertebral body, usually secondary to axial loading, sometimes with a rotatory component. Frequently there is a sagittal fracture through the body plus fractures in the posterior elements; this pattern is often seen with unstable spinal fractures

Butterfly fragment: Comminuted wedge-shaped fracture that has split off from the main fragments;

this implies high velocity of trauma from a direction opposite the fragment

Chance: A flexion distraction injury that results in compression of the vertebral body. Posteriorly there may be ligament disruption without fracture, and the disc-annulus complex may be disrupted. Alternatively, there may be transverse noncomminuted fractures of the vertebral body and neural arch. It is also known as "lap-type seat belt" fracture

Chaput: Eponym for the anterior tubercle of the distal tibia where the anterior tibiofibular ligament attaches

Chauffeur: Intra-articular oblique fracture of the styloid process of the distal radius; it is also called "backfire" or "lorry driver" or "Hutchinson" fracture

Chisel: Incomplete intra-articular fracture of the head of the radius extending distally about 1 cm from the center of the articular surface

Chopart: Fracture/dislocation of the talonavicular and calcaneocuboid joints. It is derived from Chopart's description of an amputation through these midtarsal joints

Clay-shoveler: Avulsion fracture of the spinous process of one or more of the lower cervical or upper thoracic vertebrae, most commonly at C-7. More than one vertebra may be involved

Coach's finger: Dorsal dislocation of a proximal interphalangeal joint

Colles': Transverse fracture of the distal radial metaphysis proximal to the joint with dorsal displacement of the distal fragment and volar angulation. The ulnar styloid may also be fractured. It is also known as "Pouteau fracture"

Colles', "Reverse": See Smith fracture

Cotton: Trimalleolar ankle fracture

Dashboard: Fracture of the posterior rim of the acetabulum caused by impact through the knee, driving the femoral head against the acetabulum. It is frequently associated with a posterior cruciate ligament injury, a femoral shaft fracture, or patellar fracture

De Quervain: Fracture of the scaphoid with volar dislocation of a scaphoid fragment and the lunate

Desault: Various dislocations of the distal radioulnar joint

Descot: A fracture of the "third malleolus" (i.e., the posterior lip of the tibia)

Dome: A fracture involving the weight-bearing surface of the acetabulum or the upper articular surface of the talus

Dropped: See Baseball Finger

Dupuytren: Fracture of the fibula 2½ inches above the tip of the lateral malleolus caused by a pronation-external rotation injury. It is associated with tear of the tibiofibular ligaments and the deltoid ligament (or fracture of the medial malleolus)

Duverney: Isolated fracture of the iliac wing

Essex-lopresti: Comminuted fracture of the head of the radius with dislocation of the distal radioulnar joint

Fender: See Bumper fracture

Ferguson: A type of spinal fracture

Fielding: A classification of subtrochanteric hip fractures based on the distance from the lesser trochanter (I–III)

Frykman: A classification of distal radius fractures based on involvement of the radiocarpal/radioulnar joints with or without ulnar styloid fracture

Galeazzi: Fracture of the radius at the junction of the middle and distal thirds with associated dislocation or subluxation of the distal radioulnar joint. Also called a "reverse Monteggia fracture"

Gamekeeper: Partial or total disruption of the ulnar collateral ligament at the metacarpophalangeal joint of the thumb. It may also have an avulsion fracture from the base of the proximal phalanx

Garden: A classification of femoral neck fractures. Types I, II, III, and IV are based on the displacement present

Gosselin: A V-shaped fracture of the lower third of the tibia that extends distally into the tibial plafond

Greenstick: An incomplete fracture of the shaft of a long bone, with disruption on the tension side and plastic deformation on the compression side

Hangman: Traumatic spondylolisthesis with fracture through the pedicles or lamina of C-2 secondary to a distraction-extension force

Hawkins: A classification of talar fracture-dislocations

Hawkins sign: Radiolucent line in the dome of the talus indicating that the talus fracture will heal without osteonecrosis. This subchondral osteoporosis can develop only if the blood supply of the talus is intact

Henderson: Trimalleolar fracture of the ankle

Hill-Sachs: Posterolateral defect of the humeral head caused by anterior shoulder dislocation and "implosion" fracture

Hill-Sachs, "Reverse": Anterior defect of the humeral head secondary to posterior shoulder dislocation

Hip pointer: An impaction fracture of the superior iliac wing

Hoffa: Coronal fracture of the medial femoral condyle

Holstein-Lewis: Fracture of the humerus at the junction of the middle and distal thirds where the radial nerve is tethered by the lateral intermuscular septum. Thus, it is associated with radial nerve palsy

Horseback rider's knee: Dislocation of the fibular head caused by a bump against the gatepost

Hutchinson: See Chauffeur fracture

Jefferson: A burst fracture of the ring of the atlas, with fractures both anterior and posterior to the facet joints. It is secondary to an axial load on top of the head. There are usually four breaks in the ring and lateral spread of the lateral masses

Jones: A term sometimes applied to both extra- and intra-articular fracture of the base of the fifth metatarsal

Kocher: Intra-articular fracture of the capitellum of the humerus

Kohler: Fracture of the tarsal navicular with aseptic necrosis (in children)

Lauge-Hanson: A classification of ankle fractures, based on the mechanism of injury

Laugier: Fracture of the trochlea of the humerus

LeFort (fibula): Avulsion fracture of the fibular attachment of the anterior tibiofibular ligament

Lisfranc: Fracture-dislocation through the tarsometatarsal joints, commonly associated with disruption of the second tarsometatarsal joint and lateral dislocation of the second through fifth tarsometatarsal joints. It may also show other patterns of tarsometatarsal disruption. It is named for Lisfranc's description of an amputation through the tarsometatarsal joints

Little-leaguer's elbow: Avulsion of the medial epicondyle of the elbow secondary to valgus stress

Lorry driver: See Chauffeur fracture

Maisonneuve: Fracture of the proximal third of the fibula with tear of the distal tibiofibular syndesmosis and the interosseous membrane. It may also have fracture of the medial malleolus or tear of the deltoid ligament

Malgaigne (of humerus): Extension-type supracondylar fracture

Malgaigne (of pelvis): Fracture-dislocation of one side of the pelvis. This is an unstable injury with two vertical fractures produced by a vertical shear force. The anterior fracture is in the superior and inferior rami of the pubis, and the posterior fracture or dislocation is in the ilium, the sacrum, or the sacroiliac joint. This makes the lateral fragment (containing the acetabulum) unstable

Mallet: See baseball finger

March: Stress or fatigue fracture of the metatarsals. (Other bones may have stress or fatigue fractures)

Mason: A classification of radial head fractures based on the amount of articular surface involved (I–IV)

Mechanical bull thumb: Fracture at the base of the first metacarpal

Midnight: Oblique fracture of the proximal phalanx of the fifth toe

Monteggia: Fracture of the proximal third of the ulna with an anterior dislocation of the radial head. Other types of ulnar shaft fractures and radial head dislocations are sometimes included. The classification of these fractures by Bado:

    I: ulnar shaft fracture with anterior radial head dislocation

    II: ulnar shaft fracture with lateral radial head dislocation

    III: ulnar shaft fracture with posterior radial head dislocation

    IV: both forearm bones fractured with radial head dislocation

Monteggia, "reverse": See Galeazzi fracture

Montercaux: Fracture of the fibular neck associated with diastasis of the ankle mortise

Moore: Colles' fracture of the distal radius with fracture of the ulnar styloid and dorsal subluxation of the distal ulna

Mouchet: Fracture of the capitellum of the humerus

Nightstick: Single bone fracture of the ulnar shaft due to a direct blow without disruption of the interosseous membrane or either of the radioulnar joints

Nursemaid elbow: Dislocation of the radial head in a toddler with an intact annular ligament. It is difficult to prove with x-ray because the radial head may not be ossified. The dislocation may be reduced by supination during the x-ray examination

Parachute jumper: Anterior dislocation of the fibular head

Paratrooper: Fracture of the distal tibial and fibular shafts

Pauwels: Fracture of the proximal femoral neck. Types I, II, and III designate the angle of the fracture

Piedmont: Oblique distal radius fracture without disruption of the distal radioulnar joint. It is difficult to control by closed means. It was described at a Piedmont Orthopaedic Society Meeting

Pilon: Comminuted, intra-articular fracture of the distal tibia with a long oblique component, secondary to axial loading and impaction of the talus into the tibial plafond

Pipkin: A classification of fibular head fractures based on the amount of head fractured (I–III)

Plafond: Fracture through the articular surface (*plafond* = Greek for "ceiling") of the distal tibia

Posada: Transcondylar fracture of the distal humerus with anterior flexion of the condylar fragment and posterior dislocation of the radius and ulna

Pott: A misnomer applied to bimalleolar fractures of the ankle; originally used to describe an abduction injury with fracture of the distal fibula and disruption of the medial ankle ligaments

Pouteau: See Colles' fracture

Ring: Fracture involving at least two parts of the pelvic circumference

Rolando: Severely comminuted form of Bennett fracture through the base of the first metacarpal

Salter-Harris: A classification of growth plate injuries. Stage I = epiphyseal plate fracture; II = I + metaphyseal fragment (Thurston-Holland sign); III = I + epiphyseal fragment; IV = II + III; V = I + severe comminution

Seat belt fracture: See Chance fracture

Segond: Avulsion fracture of the lateral tibial condyle at the site of attachment of the iliotibial band on Gerdy's tubercle. It is often associated with anterior cruciate ligament injury

Segmental fracture: Fracture dividing the long bone into several segments

Shepherd: Fracture of the lateral tubercle of the posterior process of the talus (which may simulate an os trigonum)

Sideswipe: Comminuted fracture of the distal humerus. It may include fracture of the radius and ulna

Sinegas: A classification of acetabular fractures

Ski boot: See boot-top fracture

Ski pole: Fracture of the base of the first metacarpal. It may be intra-articular

Smith: Transverse fracture of the distal radial metaphysis with anterior displacement of the distal fracture fragment. The fracture may be intra-articular. It is also called "reverse Colles" or "reverse Barton" or "Smith-Goyrand" fracture

Sprinter: Fracture of the anterior-superior or the anterior-inferior spine of the ilium with a fragment of bone being avulsed by sudden muscular pull

Stieda: Avulsion fracture of the medial femoral condyle at the origin of the tibial collateral ligament. It is also used in the term "Pellegrini-Stieda disease," which describes ossification in the tibial collateral ligament at the margin of the medial femoral condyle from chronic trauma

Straddle: Bilateral fractures of the superior and inferior pubic rami

Swan neck deformity: Hyperextension of the proximal interphalangeal joint of the finger secondary to disruption of the volar plate or contracture of the intrinsic muscles

Teardrop: Comminuted vertebral body fracture with a displaced anterior fragment. It is caused by an axial compression force with flexion of the mid-cervical spine. The same term sometimes is applied to an extension injury. It implies possible instability with posterior displacement of the vertebral body producing spinal cord damage

Thurston-Holland: A metaphyseal fracture "sign" in association with an epiphyseal fracture (Salter-Harris II fracture)

Tillaux-Kleiger: Intra-articular fracture of the anterolateral part of the distal tibial epiphysis (tubercle of Chaput) in children aged 12–14 years

Tongue: Horizontal fracture of the posterior-superior surface of the calcaneus

Torus: Compression fracture of a long bone in or near the metaphysis. It is usually an incomplete fracture and occurs in young children. It is derived from the Greek term for the "bulge" in an architectural column

Trimalleolar: Fracture of the medial and lateral malleoli and the posterior articular lip of the distal tibia. The term was coined by Henderson

Triplane: Fracture of the distal tibia involving the growth plate in early adolescence. It is of the Salter-Harris IV type

Turf toe: Hyperextension injury to the capsule of the first metatarsal phalangeal joint

Wagon wheel: Traumatic separation of the distal femoral epiphysis

Wagstaffe-LeFort: Avulsion of the distal fibula at the site of attachment of the anterior inferior tibiofibular ligament

Walther: Transverse ischioacetabular fracture. The fracture line passes through the ischiopubic junction, the acetabular cavity, and the ischial spine

Weber: A classification of ankle fractures

Wilson: Fracture of the volar plate of the middle phalanx of a finger

REFERENCES

1. Greenspan, A: Orthopedic Radiology: A Practical Approach, ed 2. Raven Press, New York, 1992, p 2.1.
2. Ibid, p 4.7.
3. Daffner, RH: Clinical Radiology: The Essentials. Williams & Wilkins, Baltimore, 1993, p 311.
4. Schultz, RJ: The Language of Fractures, ed 2. Williams & Wilkins, Baltimore, 1990, p 4.
5. Gozna, ER and Harrington, IJ: Biomechanics of Musculoskeletal Injury. Williams & Wilkins, Baltimore, 1982, p 21.
6. Greenspan, p 4.7.
7. Ibid, p 4.9.
8. Schultz, p 4.7.
9. Gustilo, RB: The Fracture Classification Manual. CV Mosby, St Louis, 1991.
10. Schultz, pp 5, 22.
11. Greenspan, p 4.8.
12. Schultz, pp 25–27.
13. Ibid, pp 8–9.
14. Greenspan, p 4.10.
15. Schultz, pp 17–23.
16. Greenspan, p 4.10.
17. Ibid.
18. Ibid, p 4.11.
19. Schultz, pp 23–25.
20. Rockwood, CA, Wilkins, KE, and King, RE: Fractures in Children, Vol 3. JB Lippincott, Philadelphia, 1984, p 5.
21. Schultz, p 36.
22. Rockwood, p 10.
23. Ibid, p 7.
24. Ibid, p 14.
25. Ibid, p 116.
26. Ibid, p 115.
27. Greenspan, p 4.11.
28. Rockwood, pp 120–123.
29. Schultz, pp 27–30.
30. Rockwood, CA and Green, DP: Fractures in Adults, Vol 1. JB Lippincott, Philadelphia, 1984, pp 189–198.
31. Ibid, p 189.
32. Schultz, pp 30–32.
33. Kilcoyne, RF and Farrar, E: Handbook of Radiologic Orthopedic Terminology. Yearbook Medical Publishers, Chicago, 1986, p 25.
34. Greenspan, p 4.18.
35. Schultz, pp 34–35.
36. Rockwood, Vol 1, p 148.
37. Ibid, pp 152–155.
38. Kilcoyne, pp 8–19.

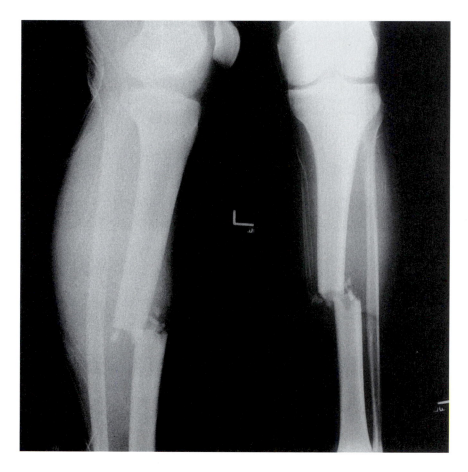

SELF-TEST

Chapter 3

1. Identify the <u>two projections</u> of this patient's lower leg.

2. Describe the <u>anatomic site</u> of the fracture.
3. Is the fracture <u>complete</u> or <u>incomplete</u>?
4. Describe the alignment of the fracture fragments in regard to <u>angulation</u> and <u>displacement.</u>
5. Describe the <u>direction of the fracture line.</u>

CHAPTER **4**

Cervical Spine

The cervical spine region is one of the most common areas of dysfunction treated by clinicians. Patient conditions that result from not only acute trauma, but also from degenerative disorders and chronic postural strains, can cause pain and debilitation that necessitate therapeutic or surgical intervention. Important to the clinical evaluation in any of these patient groups is an understanding of the underlying degenerative changes of the spine revealed on radiograph. The degree of severity of degeneration will affect the ability of the spine to withstand trauma, assume postural changes, and make functional gains in mobility and movement patterns.

In radiology the cervical spine is also one of the most frequently evaluated body segments. A busy emergency department frequently evaluates the cervical spine for direct trauma and also screens for indirect trauma if the patient has been in a severe fall or accident. The mobility of the cervical spine allows for protection of the neural contents but at the same time predisposes it to certain types of injury. The injury potential of this vulnerable area of the body should never be underestimated if some trauma has occurred, even if the trauma is at a site in the body far from the neck. Clinicians should review the radiologist's consultation prior to initiating the evaluation of a patient

who has suffered a cervical spine injury. Equally important, the clinician should never rely on the results of any diagnostic study alone. Physical evaluations, including ligamentous stability tests, are also very important and should be performed on every patient who has sustained a cervical trauma. The determination of treatment is based on all components of the examination—the history, clinical evaluation, and laboratory tests, as well as the radiographic findings.

The goals of this chapter are first to present an anatomy review, focusing primarily on osseous radiographic anatomy. A brief review of ligaments and cervical spine joint mobility is presented to assist the reader in understanding the mechanics of common injury patterns sustained in this region. The routine radiographic evaluation of the cervical spine follows, and the reader has an opportunity to learn radiographic anatomy by tracing the radiograph using a marker and transparency sheet and then comparing it with the artist's tracing. An overview of clinical information and radiographic findings pertaining to common injury patterns, common degenerative processes, and common anomalies completes the chapter. The summary is arranged as a series of practical points that highlight the clinical aspects of the chapter. The Self-Test challenges the reader's visual interpretation skills.

RADIOGRAPHIC ANATOMY

Osseous Anatomy[1]

The cervical spine (Fig. 4–1) consists of seven vertebrae positioned in a lordotic curve. The *atlas (C1)* (Fig. 4–2) and *axis (C2)* (Fig. 4–3) have unique characteristics. The remaining vertebrae, *C3* (Fig. 4–4) through *C7* (Fig. 4–5), share common osseous features.

Atlas, so named for the mythical figure, supports the globe of the head. Atlas is composed of *anterior* and *posterior arches* united by *lateral masses* and forming a bony ring. Long, perforated *transverse processes* extend from the lateral masses and are easily palpated behind the angles of the mandible. The anterior arch has a midline *anterior tubercle* on its outer surface and a midline *facet* on its inner surface for articulation with the superiorly projecting *odontoid process* or *dens* of C2. The posterior arch has a midline *tubercle* that is a rudimentary spinous process. The lateral masses support large, concave, medially inclined facets that articulate with the *occipital condyles*, forming the *atlanto-occipital joint* (Fig. 4–6). The inferior facets lie in a relatively transverse plane and articulate with the superior facets of C2, forming the *atlantoaxial joint* (Fig. 4–7).

Axis is so named as it is the pivot on which the head rotates. Axis is composed of a small *body* with the distinctive *dens* arising from the anterior portion. The dens has two articulating facets. The anterior surface of dens articulates with the inner anterior arch of atlas, and the posterior surface articulates with the *transverse ligament of atlas*. Short, thick *pedicles* extend laterally from the body and provide support for the *superior and inferior articulating processes* and associated *facets*. The inferior articulating facets are offset posteriorly from the superior pair and lie in a plane common to the remainder of the cervical facet joints. *Transverse processes* are small and not bifid at this level. The *laminae* project medially and unite in a *bifid spinous process*.

C3 through C7 are each characterized by the presence of a *vertebral body*, stout *pedicles*, paired *superior and inferior articulating processes*, bifid *transverse processes*, and *laminae* uniting in *bifid spinous processes*. All of the cervical vertebrae have large *vertebral foramina* for passage of the *spinal cord*, *transverse foramina* for transmission of the *vertebral artery and vein*, and grooves on the superior surfaces of the transverse processes for transmission of the *spinal nerves*. *Intervertebral discs* are present beginning at the C2–C3 interspace (Fig. 4–8). *Uncinate processes* project from the superolateral margins of the bodies articulating with adjacent bodies to form small *uncovertebral joints* that offer some stability to the interposed discs (Fig. 4–9). The cervical *facet joints*, also known as *apophyseal joints* or *zygapophyseal joints*, are formed by the articulating processes of adjacent vertebrae. The expanse of bone that encompasses the superior and inferior articulating processes is referred to as the *articular pillar* and is distinct from the pedicle.[1a] The expanse of bone between the supe-

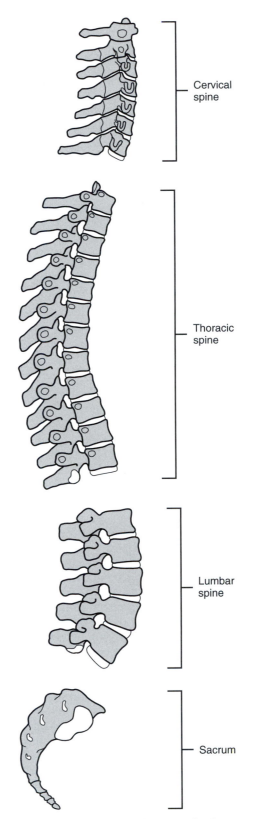

FIGURE 4–1. Divisions of the spinal column.

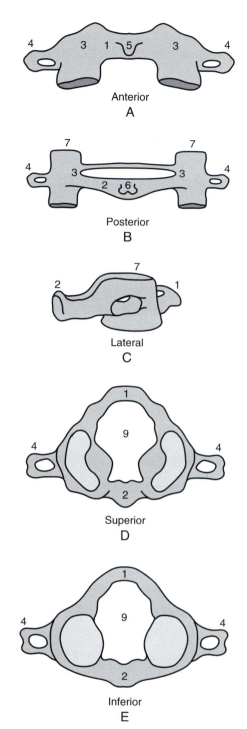

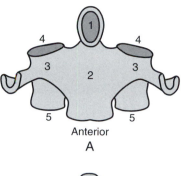

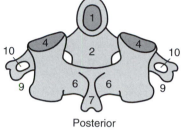

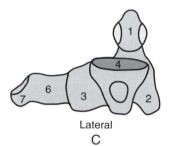

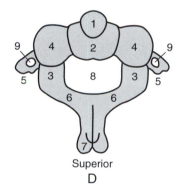

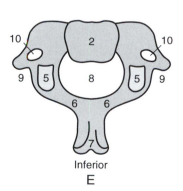

FIGURE 4–2. (*A–E*). Atlas (C1). 1 = anterior arch; 2 = posterior arch; 3 = lateral mass; 4 = transverse process; 5 = anterior tubercle; 6 = posterior tubercle; 7 = occipital condyles; 8 = inferior facets; 9 = vertebral foramen.

FIGURE 4–3. (*A–E*). Axis (C2). 1 = dens; 2 = body; 3 = pedicles; 4 = superior articulating processes; 5 = inferior articulating processes; 6 = laminae; 7 = bifid spinous process; 8 = vertebral foramen; 9 = transverse processes; 10 = transverse foramen.

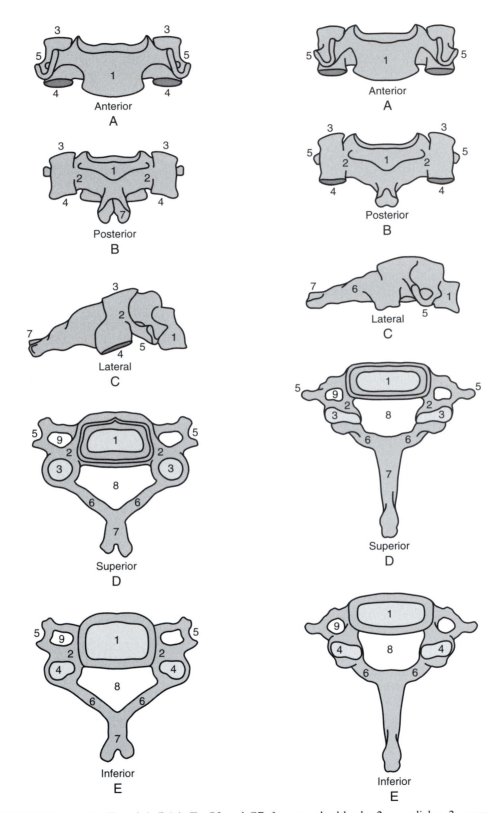

FIGURES 4–4 (*A–E*) and **4–5** (*A–E*). C3 and C7. 1 = vertebral body; 2 = pedicles; 3 = superior articulating processes; 4 = inferior articulating processes; 5 = transverse processes; 6 = lamina; 7 = spinous process; 8 = vertebral foramen; 9 = transverse foramen.

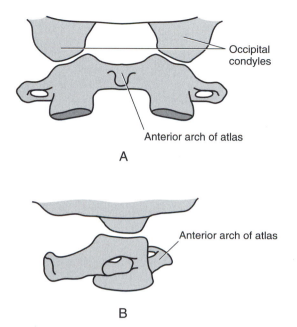

FIGURE 4–6. (*A*) Anterior and (*B*) lateral views of the atlanto-occipital joints.

rior and inferior articulating processes is known as the *pars interarticularis*.

Muscles of the cervical region work in concert with the ligaments to support the head and stabilize the flexible spine. A complete description of muscle anatomy is beyond the scope of this text. The primary ligaments of this region are reviewed to assist in the understanding of mechanisms of injury and the resultant instabilities. Although ligaments are of water density and generally do not possess enough radiodensity to

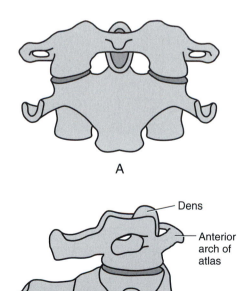

FIGURE 4–7. (*A*) Anterior and (*B*) lateral views of the atlantoaxial (C1–2) joint.

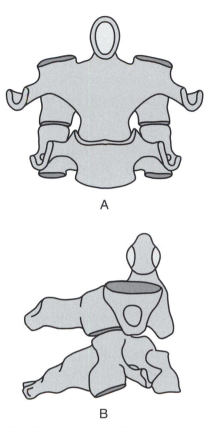

FIGURE 4–8. (*A*) Anterior and (*B*) lateral views of C2–3 joint articulation.

be visible on radiographs, the articular relationships that intact ligaments provide can be evaluated on films. Loss of normal articular relationships infers a possible loss of ligamentous support.

Ligamentous Anatomy[2]

The *cervicocranial ligaments* intricately support the articulating relationship among the occiput, atlas, and axis (Fig. 4–10). The principal ligamentous stabilizers are (1) the *alar ligaments*, extending upward and outward from the superiolateral surfaces of the dens to

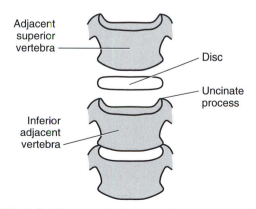

FIGURE 4–9. Uncovertebral joint, distracted, to illustrate anatomy.

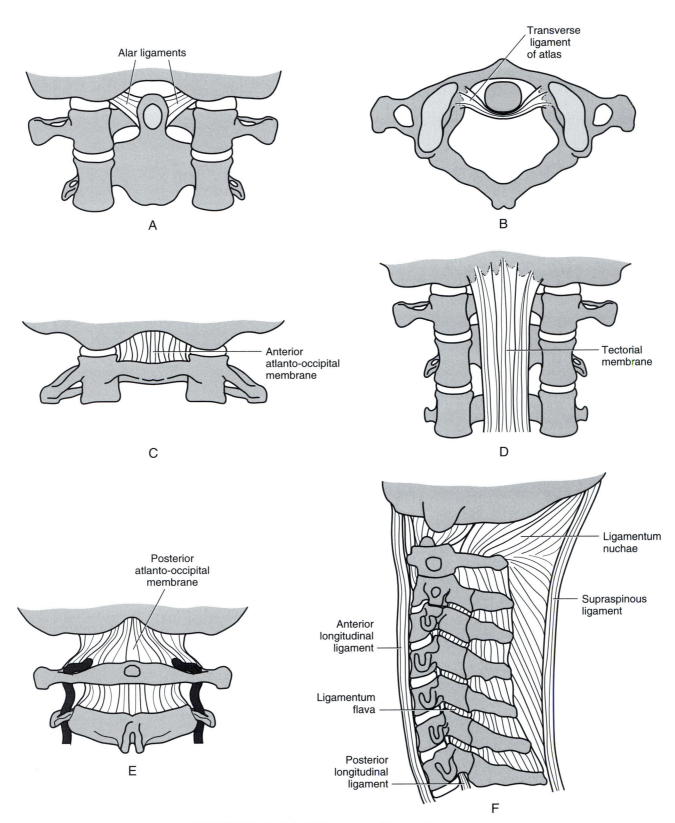

FIGURE 4–10. (*A–F*) Ligaments of the cervical spine.

the occiput, providing a restraint against excessive rotation at the atlanto-occipital joint, (2) the *transverse ligament of atlas*, extending horizontally across the dens and attached to the lateral masses of atlas, securing the articulation between these two bones, (3) the *anterior and posterior atlanto-occipital ligaments*, extending from the superior margins of atlas to the foramen magnum, and (4) *the tectorial membrane*, extending from the posterior body of axis and attached to the anterior margins of the foramen magnum, providing support to the subcranial region.

The lower cervical vertebrae are supported posteriorly by the (1) *ligamentum nuchae* stretching from the occipital crest to the spinous processes; (2) the *ligamenta flava*, joining the laminae of adjacent vertebrae; (3) the *interspinous ligaments*, joining adjacent spinous processes; and (4) the *posterior longitudinal ligament*, located within the vertebral canal and attached to the discs and posterior vertebral bodies. All of these ligaments assist in limiting forward flexion and rotation of the cervical spine. The *anterior longitudinal ligament* stretches from the occiput to the sacrum, attaching to the anterior discs and margins of the vertebral bodies and limiting backward bending.

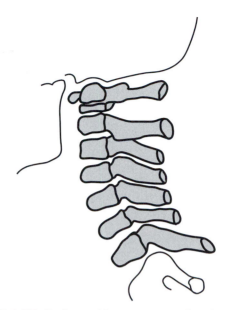

FIGURE 4–11. Radiographic appearance of newborn cervical spine.

MOBILITY[3]

The cervical spine possesses great mobility, allowing for a wide range of movements for the head. Combined motions at all cervical joints produce about 145 degrees of flexion and extension, 180 degrees of axial rotation, and 90 degrees of lateral flexion. The unique structural anatomy of the upper cervical joints produces unique functional mobility. The cervical joints below C2 are similar in their functional contributions to cervical mobility.

Approximately 10 to 15 degrees of both flexion and extension are possible at the atlanto-occipital joint. Less than 10 degrees of lateral flexion is possible to each side, and very minimal or no rotation occurs at this articulation.

The atlantoaxial joint is the most mobile segment of the cervical spine. Approximately 50 degrees of rotation is possible to each side, accounting for half of the rotation mobility present in the entire cervical spine. Less than 10 degrees of both flexion and extension takes place, and minimal or no lateral flexion exists.

All the cervical joints below C2 allow for flexion, extension, rotation, and lateral flexion. Dispersed between C3 and C7 are approximately 40 degrees of flexion, 25 degrees of extension, 45 degrees of rotation to either side, and 50 degrees of lateral flexion to either side.

GROWTH AND DEVELOPMENT[4–6]

The process of ossification of the vertebrae begins in the sixth week of fetal life. At birth at least three pri-

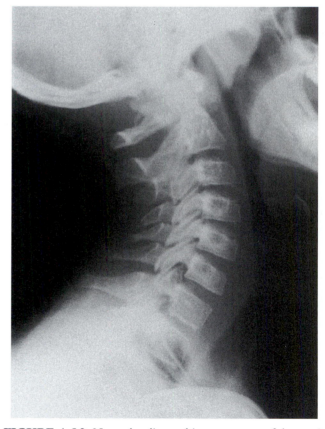

FIGURE 4–12. Normal radiographic appearance of the cervical spine of an 11-year-old female, lateral view. The vertebrae exhibit their gross adult form, although the anterior vertebral bodies still show some slight wedging. The tips of the spinous processes have just begun to fuse.

mary ossification centers are present at each vertebral level. (See the radiograph of an infant skeleton, Fig. 6–7.)

The anterior arch of atlas is completely cartilaginous at birth (Fig. 4–11). Complete fusion of the synchondroses will unite the anterior arch by age 8, and the posterior arch by age 4. The odontoid process is formed by two vertically positioned ossification centers. The odontoid fuses inferiorly to the vertebral body between the ages of 3 and 6. The superior tip fuses by age 12.

The bodies of axis and the lower vertebrae are ossified at birth. The neural arches and spinous processes fuse by the age of 2 or 3. The posterior spinal elements then fuse with vertebral bodies between the ages of 3 and 6. The vertebral bodies are wedge shaped anteriorly until they take on a more squared-off shape by age 7. After age 8 the cervical spine has attained its gross adult form (Fig. 4–12).

Continued vertebral growth throughout childhood occurs via periosteal apposition, similar to the periosteal growth of long bones. At puberty, secondary centers of ossification develop in the superior and inferior endplates of the vertebral bodies. Secondary ossification centers also appear for the bifid spinous processes, transverse processes, and articular processes at this age. Each of these structures completes fusion by age 25.

The uncovertebral joints are not present in early life and appear to be the result of degenerative fibrotic changes associated with normal aging.[7]

Postural Development

At birth the spinal column exhibits one long curve that is convex posteriorly, the *primary curve* of the spine. As the baby learns to lift its head from prone lying the *secondary curve* of *cervical lordosis* begins to develop (Fig. 4–13). The onset of walking develops the secondary curve of *lumbar lordosis*. These secondary curves continue to develop until the growth of the vertebral column matures post puberty.[8,9]

Postural changes in the spine throughout adult life appear to be influenced by multiple factors including genetics, health, occupation, and type of recreational activities (Fig. 4–14). Degenerative conditions and disease processes often render characteristic alterations in spinal posture. Trauma to the spine or any extremity may affect spinal posture as the body attempts compensatory strategies to lessen pain. The cervical spine appears to adapt with the additional goal of maintaining the eyes to a forward and horizontal orientation.[10]

ROUTINE RADIOGRAPHIC EVALUATION OF THE CERVICAL SPINE

Basic: AP Open Mouth
AP Lower C-Spine
Lateral

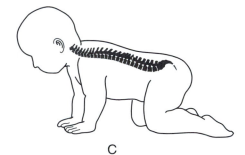

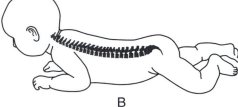

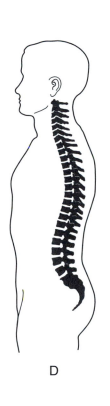

FIGURE 4–13. (*A–D*) Postural development of spinal curvatures progresses from the primary convex curve of the newborn (*A*) to the secondary concavities of the cervical and lumbar spines in the adult (*D*).

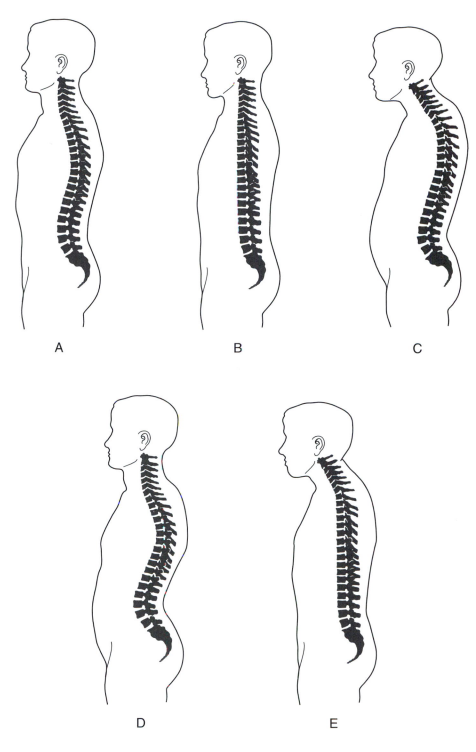

A   B   C

D   E

FIGURE 4–14. (*A–E*) Variations in postural curves.

R Oblique
L Oblique
Optional: Lateral Flexion and Extension Stress Films

The routine radiologic evaluation of the cervical spine includes five views. The patient is usually erect, either sitting or standing. If a patient's condition warrants, the series may be obtained from the supine position.

The routine evaluation is indicated for typical complaints and for less severe acute conditions. The radi-ographs are reviewed by the physician before any special views or additional imaging studies are ordered.

The lateral flexion-extension stress films are done under the supervision of a radiologist if there is radiologic, clinical, or historic evidence of possible ligamentous injury. Radiographs of the cervical spine taken while the spine is positioned in full flexion and in full extension may expose unstable joint segment positioning if ligamentous laxity or tears are present.[22] A "limited" supine cervical radiologic evaluation is indicated in severe trauma cases to prevent undue movement of the patient. This examination usually consists of a cross-table lateral view to screen for fractures or dislocations.

Anteroposterior Open Mouth (Figs. 4–15, 4–16, 4–17)

This view demonstrates the articulation of C1 and C2, the atlantoaxial joint. The patient is positioned with the mouth wide open to remove the superimposition of the density of the mandible from obscuring the upper cervical spine. The important observations are:

1. The atlas is positioned symmetrically on axis.
2. The dens is positioned symmetrically between the lateral masses of atlas.
3. The bilateral joint spaces at the lateral atlantoaxial facet articulations are of equal height.
4. The C2 spinous process is positioned in midline.

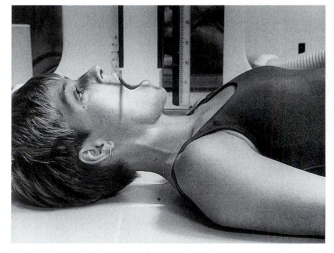

FIGURE 4–15. Patient position for AP open-mouth cervical spine radiograph.

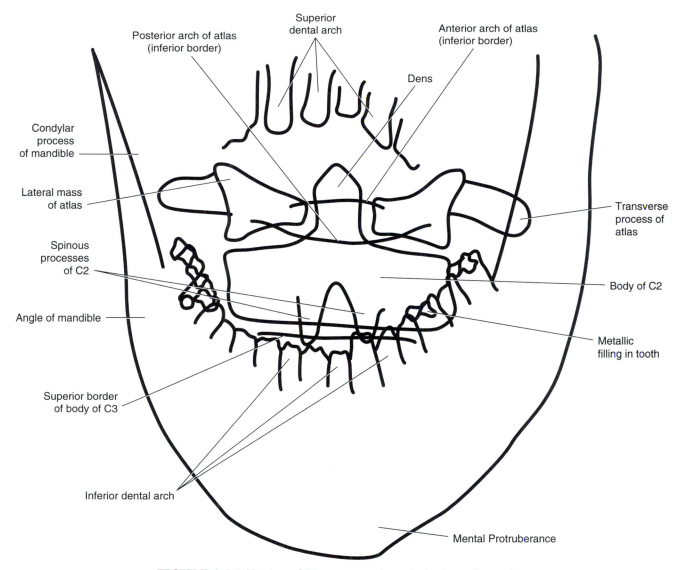

FIGURE 4–16. Tracing of AP open-mouth cervical spine radiograph.

Alterations in these landmarks may be indicators of ligamentous laxity or tear, fracture, or dislocation, relative to the atlanto-occipital and atlantoaxial articulations.

5. The dens is superimposed with both the anterior and posterior arches of atlas. The borders of the arches image as lines that cross over the dens. Do not mistake these for fracture lines.

Clinical Objectives

1. Trace the large curvilinear line that is the base of the occiput.
2. Trace the angle of the mandible.
3. Trace the dens and body of C2.
4. Trace the anterior arch of atlas.
5. Trace the posterior arch of atlas.
6. Trace the lateral atlantoaxial facet joints.
7. Trace the transverse processes of atlas.
8. Trace the bodies and spinous processes of C2 through T1.

Anteroposterior Lower Cervical Spine (Figs. 4–18, 4–19, 4–20)

This view demonstrates the five lower cervical vertebrae, the upper thoracic vertebrae and associated ribs, the medial thirds of the clavicles, and the trachea.

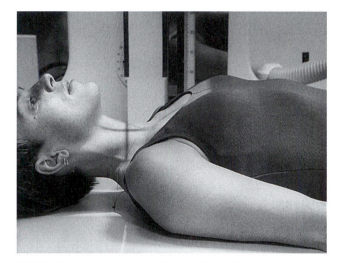

FIGURE 4–18. Patient positioning for AP lower cervical spine radiograph.

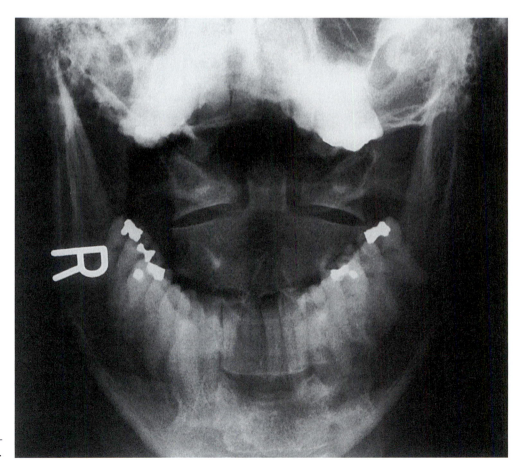

FIGURE 4–17. Anteroposterior open-mouth cervical spine.

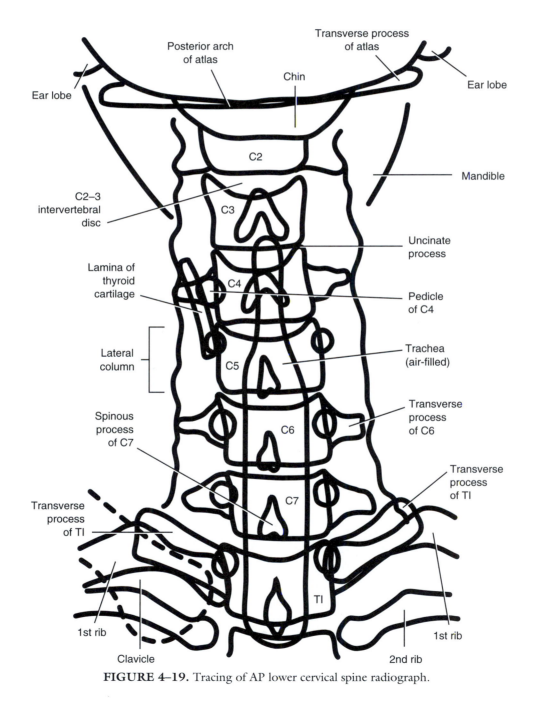

FIGURE 4–19. Tracing of AP lower cervical spine radiograph.

The superimposition of the mandible and skull will obscure the upper cervical vertebra. When identifying the level of cervical vertebrae, remember that C2–C3 possesses the first intervertebral disc and T1 possesses the first rib articulation. The important observations are:

1. The cervical and thoracic vertebral bodies are aligned in a relatively vertical column.
2. The spinous processes are positioned in midline throughout the spine. Note normal irregularities in the shape of the processes.
3. The superimposition of the overlapping facet joints and articular pillars creates a radiographic illusion of one smoothly undulating column of bone on either side of the vertebral bodies, the "lateral column."
4. The transverse processes are mostly within the image of this lateral column. The superimposed densities of the lateral column make the transverse processes difficult to discern.
5. The pedicles are also somewhat superimposed by the lateral column image but can be identified by their radiodense oval-like cortical outline. Similar to the spinous processes, this image is analogous to the image created by the cylinder radiographed end-on (see Fig. 1–9A).
6. The disc spaces are not evaluated in this frontal view as the sagittal plane of the lordosis and the angled x-ray tube tilt prohibit true dimensions of

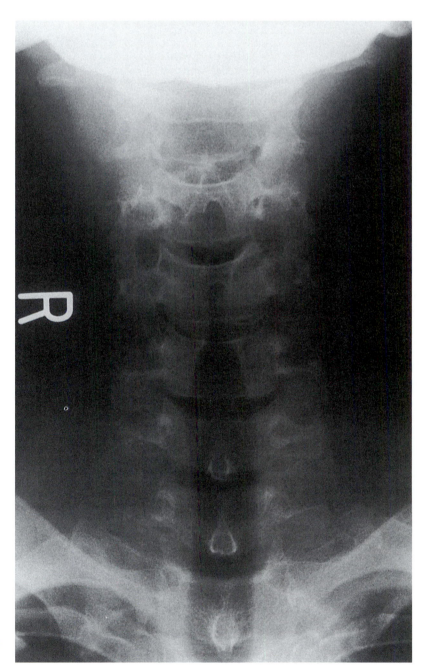

FIGURE 4–20. Anteroposterior lower cervical spine.

the disc spaces from visualization. The lateral view best demonstrates disc spaces.

7. Note the uncinate processes extending from the superior vertebral bodies and the formation of uncovertebral joints at some levels.

8. Note the radiolucent image of the air-filled trachea overlying the cervical spine at midline.

9. The clavicles are farthest from the film plate and thus are imaged with the greatest amount of size distortion in comparison to the other structures. Note the *magnification* of the radiographic image of the clavicles.

Clinical Objectives

1. Trace the vertebral bodies of C3 through T1. Note the presence of *uncinate processes* at some levels.
2. Trace the spinous processes of C3 through T1.
3. Trace the large transverse process of T1.
4. Trace the first ribs and costotransverse joints.
5. Trace the clavicles.
6. Trace the air-filled trachea.

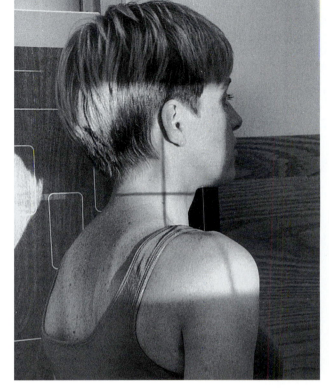

FIGURE 4–21. Patient position for lateral cervical spine radiograph.

Lateral (Figs. 4–21, 4–22, 4–23)

This view demonstrates the seven cervical vertebrae, intervertebral disc spaces, articular pillars and facet joints, spinous processes, and prevertebral soft tissues. The important observations are:

1. The alignment of the lateral cervical spine can be imagined as three roughly parallel lines. *In a normal spine the spatial relationship of these lines will remain constant whether the neck is positioned in neutral, flexion, or extension*[23–25] (Fig. 4–24). Disruption of this spatial relationship may be due to fracture, dislocation, or severe degenerative changes.

   Line 1. The anterior borders of the vertebral bodies normally align in a lordotic curve. Osteophytes may project anteriorly and are thought to be traction spurs from tension at the attachment of the anterior longitudinal ligament, or related to degenerative intervertebral disc changes. They are ignored in evaluating the *spatial* relationships of these lines.

   Line 2. The posterior borders of the vertebral bodies normally follow the same curve as the anterior bodies. Osteophytes that project from this line encroach upon the spinal canal and intervertebral foramina and have

the potential to compress the spinal cord or nerve roots.

   Line 3. The spinolaminar line is the junction of the lamina at the spinous processes. This line represents the posterior extent of the central spinal canal. The spinal cord lies between lines 2 and 3.

2. The vertebral bodies are boxlike in appearance with distinct smoothly curved osseous margins. Note any osteophyte formation as described earlier.

3. The intervertebral disc spaces are well preserved in height at each level.

4. The articular pillars and facet joints are superimposed as a pair at each level. The facet joints can be individually defined on the oblique views, but the lateral view is best for visualizing joint margins and joint spaces.

5. The bursa between the dens and its articulating facet on atlas is represented by the dark radiolucent line anterior to dens. This *atlantodental interface* or *predental space* is a distance kept constant by the transverse ligament of atlas during all neck ranges of motion.[26,27] See the lateral flexion-extension films for more information regarding this point.

6. The transverse processes are superimposed over the vertebral bodies.

7. The prevertebral soft tissues will cast a shadow roughly parallel to the spine. Distention of the soft

tissue shadow is often due to hemorrhage or effusion and is a sign of trauma.

Right and Left Obliques (Figs. 4–25, 4–26, 4–27)

This view demonstrates the intervertebral foramina, uncovertebral joints, facet joints, and pedicles of the cervical vertebrae. Both right and left obliques are obtained so that each of these structures is viewed individually, as opposed to the lateral view, which superimposes the posterior vertebral elements. The important observations are:

1. In this view the head and body are in neutral alignment and rotated as a unit 45 degrees from the lateral view. The 45-degree rotation may be to either side of the lateral, depending on the preference of the facility. A left anterior oblique (LAO) projection (meaning the patient's left anterior neck is closest to the film plate) will image the *open left intervertebral foramina*, and the right anterior oblique (RAO) will image the *open right intervertebral foramina*. Conversely, the left posterior oblique (LPO) projection (meaning the patient's left posterior neck is closest to the film plate) images the right intervertebral foramina, and the right posterior oblique (RPO) images the left intervertebral foramina. The images are alike for either view, but the projection must be understood to know which side of the joint is being defined.[28] See Chapter 1 for positioning diagrams.
2. The intervertebral foramina, through which the spinal nerves exit, are normally imaged as radiolucent ovals. Narrowed, ragged margins of the ovals may indicate bony encroachment on the spinal nerves. The contralateral foramina are not seen. The inter-

vertebral foramina are named by spinal segment (e.g., the *C4–C5* foramina or the *C5–C6* foramina).
3. The pedicles are viewed *en face*. The contralateral pedicles are superimposed behind the vertebral bodies and image as cylinders seen end-on.
4. The irregular shape of the laminae, becoming larger in descending vertebrae, is normal. They too image as a structure seen end-on.

Optional Projections: Lateral Flexion and Extension Stress Films (Figs. 4–28, 4–29, 4–30)

These projections are not part of the routine radiographic examination of the cervical spine but are common optional projections. The purpose of these projections is to observe joint alignment while the supporting soft tissue structures are stressed by gross neck flexion or extension positions. Thus, these views are also referred to as **stress** films or **functional** studies, as they examine the joints at the end ranges of voluntary flexion and extension. Joint instabilities that were not apparent on the routine lateral view may effectively be demonstrated here. The important observations are:

1. As noted on the routine lateral projection, the spatial relationship of the three parallel lines designating normal cervical spine alignment will, under normal conditions, remain constant through any degree of flexion or extension. Note the preservation of this relationship on these normal films. Disruption of this spatial relationship may be due to fracture, dislocation, or severe degenerative changes.
2. The cortical outlines of the vertebral bodies, articular pillars, and spinous processes appear as on the routine lateral projection. The joint positions will change slightly on these views, however. In *flexion*, the anterior intervertebral disc spaces narrow and the posterior intervertebral spaces and interspinous spaces widen. In *extension*, the anterior interverte-

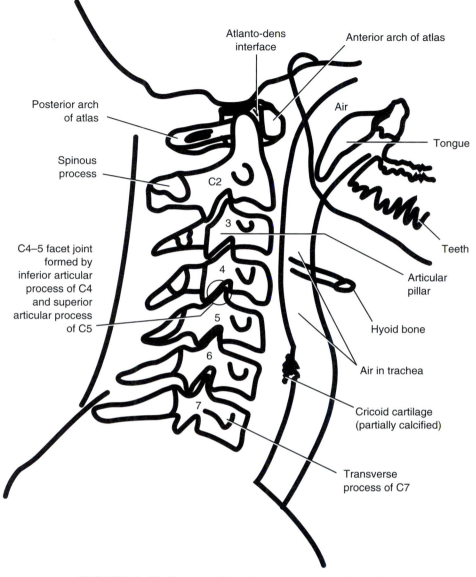

FIGURE 4–22. Tracing of lateral cervical spine radiograph.

bral spaces widen and the posterior intervertebral spaces and interspinous spaces narrow.

3. The *atlantodental interface*, represented by the radiolucent line anterior to the articulating facet of the dens, is recognized as seen on the routine lateral view. The width of this space will, under normal conditions, remain constant in any degree of flexion or extension. An increase in this distance to more than 3 mm indicates C1–C2 subluxation. (See Fig. 2–30A, B, and C for a radiographic example of an increased atlantodental interface representing C1–C2 joint instability.)

CERVICAL SPINE TRAUMA

Trauma Radiography[29-35]

The *lateral view* is the first radiograph filmed and evaluated if the patient has a history of trauma. The significance of the lateral view is that normal cervical alignment is easily evaluated in the aforementioned series of parallel line images (see description on the routine lateral view). Discontinuity or obvious step-offs in the bony alignment may indicate the presence

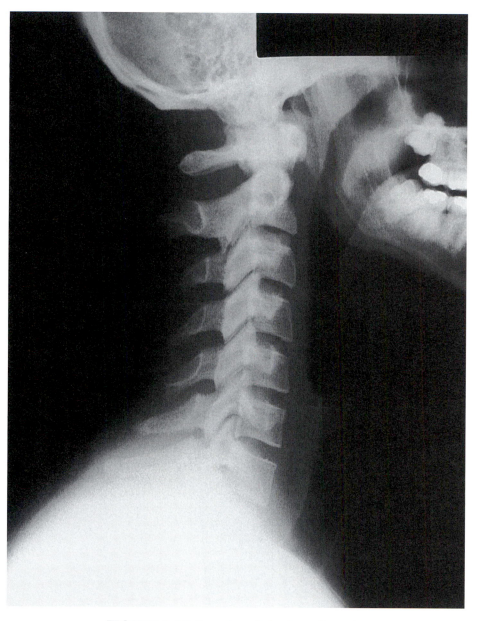

FIGURE 4–23. Lateral cervical spine radiograph.

of fracture or dislocation. In severe trauma cases the lateral view functions as a preliminary diagnostic screen and is performed on the supine patient. This ''cross-table lateral'' prevents undue movement of the patient. The majority of cervical spine injuries can be grossly identified on the lateral view.

The lateral flexion and extension views are stress radiographs done to expose excessive segmental motion due to degeneration or ligamentous rupture. At times there are sufficient historical evidence and patient symptoms to support the presence of serious injury but little radiographic evidence of such. Further imaging studies are then warranted.

Evaluation of radiographs for significant signs of cervical trauma includes examination of the soft tissues, vertebral alignment, and joint characteristics[36] (Table 4–1):

Abnormal soft tissues signs are (1) widened retropharyngeal or retrotracheal spaces, (2) displacement of the trachea or larynx, and (3) displacement of the prevertebral fat pad. Any of these signs suggest the presence of edema or hemorrhage, indicating associated pathology.

Abnormal vertebral alignment signs include (1) loss of the parallel lines as outlined for the lateral view indicating fracture, dislocation, or severe degenerative changes; (2) loss of lordosis, indicating muscle spasm in response to underlying injury; (3) acute kyphotic angulation with a widened interspinous space, indicating rupture of the posterior ligaments; and (4) rotation of a vertebral body, indicating unilateral facet dislocation, a hyperextension fracture, muscle spasm, disc, or capsular injury.

Abnormal joint signs are (1) widened atlantodental interface indicating degeneration, stretching, or rupture of the transverse ligament; (2) widened interspinous process space (known as "fanning"), indicating rupture of interspinous and other posterior ligaments; (3) widened intervertebral disc space, indicating posterior ligament rupture; (4) narrowed intervertebral disc space indicating rupture of disc and extrusion of nuclear material; and (5) loss of facet joint articulation, indicating dislocation.

Incidence of spine injuries has increased in recent decades primarily due to the increase in motor vehicle accidents and sporting activities.[37] Although fractures may occur at any level in the spine, the lower cervical, lower thoracic, and upper lumbar regions are the most frequent sites of injury. The cervical spine, however, has the greatest potential risk for spinal cord damage.[38,39] Approximately two-thirds of spinal cord injuries occur in the cervical spine. Adults characteristically injure their lower cervical spine, and children more frequently injure their upper cervical spine.[40–42]

Injuries to the cervical spine are first broadly classified as *stable* or *unstable* injuries, in reference to the *immediate or subsequent potential risk to the spinal cord and*

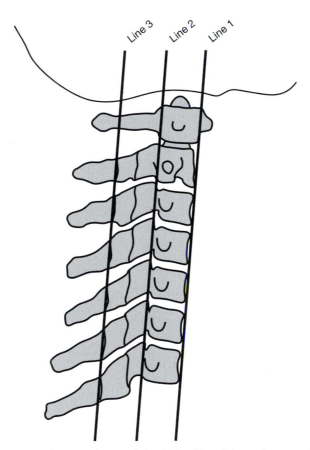

FIGURE 4–24. In a normal spine, the *spatial relationship* of these three parallel lines will remain constant in any degree of flexion or extension. Line 1 = anterior borders of the vertebral bodies. Line 2 = posterior borders of the vertebral bodies. Line 3 = the spinolaminar junctions.

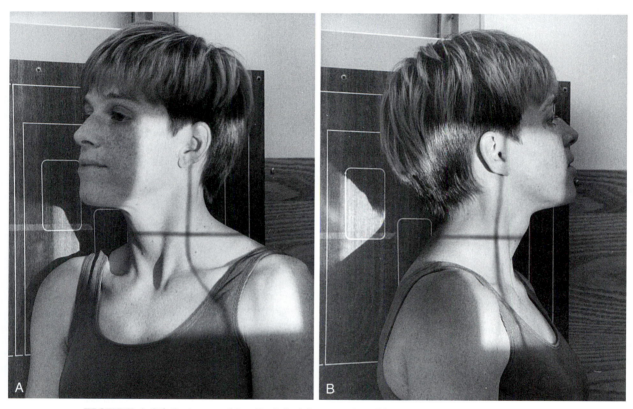

FIGURE 4–25. Patient position for (*A*) right posterior oblique and (*B*) left posterior oblique cervical spine radiograph.

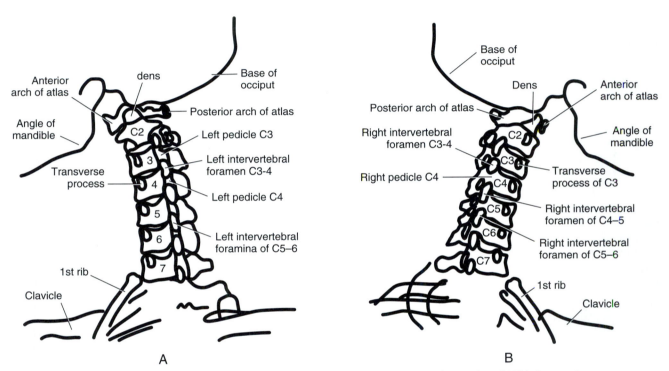

FIGURE 4–26. (*A*) Tracings of right posterior oblique cervical spine radiograph and (*B*) left posterior oblique cervical spine radiograph.

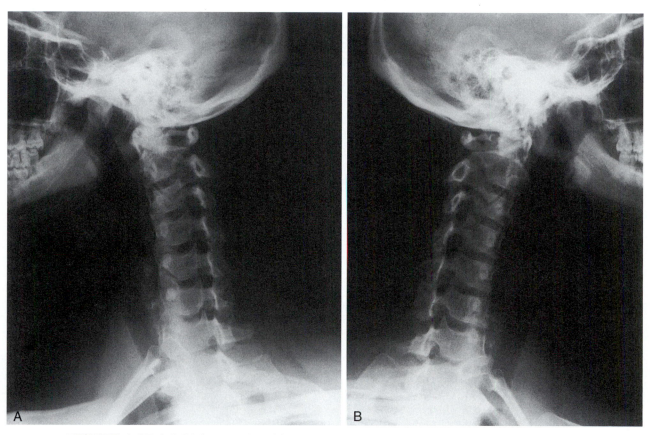

FIGURE 4–27. (*A*) Right posterior oblique cervical spine radiograph. (*B*) Left posterior oblique cervical spine radiograph.

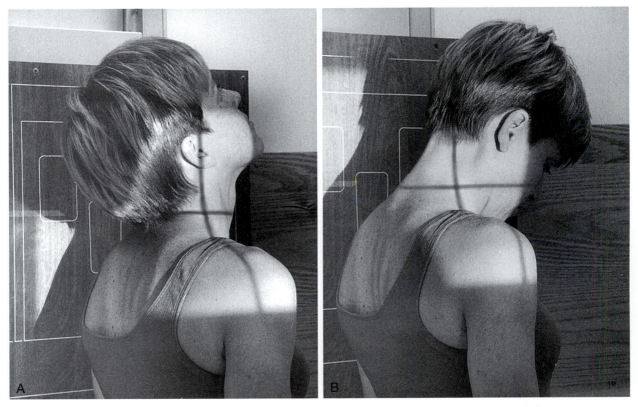

FIGURE 4–28. Patient position for lateral views of cervical spine in (*A*) extension and (*B*) flexion.

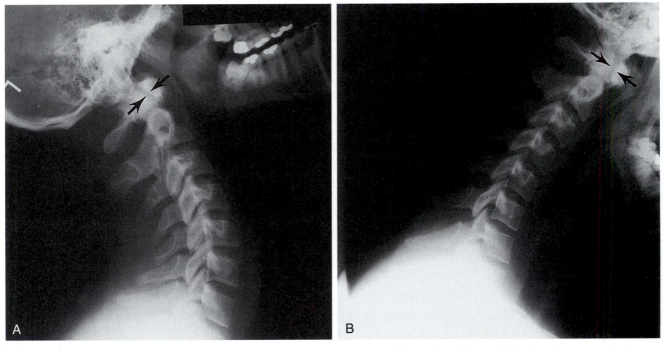

FIGURE 4–29. (*A*) Lateral extension and (*B*) flexion stress radiographs of the cervical spine. Arrows indicate the atlantodental interface, which has remained at a constant distant in either radiograph.

nerve roots. Stable injuries are protected from significant bone or joint displacement by intact posterior spinal ligaments. Examples of stable injuries are compression fractures, traumatic disc herniations, and unilateral facet dislocations. Unstable injuries may show significant displacement initially or have the potential to become displaced with movement. Examples of unstable injuries are fracture-dislocations and bilateral facet dislocations.[43,44]

The mechanism of injury is broadly classified as either being direct force, such as in a blow to the head, or indirect force, such as the rapid acceleration and deceleration of the body in a motor vehicle accident. Mechanisms of injury are further defined by the motion or position of the neck during the injury. The cervical spine will suffer injury when forced past the extreme end ranges of extension, flexion, lateral flexion,

or rotation or when axially loaded by compression. A summary of the injuries that can happen as a result of these mechanisms is presented in Table 4–2.

Fractures

Two types of fractures are often seen in the cervical spine: *avulsion fractures* and *compression or impaction fractures*. Avulsions occur as a bone fragment is pulled off by violent muscle contraction or, more commonly, by the passive resistance of a ligament applied against an oppositely directed force. For example, an avulsion of the C7 spinous process may occur as a result of forceful contraction of the rhomboids and trapezius, or of the resistance of the supraspinous and interspinous ligaments during hyperflexion. Compression or impaction fractures will result when two vertebrae are forced together. For example, an axial compression force will cause a comminuted or "burst" fracture of the impacted vertebral body. A flexion force will compress the impacted vertebral body into an anterior wedge shape. An extension force will fracture and compress the articular pillars.

Descriptions of some common fractures specific to levels in the cervical spine follow.

ATLAS

A common fracture at atlas is a *posterior arch fracture*, sustained during a hyperextension force that compresses the arch between the occipital condyles and posterior elements of axis. A less common fracture occurs through both the anterior and posterior arches of atlas, called a *Jefferson fracture*. The mechanism is axial compression that forces the occiput onto atlas. Diving into shallow water head first and auto accidents are the usual causative actions.[45]

TABLE 4–1 Radiologic Signs of Cervical Trauma

Abnormal Soft Tissues
   Widened retropharyngeal space
   Widened retrotracheal space
   Displacement of prevertebral fat pad
   Tracheal displacement
   Laryngeal displacement
Abnormal Vertebral Alignment
   Reversal of lordosis
   Acute kyphotic angulation
   Rotation of vertebrae
   Widened intervertebral space
   Step-offs in vertical alignment
Abnormal Joint Relationships
   Widened atlantodental interspace
   Widened interspinous space
   Widened intervertebral disc space
   Narrowed intervertebral disc space
   Facet disarticulation

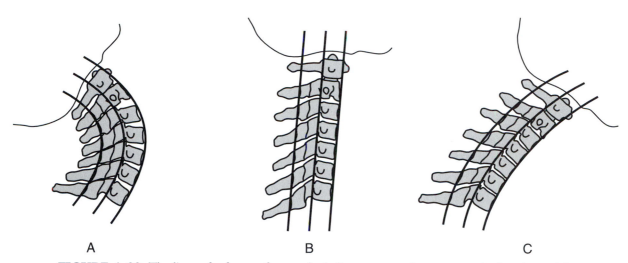

A   B   C

FIGURE 4–30. The lines of reference for vertebral alignment remain constant whether the neck is positioned in (*A*) extension, (*B*) neutral, or (*C*) flexion.

TABLE 4–2 Cervical Spine Injuries

Structures Involved	Mechanism	Appearance	Stable +/−
Hyperflexion sprain: Disruption of superficial posterior ligaments and capsules with transient anterior subluxation of vertebral joints	Hyperflexion		+
Bilateral facet joint dislocation	Hyperflexion		−
Disruption of alar, apical, and transverse ligaments; possible C1–C2 dislocation; possible odontoid fracture	Hyperflexion		−
Avulsion fracture of spinous process, "clay shoveler's fracture"	Hyperflexion		+
Unilateral facet dislocation	Hyperflexion + Rotation		+
Anterior vertebral body compression fracture "wedge fracture"	Hyperflexion ± compression		+
Anterior inferior vertebral body fracture with posterior displacement of the rest of the vertebrae; "flexion teardrop fracture"	Hyperflexion ± Compression		+/−
Fracture-dislocation at C1–C2	Hyperflexion ± compression		−
Fracture-dislocation at any other vertebral segments C3–C7	Rotation		−
Unilateral facet dislocation	Rotation		+

TABLE 4–2 Cervical Spine Injuries *(continued)*

Structures Involved	Mechanism	Appearance	Stable +/−
Dislocation of C1 on C2	Rotation		−
Odontoid fracture	Rotation		+/−
Fracture of anterior and posterior arches of C1; "Jefferson fracture"	Axial Compression		−
Comminuted fracture of vertebral body "burst fracture"	Axial Compression		+/−
Hyperextension sprain: disruption of anterior ligaments and soft tissues with transient posterior subluxation	Hyperextension		+
Anteroinferior vertebral body fractures	Hyperextension		+/−
Posteriorly displaced odontoid fractures	Hyperextension		−
Avulsion fracture of the anterior arch of C1	Hyperextension		+
Fracture of the posterior arch of C1	Hyperextension		+
Fracture of the pedicles of C2 with dislocation of the body of C2 on C3; "hangman's fracture"	Hyperextension		−
Fracture of the uncinate process	Lateral flexion		+

TABLE 4–2 Cervical Spine Injuries (*continued*)

Structures Involved	Mechanism	Appearance	Stable +/−
Avulsion fracture of transverse process	Lateral flexion		+
Lateral compression fracture of vertebral body	Lateral flexion		+
Compression fracture of articular pillar	Lateral flexion		+

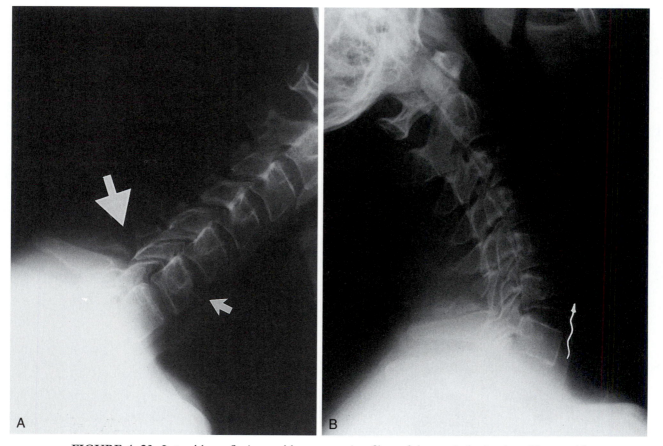

FIGURE 4–31. Lateral hyperflexion and hyperextension films of the cervical spine in a 38-year-old female involved in a motor vehicle accident. (*A*) Upon flexion, a wide interspinous space is noted at C6–7 (large arrow). A compression fracture is present at the anterior superior corner of the vertebral body of C6 (small arrow). Hyperextension film shows widening of the C6–7 interspace (wavy arrow). The wide interspaces are signs of ligamentous disruption at that segment.

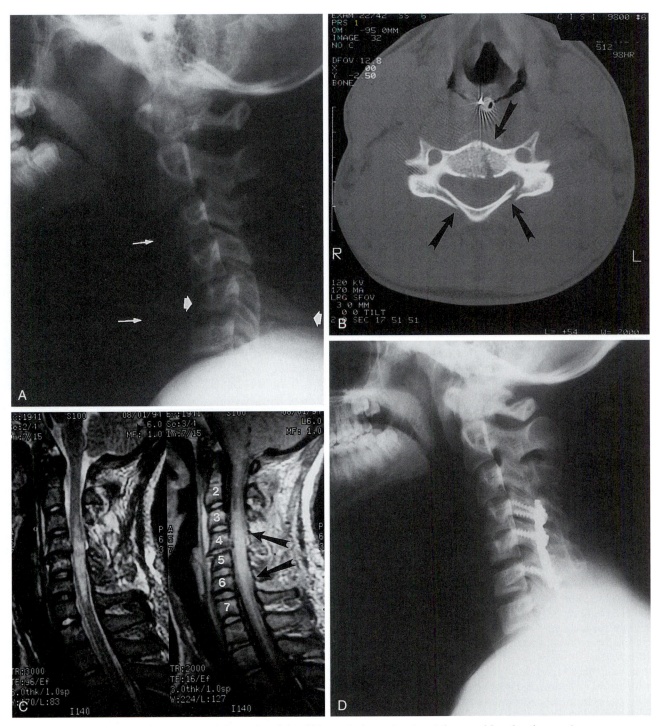

FIGURE 4–32. Fracture-dislocation of the fifth cervical vertebra in a 15-year-old male who was in a motor vehicle accident. (*A*) Plain film, lateral view, shows the posterior displacement of the C5 vertebra (wide arrows). Small arrows point to the prevertebral shadow (normal soft tissue image of the anterior neck), which is displaced anteriorly because of swelling and edema. (*B*) CT axial view of C5 shows a burst fracture of the vertebral body and fractures of both laminae (arrows). (*C*) MRI, sagittal plane, reveals edema of the spinal cord from the level of C3 through C7 (arrows). (*D*) Plain film, lateral view, of internal fixation restoring vertebral alignment and stabilizing the spinal segments.

AXIS

A common fracture of axis is the bilateral fracture of the pedicles causing a dislocation of C2 on C3. This dislocation is called a **traumatic spondylolisthesis**, or a **hangman's fracture** as it bears a pathological skeletal resemblance to the fatal characteristics of a judicial hanging. The precipitating mechanism is hyperextension, often due to auto accidents. **Odontoid process fractures** are common traumatic injuries of the cervical spine and are divided into type I, an avulsion of the tip caused by alar or apical ligament stress; type II, a fracture at the junction of the dens to the body, most common and most difficult to heal; and type III, a fracture deep below the junction, which heals readily. The mechanism for these fractures is excessive rotation.[46,47]

MID AND LOWER CERVICAL VERTEBRAE[48-50]

Fractures of the remaining vertebrae may occur at any site on the vertebral structure. Some of the more commonly seen fractures are:

- *Wedge fracture:* This fracture occurs when an interposed vertebra is compressed anteriorly by two adjacent vertebrae, owing to hyperflexion forces. Two-thirds of these fractures in the cervical spine occur at C5, C6, or C7. This fracture is stable because of at least partially intact ligamentous structures (Fig. 4–31).
- *Burst fracture:* This fracture occurs when an intervertebral disc is axially compressed, and the nucleus pulposus is driven through an adjacent vertebral endplate, causing a literal bursting apart of the vertebral body resulting in comminution. This fracture may be stable or unstable, depending on the fracture configuration (Figs. 4–32, 4–33).
- *Teardrop fracture:* This fracture occurs when a triangular fragment of bone is separated from the anteroinferior corner of the vertebral body because of either an avulsion force sustained during hyperextension or a compressive force sustained during hyperflexion. The force necessary to cause this fracture is often associated with additional injury such as intervertebral disc tearing, ligament rupture, and facet dislocation, rendering this a potentially unstable injury.
- *Articular pillar fracture:* The articular pillar, the rhomboidal structure composed of the superior and inferior articulating processes, is fractured by a compressive hyperextension force, combined with a degree of lateral flexion. This fracture occurs most frequently at C6 and is usually a stable injury.
- *Clay shoveler's fracture:* This fracture is an avulsion fracture of the spinous process produced by hyperflexion forces or forceful muscular contraction of the trapezius and rhomboids often associated with the repetitive heavy labor of the upper extremities, as seen in shoveling. Occurring most frequently at C6, C7, and T1, this fracture is stable (see Fig. 4–31).

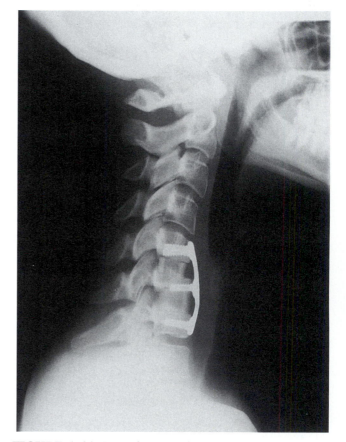

FIGURE 4–33. Burst fracture of C6. Lateral view, postoperative film demonstrates internal fixation and donor bone graft stabilizing a C6 burst fracture. Patient is a 28-year-old female who fractured her neck in a fall while skiing.

- *Transverse process fracture:* This uncommon fracture, when present, usually occurs at the largest transverse process in the cervical spine, C7. This fracture usually results from lateral flexion forces causing an avulsion at the tip of the contralateral side transverse process.

Dislocations[51,52]

The most serious and life-threatening injuries to the cervical spine are *fracture-dislocations*. In the upper cervical spine, a fracture through the base of the dens combined with a ligament rupture will cause a fracture-dislocation of the atlantoaxial joint, C1–C2. The hangman's fracture of axis described earlier is usually associated with anterior dislocation of C2 on C3. At any lower vertebral level, fractures of the posterior vertebral structures combined with tears of the posterior ligaments may cause a vertebral body to displace anteriorly, transecting or contusing the spinal cord. Note that dislocations in the spine are described by the direction that the superior vertebrae of the segment moved. For example, an anterior dislocation of C2–C3 indicates that C2 displaced anteriorly on C3.

Dislocations *not* associated with fractures may be either *complete* or *self-reducing dislocations* and *are in reference to the facet joints.* Complete facet joint dislocation may occur *unilaterally* at a segment due to a rotary force, or *bilaterally,* due to a hyperflexion force. In either case, the inferior articulating process of the uppermost vertebrae will come to lie in front of the superior articulating process of the subjacent vertebrae, locking the joint out of normal articulation, hence the term "*locked facets.*"

In self-reducing dislocations, a force momentarily disengages the articulations, which then return to normal alignment once the force dissipates. These momentary dislocations are also referred to as *transient dislocations* or *subluxations.*

Hyperflexion and Hyperextension Sprains[53-55]

Cervical sprains are injuries to the ligaments of the spine. *Hyperflexion* and *hyperextension sprains* more accurately define the mechanism of injury, direction of force, and the ligaments susceptible to disruption. A mention of the layperson's term "whiplash," so often incorrectly used to encompass all soft tissue injuries to the neck, is warranted.

The common usage of "whiplash" persists despite its lack of clear definition. Commonly associated with auto accidents, the term is at best an emotional one, with no value in defining the injury. To its credit, use of the term began somewhat logically in an attempt to describe the action of the heavy head on the flexible cervical spine during sudden deceleration or acceleration of the trunk. Unfortunately, however, it became synonymous with a host of unspecified cervical soft tissue injuries and gained enduring popularity as a general description of the state of the patient's neck. As this word is vague and nonanatomic, it neither assists in accurate evaluation or treatment determination nor has any useful place in professional vocabulary.

Hyperflexion sprains disrupt the posterior ligament complex. The posterior ligament complex includes all of the posterior ligaments and the facet joint capsules. With extreme force, injury to the posterior annulus fibrosus and posterior aspect of the intervertebral disc, transient facet dislocations and avulsion fractures may occur. The magnitude of the force, direction, and degree of flexion determine the injury severity and number of structures compromised.

Tears of the posterior ligaments allow the superior vertebra of a segment to rotate or translate anteriorly on its subjacent vertebra. That vertebral segment will no longer align in a normal lordotic curve and will instead show a *hyperkyphotic angulation* on the lateral radiograph. Thus, the injured segment appears to be *flexed,* whereas the remainder of the spine is in relatively neutral alignment (Fig. 4–34).

At times the posterior complex may be torn, but the lateral radiograph does not reveal any signs of joint

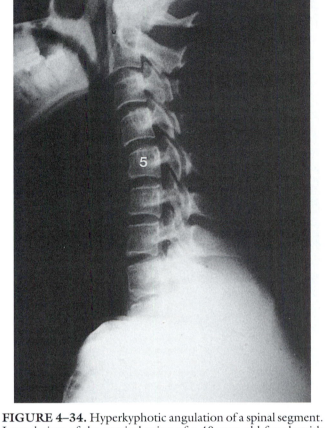

FIGURE 4–34. Hyperkyphotic angulation of a spinal segment. Lateral view of the cervical spine of a 40-year-old female with complaints of chronic neck pain. The only history of injury was an incident 5 years earlier whereby the patient ran into a wall while playing racquetball. The most striking feature is the loss of cervical lordosis and the hyperkyphotic angulation of the C4–5 and C5–6 segments. Assuming that there were no professional errors in positioning the patient for this view, one possible assumption is that a ligmentous injury occurred at one or more segments in the past, and adaptive shortening of the soft tissues has occurred over time. Lateral hyperflexion and hyperextension films would provide valuable information regarding the segmental mobility available.

instability. If there is a history of trauma and joint instability or hypermobility or if either is clinically suspected or needs to be ruled out, lateral flexion and extension *stress* films should be obtained. These two films are then evaluated to identify joint hypermobility revealed by misalignment (excessive angulation or excessive glide) of the injured segment. Misalignment is judged by referencing the anatomic spatial relationship of the lines described on the routine neutral lateral film (Fig. 4–35).

Hyperextension sprains result from forcing the neck past the extreme end ranges of extension. Hyperextension injuries may happen in a rebound action of the head and neck following hyperflexion, or in isolation. Disruption of the anterior ligaments and soft tissues may cause a transient posterior subluxation of the vertebral segment. Lateral flexion and extension stress

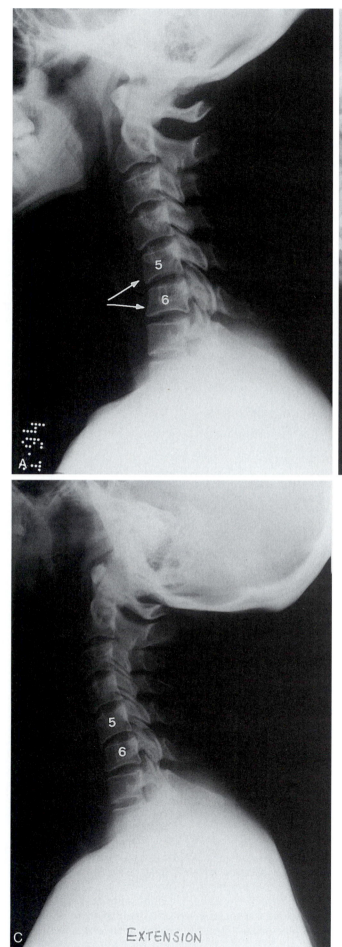

FIGURE 4–35. Cervical sprain. This 22-year-old female sustained a hyperflexion-hyperextension sprain to her cervical spine while driving in a demolition derby contest. (*A*) Plain film, lateral view shows a loss of cervical lordosis and hyperkyphotic angulation at C5–6. (*B*) Lateral flexion film shows slight anterior displacement of C5 on C6 (arrow) and widening of the C5-6 interspinous space. (*C*) Extension film shows reluctance or inability of patient to hyperextend the neck and a persistent hyperkyphotic angulation of the C5–6 segment. These findings suggest ligamentous disruption at the C5–6 segment.

views are obtained to evaluate joint stability. Increased magnitude of the extension force can cause compressive injuries to the spine. Compression during hyperextension is due to the parallel pull of the neck flexor muscles on the spine while the vertebrae are already in bony approximation.

Acute Intervertebral Disc Herniations[56]

Acute disc herniation in a posterolateral direction causing nerve root compression is uncommon in the cervical spine, owing to inherent anatomic protection. The anteriorly positioned nucleus pulposus, posteriorly reinforced annulus fibrosus, wide and double-layered posterior longitudinal ligament, and uncovertebral joints offer security to the discs lacking in the more commonly herniated lumbar intervertebral discs. Traumatic injury to the cervical spine may, however, cause a posterior or lateral disc herniation that results in neural compression. Plain film radiographs are of little diagnostic value in the diagnosis of cervical disc herniation. Myelography, computed tomography (CT)-myelography, and magnetic resonance imaging (MRI) are used, often in combination, to assist in determining treatment protocols or necessity for surgery (Fig. 4–36).

CERVICAL SPINE JOINT DISEASES[57-59]

Degenerative Disc Disease

Evidence of *degenerative disc disease* is seen radiographically in most persons over age 60.[58] Degenerative changes in the disc may include dehydration, nuclear herniation, annular protrusion, and fibrous replacement of the annulus. The different degenerative changes within the disc all cause a decrease in disc height. As the intervertebral space decreases, the vertebral endplates approximate. Uncinate processes approximate with the superadjacent vertebrae, forming uncovertebral joints. Excessive friction at these joints leads to osteophyte formation at this site and eventually around the entire osseous margin of the endplates.

The radiographic indication of degenerative disc disease is seen in the decreased height of the disc spaces on the lateral view[60] (Fig. 4–37).

Spondylosis/Foraminal Encroachment

Cervical spine spondylosis is the formation of osteophytes in response to degenerative disc disease. Os-

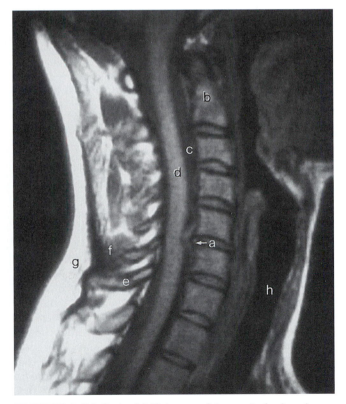

FIGURE 4–36. Sagittal MR image of the cervical spine. A posterior intervertebral disk herniation is present at C5–6 (a). Other structures are dense (b), cerebrospinal fluid (c), spinal cord (d), spinus process of C6 (e), muscle (f), skin, and fat (g), and trachia (h).

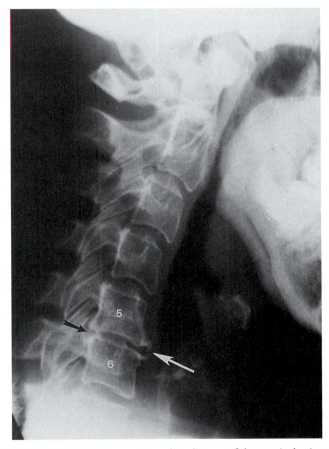

FIGURE 4–37. Degenerative disc disease of the cervical spine. On this lateral view decreased disc space is evident at C5–6. Note the osteophyte formation both anteriorly (white arrow) and posteriorly (black arrow).

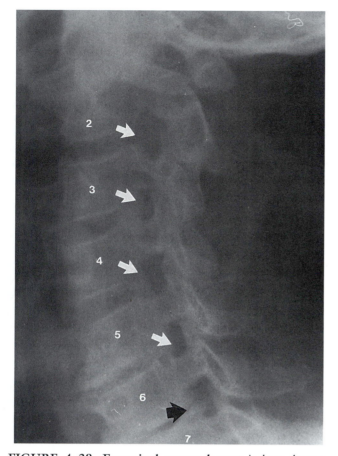

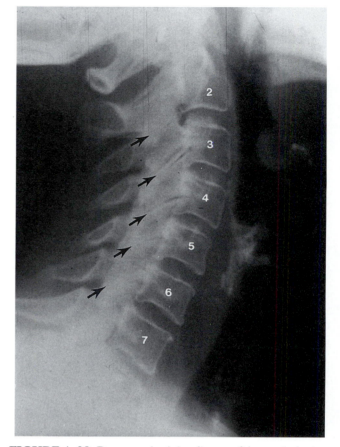

FIGURE 4–38. **Foraminal encroachment** is best demonstrated on the oblique view of the cervical spine. Arrows indicate the foramina. Note the foramen of C2–3 not constricted by any osteophyte (spur) formation. The remaining foramina show varying amounts of encroachment. The most severely compromised level is C6–7 (black arrows). Note the large osteophytes projecting from the posterior bodies of these two vertebrae.

FIGURE 4–39. Degenerative joint disease of the cervical spine. On this lateral view of the cervical spine the black arrows indicate the facet joint spaces. Note the narrowing of the joint spaces and sclerosis of the articular surfaces at all levels. Note also that the disc spaces at all levels are well preserved and without degenerative changes. This is true degenerative joint disease of the cervical spine; that is, the facet joints show the clasic hallmarks of osteoarthritis.

teophyte formation has been shown to be most predominant at the points in the curvatures of the spine farthest from the center line of gravity, or at the apices of the concavities, as a result of greater segmental mobility. In the cervical spine these sites are at C4–C5 and C5–C6. Osteophyte formation may be the body's attempt to repair friction damage or to protect from friction damage, but osteophytes can become a source of friction themselves. Osteophyte protrusion into the intervertebral foramina will narrow the passageway of the spinal nerves, causing potential for neural deficits. This *foraminal encroachment* is best seen on the oblique radiograph (Fig. 4–38).

Degenerative Joint Disease

Degenerative joint disease (DJD) of the cervical spine refers to osteoarthritic changes of the facet joints.[62] The facet joints are vulnerable to DJD because of the great mobility of the cervical spine, postural strains, and re-

petitive occupational or recreational actions that contribute to the abnormal tissue and joint biomechanics and biochemistry. Like degenerative joint disease elsewhere in the body, facet joints undergo articular cartilage thinning, subchondral bone sclerosis, and development of osteophytes at joint margins. Significant in facet DJD, however, is the susceptibility of the intervertebral foramina to encroachment from osteophytes at the facet joint margins. Facet DJD is observed on either the lateral view or oblique view (Fig. 4–39).

Cervical DJD may develop in isolation or concomitantly with degenerative disc disease and cervical spondylosis. Indeed, one process often predisposes or accelerates the joint's development of the other process. Significant for the clinician to appreciate is that these processes are slow and the body has time to adapt. However, the body may at some time reach limits in its ability to adapt. At this point the cervical spine may become symptomatic to even minor trauma. The normal spine has a margin of safety in its elastic capsules, resilient and flexible ligaments, hydrated and cushioning discs and cartilage, and wide open foram-

TABLE 4–3 Cervical Anomalies

Anomaly	Clinical Considerations	Radiographic Features	Appearance
Atlas			
Occipitalization of C1	No motion possible at AO joint. Excessive compensatory motion at subjacent joints with resultant degenerative joint changes.	Lateral film: see decreased or absent space between occiput and posterior arch.	
Agenesis of posterior arch of C1	Transverse ligament integrity may be compromised; possible AA instability.	Lateral film: absent posterior neural arch, enlarged anterior arch (from stress), enlarged C2 spinous process representing fusion of rudimentary post. arch with sp. p.	
Absence of transverse ligament	AA joint instability; possible cord compression.	Lateral flexion film: required to determine AA stability.	
Axis			
Dens anomalies: Ossiculum terminale—failure of tip of dens to unite	Usually no clinical significance.	View dens anomalies on AP open-mouth films: cephalic portion of dens separate from peg, bounded by smooth osseous margins.	
Os odontoideum—failure of dens to unite with body of C2	Possible AA joint instability. Associated with Klippel-Feil and Morquio syndromes; present in 20% of Down's syndrome cases.	Dens separated from body by a radiolucent cleft. Lateral flexion film required to determine AA joint stability.	
Hypoplastic dens— abbreviated development	Possible AA instability.	Small, malformed dens. Lateral flexion film required to determine AA stability.	
Cervical vertebrae			
Block vertebrae—two adjacent vertebrae fused at birth. Partial or complete fusion of bodies, facets, spinous processes	No motion at fused segment. Excessive compensatory motion at adjacent free joints with resultant degenerative changes. Most common at C5–6, C2–3; associated with Klippel-Feil syndrome.	Lateral film: Small AP diameter of bodies with indented "wasp-waist" fused intervertebral disc space. Facets fused in 50% of cases. Spinous processes may be fused or malformed.	
Sprengel's deformity— congenital elevation of scapula	Present in 25% of Klippel-Feil syndrome cases; frequently associated with scoliosis, block vertebrae, spina bifida occulta, hemivertebrae, and cervical ribs.	AP film: 30–40% of cases have an omovertebral bone appearing as a bony bar projecting from the lamina of C7 to the vertebral border of the scapula.	

TABLE 4–3 Cervical Anomalies *continued*

Anomaly	Clinical Considerations	Radiographic Features	Appearance
Axis			
Cervical ribs—extra bone projecting from and sometimes forming a joint with transverse process	Possible source of compression in thoracic outlet syndrome. Most common at C7, less often present at C6 and C5; often bilateral but usually asymmetric in size and shape.	AP film: rib projecting caudally from cervical transverse process. (Thoracic ribs project cephalicly.) Joint may be formed at distal end of rib. When no joint is formed distally, there is sometimes a fibrous band anchoring the distal rib. A fibrous band would not appear on radiograph but could contribute to compression of the NV bundle.	
Spina bifida occulta—failure of laminae to unite and form a spinous process	Usually no clinical significance.	AP film: see a vertically oriented radiolucent cleft between the laminae. The spinous process will be absent or malformed at the involved level.	

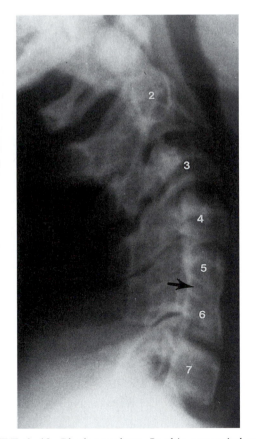

FIGURE 4–40. Block vertebrae. In this congenital anomaly the vertebrae of C5 and C6 have fused into a single unit. Note the lack of a disc space at C5–6 because of failure of segmentation (arrow), and also the fusion of the posterior elements into a single spinous process.

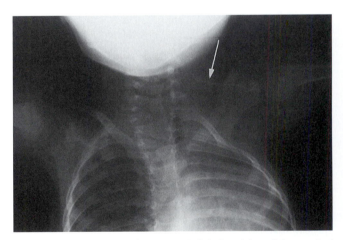

FIGURE 4–41. Multiple congenital deformities of the cervical spine and scapula in a 3-year-old boy. The left scapula is elevated (arrow points to the spine of the scapula). This condition is commonly known as Sprengel's deformity. The etiology is a failure of the scapula to descend to normal position from its high level in the early weeks of gestation. The cause of this failure is unknown. It is usually associated with other deformities as seen here. A group of deformities in the cervical spine, commonly known as Klippel-Feil syndrome is present. Note failure of the laminae to unite at midline at some levels, and synostosis of much of the lower cervical spine into one bony mass. There is an omovertebral bar connecting the scapula to the cervical spine.

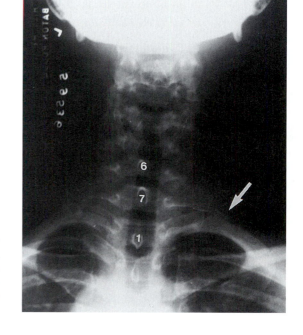

FIGURE 4–42. Cervical rib at C7. This congenital anomaly occurs most commonly at the seventh cervical vertebra. Cervical ribs are usually bilateral and when this is the case, one rib is always higher and presents a more advanced stage of development than the other as seen here. The left rib is larger and has formed an articulation with the first thoracic rib (arrow).

ina. The degenerative spine, in contrast, has lost its margin of safety and, in trauma, suffers greater dysfunction and requires longer time to heal. A review of the acute patient's radiographs, with special observation of the underlying chronic degenerative changes, is necessary to understand the patient's pain pattern and assist in developing a comprehensive treatment plan.

CERVICAL SPINE ANOMALIES[63]

Congenital or developmental anomalies of the spine appear with frequency at the transitional segments or junctions of the curvatures. The atlanto-occipital region and the lumbosacral region are common sites of anomalies. Spinal anomalies are related to a structure's (1) failure to develop, (2) arrested development, (3) de-

velopment of accessory bones, or (4) asymmetric structural development. Spinal anomalies may occur in isolation or in combination with other spinal, visceral, and soft tissue malformations.

Clinically significant in cervical spine anomalies, especially in the upper cervical region, is the potential for joint instability. Mobilization, manipulation, manual resistance, or traction applied without prior knowledge of the anomaly may result in neurologic deficit, paralysis, or even death. Although spinal anomalies are present in only a small portion of the general population, the potential devastating effects of mishandling these patients warrants the clinician's attention to any spinal structural variant.

Examples of cervical anomalies, their clinical significance, radiographic features, and appearance are presented in Table 4–3. See Figures 4–40, 4–41, 4–42, and 5–47 for film examples.

SUMMARY OF KEY POINTS

1. The routine radiographic evaluation of the cervical spine includes five projections:
   a. Anteroposterior open mouth—demonstrates the atlantoaxial or C1–C2 joint.
   b. Anteroposterior lower cervical spine—demonstrates the five lower cervical vertebrae.
   c. Lateral—demonstrates the normal alignment of all seven cervical vertebrae.
   d. Right and left obliques—demonstrate the intervertebral foramina.
2. On the lateral projection, three approximately parallel line images are constructed at (a) the borders of the anterior vertebral bodies, (b) the borders of the posterior vertebral bodies, and (c) the junctions of the laminae to the spinous processes (spinolaminar line). Discontinuity in the spatial relationships of these lines may indicate fracture or dislocation.
3. In evaluation of cervical trauma, the lateral projection is the first radiograph filmed and evaluated. Radiographic indicators of trauma include abnormal soft tissue images, abnormal vertebral alignment, and abnormal joint relationships.

4. Injuries to the cervical spine are broadly classified as stable or unstable injuries. Unstable injuries such as fracture-dislocations threaten the integrity of the spinal cord and are the most serious and life-threatening injuries in the cervical spine.
5. Cervical sprains are injuries to the ligaments of the spine. Hyperflexion sprains injure the posterior ligament complex and related soft tissues; hyperextension sprains injure the anterior ligaments and related soft tissues. The degree of severity of a sprain may range from minimal soft tissue involvement to ligamentous tearing with possible transient joint subluxations and compression fracture.
6. Acute disc herniations are not diagnosed by plain film radiography and require ancillary techniques such as myelography or MRI for diagnosis.
7. In most people over age 60 DJD disease is seen radiographically. Radiographic signs include decreased disc space height, formation of uncovertebral joints, and osteophyte formation at the margins of the vertebral body endplates.
8. Cervical spondylosis is the formation of osteophytes in response to degenerative joint disease.
9. Foraminal encroachment refers to the protrusion of osteophytes into the intervertebral foramina, narrowing the passageway of the exiting spinal nerve.
10. Degenerative joint disease of the cervical spine refers to osteoarthritic changes at the facet joints. Radiographic hallmarks of DJD are decreased joint spaces, sclerotic subchondral bone, and osteophyte formation at joint margins. Cervical spine DJD may develop in isolation or concomitantly with degenerative disc disease and cervical spondylosis.

REFERENCES

1. Netter, FH: The Ciba Collection of Medical Illustrations, Vol 8, Part I, Musculoskeletal System. Ciba-Geigy Corp, Summit, NJ, 1978, pp 9–13.
1a. Yochum, TR and Rowe, LJ: Essentials of Skeletal Radiology. Williams & Wilkins, Baltimore, 1987, p 438.
2. Netter, pp 9–13.
3. Nordin, M and Frankel, VH: Basic Biomechanics of the Musculoskeletal System, ed 2. Lea & Febiger, Malvern, PA, 1989, p 215.
4. Gehweiler, JA, Osborne, RL, and Becker, RF: The Radiology of Vertebral Trauma. WB Saunders, Philadelphia, 1980, p 54.
5. Meschan, I: An Atlas of Normal Radiographic Anatomy. WB Saunders, Philadelphia, 1960, p 396.
6. Netter, p 128–129.
7. Nordin, p 211.
8. Netter, p 136.
9. Gehweiler, p 41.
10. Yochum, pp 441–442.
11. Bontrager, KL: Textbook of Radiographic Positioning and Related Anatomy, ed 3. Mosby, St. Louis, 1993, pp 13–16.
12. Chew, FS: Skeletal Radiology: The Bare Bones. Aspen Publications, Rockville, MD, 1989, pp 64–67.
13. Fischer, HW: Radiographic Anatomy: A Working Atlas. McGraw-Hill, New York, 1988, pp 78–79.
14. Greenspan, A: Orthopedic Radiology: A Practical Approach, ed 2. Raven Press, New York, 1992, pp 10.27–10.53.
15. Harris, JH and Edeiken-Monroe, B: Radiology of Acute Cervical Spine Trauma. Williams & Wilkins, Baltimore, 1987.
16. Helms, CA: Fundamentals of Skeletal Radiology. WB Saunders, Philadelphia, 1989.
17. Krell, L (ed): Clark's Positioning in Radiology, Vol 1, ed 10. Yearbook Medical Publishers, Chicago, 1989, pp 190–194.
18. Meschan, pp 409–415.
19. Weir, J and Abrahams, P: An Atlas of Radiological Anatomy. Yearbook Medical Publishers, Chicago, 1978, p 93.
20. Wicke, L: Atlas of Radiologic Anatomy, ed 5. Lea & Febiger, Malvern, PA, 1994, p 262.
21. Yochum, pp 13–16, 179, 216, 290.
22. Ibid, p 21.
23. Greenspan, p 10.5.
24. Helms, p 92.
25. Yochum, p 21.
26. Greenspan, pp 10.2–10.3.
27. Helms, p 93.
28. Krell, p 279.
29. Berquist, TH: Imaging of Orthopedic Trauma, ed 2. Raven Press, New York, 1989, pp 104–115.
30. Gehweiler, pp 100–101.

31. Greenspan, pp 4.1–4.32.
32. Harris, p 212.
33. McCort, JJ and Mindelzun, RE: Trauma Radiology. Churchill Livingstone, New York, 1990, p 66.
34. Rockwood, CA and Green, DP (eds): Fractures in Adults, Vol 2, ed 2. JB Lippincott, Philadelphia, 1984, pp 987–1005.
35. Yochum, p 533.
36. Ibid, p 441.
37. Ibid, p 429.
38. Ibid.
39. Greenspan, p 10.1.
40. Harris, p 65.
41. Yochum, p 110.
42. McCort, p 42.
43. Rockwood, pp 987–1005.
44. Greenspan, pp 10.1–10.26.
45. Yochum, p 430.
46. Ibid, p 432.
47. Greenspan, pp 10.20–10.22.
48. Yochum, pp 430–433.
49. Rockwood, 987–1005.
50. Greenspan, pp 10.15–10.27.
51. Rockwood, pp 987–1005.
52. Yochum, pp 430–433.
53. Cailliet, pp 65–85.
54. Gehweiler, pp 215–239.
55. Harris, p 67.
56. Yochum, pp 293–294.
57. Ibid, pp 550–553.
58. Salter, RB: Textbook of Disorders and Injuries of the Musculoskeletal System, ed 2. Williams & Wilkins, Baltimore, 1983, p 227.
59. Brashear, HR and Raney, RB: Shand's Handbook of Orthopaedic Surgery, ed 9. CV Mosby, St Louis, 1978, p 340.
60. Yochum, pp 550–553.
61. Ibid, p 308.
62. Ibid, p 551.
63. Ibid, p 112.

SELF-TEST

Chapter 4

Films A and B belong to the same patient; films C and D belong to another patient.

1. Identify which films are <u>lateral</u> projections and which films are <u>oblique</u> projections.
2. What <u>anatomic feature</u> of the cervical spine is best demonstrated on the oblique projection?
3. Identify the <u>intervertebral disc spaces</u>. Which patient, A/B or C/D, exhibits a greater degree of <u>degenerative disc disease</u>?
4. Identify the <u>apophyseal (facet) joint spaces</u>. Which patient exhibits a greater degree of <u>degenerative joint disease</u>?
5. Regarding patient A/B, what specific <u>intervertebral segments</u> exhibit <u>narrowed disc spaces</u> and <u>spur formation</u> at the margins of the vertebral bodies?
6. Regarding patient C/D, what <u>nerve root</u> is likely to be compromised by <u>foraminal encroachment</u>?
7. Considering the degenerative changes in the joints, which patient probably has the greater degree of <u>restricted range of motion</u> in the cervical spine?

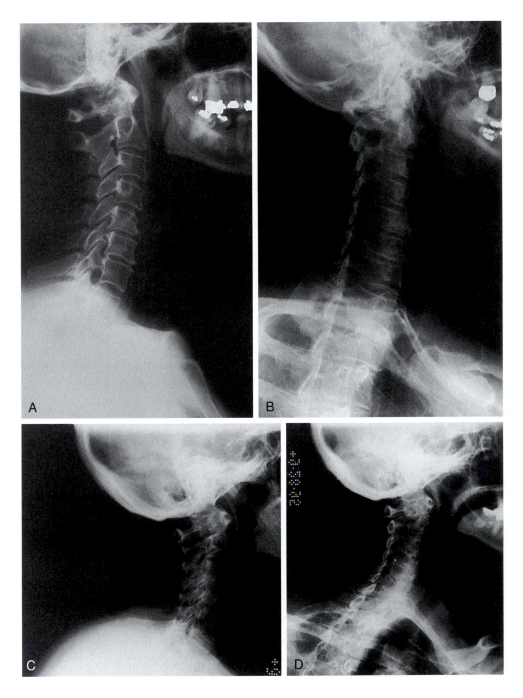

Thoracic Spine, Sternum, and Ribs

The length of the thoracic spine and its different regional vertebral characteristics result in a variety of developmental and postural deformities, fracture types, and joint dysfunctions to occur. The transitional cervicothoracic and thoracolumbar regions are prone to specific mechanical problems as these areas represent the junctions between the flexible cervical and lumbar spines with the relatively more inflexible thoracic spine.[1]

Radiographically, almost all features of the thoracic spine are accountable on the anteroposterior (AP) and lateral views. The sternum and ribs are not included in a routine thoracic evaluation and are radiographed as separate evaluations. They are included in this chapter for comprehensiveness owing to their associated articulations and sometimes associated involvement in injury, disease, and developmental processes.

The goals of this chapter are first to provide a review of osseous radiographic anatomy. A brief review of ligamentous anatomy and thoracic spine mobility is presented to assist the reader in understanding the mechanics of common injury patterns in this region. The routine radiographic evaluation of the thoracic spine follows. Here the reader has an opportunity to interact and learn radiographic anatomy by tracing a radiograph with a marker on a transparency sheet, and then comparing it with the radiographic tracing. The routine evaluations of the ribs and sternum are also pictured. Additional goals are to present the radiographic findings of common fractures of this region, the radiographic findings of osteoporosis as manifested in this region, and the radiographic evaluation of scoliosis. The summary is organized into a list of practical points highlighting the clinical aspects of this chapter. A self-test at the end of the chapter challenges the reader's visual interpretation skills.

RADIOGRAPHIC ANATOMY

Osseous Anatomy[2,3]

The bones of the *thorax* include the *12 thoracic vertebrae*, 24 ribs, and the *sternum*. The thorax forms a protective cage to house the heart, lungs, and upper abdominal viscera. The articulations of the thorax allow for flexibility to accommodate the actions of respiration and trunk mobility. Additionally, the thorax provides stability for neck and upper extremity movements.

Thoracic vertebrae are positioned in a curve convex posteriorly approximately 20 to 40 degrees (Fig. 5–1). Mild lateral curves are commonly noted and believed to be related to hand dominance. The upper thoracic vertebrae, T1–T4, exhibit some of the characteristics of cervical vertebrae, while the lower thoracic vertebrae, T9–T12, exhibit some of the characteristics of lumbar vertebrae. These *transitional vertebrae* are often referred to as components of the *cervicothoracic* and *thoracolumbar regions*, respectively. Considered typical thoracic vertebrae are T5–T8.[2]

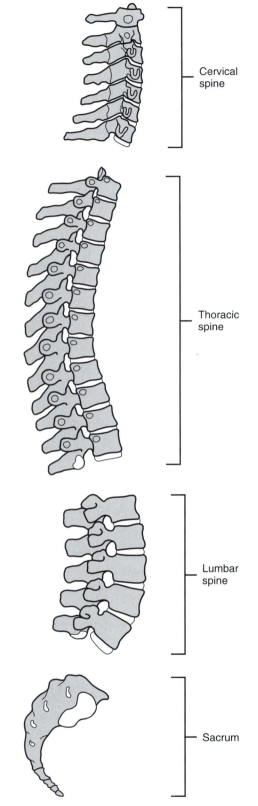

FIGURE 5–1. Divisions of the spinal column.

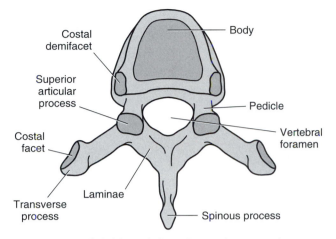

FIGURE 5–2. Typical thoracic vertebrae, top view.

Thoracic vertebrae have heart-shaped *vertebral bodies*; paired *superior and inferior costal demifacets* on the posterolateral surfaces of the bodies; round *vertebral foramina*; stout *pedicles*; short, thick *laminae* that partially overlap adjacent laminae in a shingle effect; long and downwardly inclined *spinous processes*; and long and posterolaterally inclined *transverse processes* with *costal facets* at the tips (Figs. 5–2, 5–3). The paired *superior and inferior articular processes* form *facet* or *zygapophyseal joints* with adjacent vertebrae. Typical thoracic facet joints are oriented vertically in the frontal plane, although the upper thoracic facets gradually orient to the angled frontal cervical facet plane and the lower thoracic facets gradually orient to a sagittal lumbar facet plane. Twelve pairs of *spinal nerves* exit the *intervertebral foramina* formed by co-adjacent pedicles.

Ribs are semicircular flat bones that are continuous anteriorly with hyaline costal cartilage (Fig. 5–4). Anteriorly the first rib attaches to the *sternal manubrium*, the second rib to the sternal angle, the third through sixth ribs to the *sternal body*, and the remaining ribs attach in turn to each other, forming the *costal margin*. The exceptions are the 11th and 12th ribs, the "float-

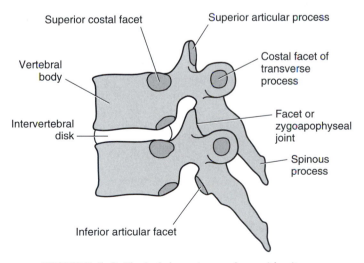

FIGURE 5–3. Typical thoracic vertebrae, side view.

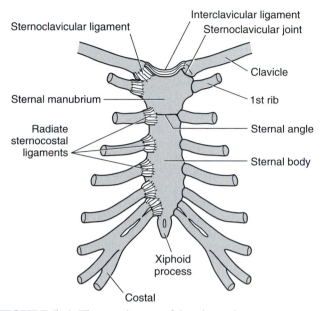

FIGURE 5–4. The attachment of the ribs to the sternum comprises the anterior portion of the thoracic cage.

ing" ribs, which are unattached anteriorly. Posteriorly the ribs attach to the thoracic spine via the synovial *costovertebral joints*. Each rib head forms a *costocentral joint* with two adjacent vertebral bodies and the interposed *intervertebral disc*. Each rib tubercle forms a *costotransverse joint* with a transverse process. The exceptions are the first rib, which forms a costocentral joint with only one vertebral body, and the 11th and 12th ribs, which also form costocentral joints with only one vertebral body and do not articulate with the transverse processes.

The sternum consists of a body joined superiorly via the sternal angle to the manubrium and joined inferiorly to the *xiphoid process*. These joints allow some movement to occur in the sternum but will generally

fuse into a rigid unit after middle age. Note the clavicle articulates to the manubrium just superior to the first rib, forming the sternoclavicular joint.

Ligamentous Anatomy

The thoracic spine is supported anteriorly by the *anterior longitudinal ligament* attaching to the anterior margins of the vertebral bodies and intervertebral discs, increasing in width as it extends downwardly from atlas to the sacrum. Posteriorly the thoracic spine is supported by (1) the *posterior longitudinal ligament*, attaching to the posterior margins of the vertebral bodies and intervertebral discs and decreasing in width as it descends from axis to the sacrum; (2) the *ligamenta flava*, joining adjacent laminae; (3) the *supraspinous* and *interspinous ligaments*, joining adjacent spinous processes; (4) the *intertransverse ligaments*, joining adjacent transverse processes; and (5) the *articular capsules*, supporting the facet joints. Together these ligaments are referred to as the *posterior ligament complex* (Fig. 5–5).

The costocentral joints of the ribs are supported by (1) the *articular capsules*; (2) the *intra-articular ligaments* blending with the fibers of the intervertebral disc; and (3) the *radiate or stellate ligaments* extending from the rib heads to the vertebral bodies and interposed discs. The costotransverse joints are supported by (1) the *articular capsules*; (2) the *middle costotransverse ligaments*, attaching the rib necks to the transverse processes; (3) the *superior costotransverse ligaments*, attaching the rib necks to the transverse processes of the vertebrae above; and (4) the *lateral costotransverse ligaments*, extending from the tips of the transverse processes to the nonarticular portion of the rib tubercle (Figs. 5–6, 5–7). Anteriorly the ribs are joined to the sternum via radiate *sternocostal ligaments*.

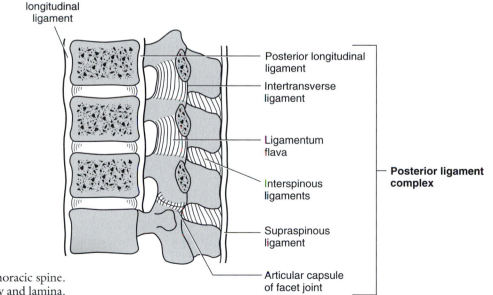

FIGURE 5–5. Ligaments of the thoracic spine. Cutaway through the vertebral body and lamina.

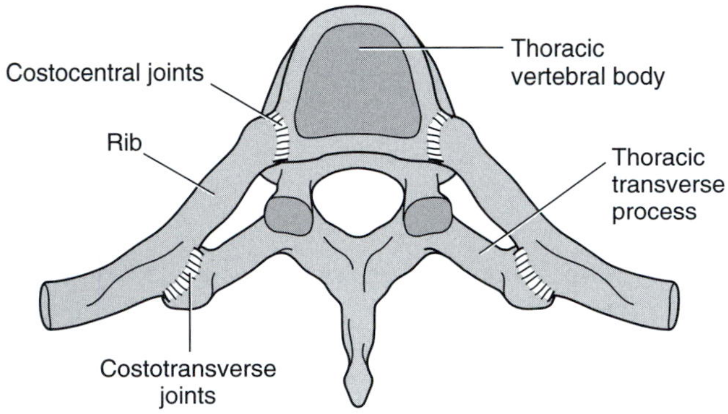

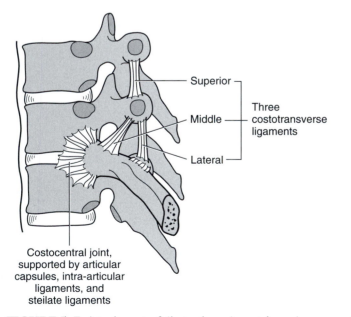

FIGURE 5–6. Attachment of ribs to thoracic vertebra via costocentral and costotransverse joints, top view.

JOINT MOBILITY[4]

The functional mobility of the thoracic vertebral segments allows for flexion, extension, lateral flexion, and rotation of the trunk to occur. The associated articulations of the bony thorax additionally play a role in orienting and restricting trunk motion. Thus the thoracic spine, rib cage, and sternum are considered as a unit during movement, as these related articulations not only limit each other but adapt in response to movement produced by each other.

Trunk flexion, extension, and lateral flexion each incur approximately 20 to 45 degrees of motion in the thoracic spine. Trunk rotation incurs approximately 35 to 50 degrees of rotation within the thoracic spine. The elasticity of the ribs and their articulations allows for adaptive increases or decreases in the intercostal spaces and the costovertebral, sternocostal, and chondrocostal angles as the spine moves.

GROWTH AND DEVELOPMENT[5–8]

Ossification of the thoracic vertebrae begins in the sixth week of fetal life. At birth the bodies of the vertebrae are ossified and at least three ossification centers are present at each vertebral level to continue development of the body and posterior structures (see radiograph of newborn skeleton in Figure 6–7). Fusion of the neural arches to the spinous processes occurs by age 2 or 3, and these posterior elements fuse to the vertebral body by ages 3 to 6. At puberty secondary centers of ossification appear at the vertebral endplates and the spinous, transverse, and articular processes. These structures complete ossification by age 25.

At birth the shape of the thoracic and lumbar bodies is rounded. Radiographically the superior and inferior aspects of the vertebral bodies show dense calcification, appearing as clearly defined white margins with relatively darker, more radiolucent bodies. Occasionally the opposite will be seen, and the centrum of the bodies will appear densely calcified, causing a ''bone-within-bone'' radiographic image. The middle anterior aspects of the vertebral bodies will also show indentations, which are grooves for vertebral veins (Fig. 5–8). Single or double grooves may also be seen on the posterior aspects of the vertebral bodies, and these may persist into adulthood.

At approximately age 6, *vertebral ring apophyses* appear on the anterolateral superior and inferior surfaces of the mid and lower thoracic and upper lumbar vertebrae (Fig. 5–9). Less often the cervical and upper thoracic vertebrae share in this development. Radiographically these apophyses will appear as thin rims of bone slightly separated from the vertebral body. Ossification of the apophyses to the bodies is most pronounced at age 13, and fusion is usually complete by age 18. These apophyses are outside of the true epiphyseal plates and do not contribute to vertebral growth.

FIGURE 5–7. Attachment of ribs to thoracic vertebrae via costocentral and costotransverse joints, side view.

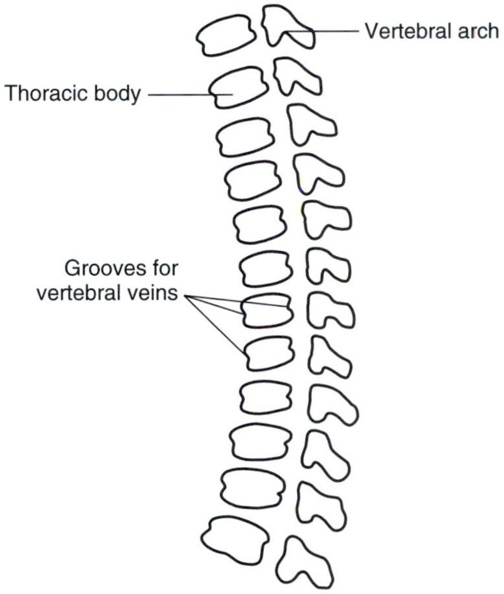

FIGURE 5–8. Radiographic appearance of ossified structures in the newborn thoracic spine.

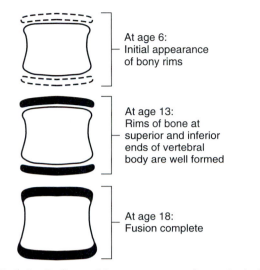

At age 6:
Initial appearance
of bony rims

At age 13:
Rims of bone at
superior and inferior
ends of vertebral
body are well formed

At age 18:
Fusion complete

FIGURE 5–9. Radiographic appearance of vertebral ring apophyses.

The significance of these structures is that they represent a radiographic indicator of skeletal *bone age* or *physiologic age*. Determination of the time frame available to effectively brace and correct a scoliotic curve, for example, is largely predicated on this reliable sign of skeletal maturity.[8a]

The normal *thoracic kyphosis* increases with postural maturity from approximately 20 degrees in childhood to approximately 30 to 40 degrees in adulthood. Females tend to show increased kyphosis with maturity. Excessive kyphosis can result from numerous and highly variable conditions such as the degenerative changes associated with osteoporosis, genetic predisposition, postural habits, congenital anomalies, paralysis, tuberculosis, arthritis, ankylosing spondylitis, vertebral epiphysitis (Scheuermann's disease), Paget's disease, osteomalacia, or rickets.[8–10]

Ossification of the sternum and ribs begins in the eighth to ninth week of fetal life. At birth the sternum is largely cartilaginous with vertically positioned ossification centers at each sternebra. Fusion of the sternebrae takes place after puberty. At birth the xiphoid process is cartilaginous, and its ossification center does not appear until 3 years of age. The xiphoid process remains cartilaginous into young adulthood. The chondrocostal extensions of the ribs gradually undergo ossification throughout late adulthood, progressively limiting flexibility of the rib cage and in turn limiting flexibility of the thoracic spine.

ROUTINE RADIOGRAPHIC EVALUATION

Thoracic Spine[11–17]

Basic: Anteroposterior
Lateral
Optional: Oblique

The routine radiologic evaluation of the thoracic spine includes an anteroposterior and a lateral projection. Most structures of the thoracic vertebrae are well-demonstrated on these two views. The oblique view is not common in the basic evaluation and is considered an optional view, done for additional visualization of the facet joint articulations.

ANTEROPOSTERIOR (FIGS. 5–10, 5–11, 5–12)

This view demonstrates the thoracic vertebral bodies; the intervertebral disc spaces; alignment of the pedicles, spinous processes, transverse processes, and articular processes; and the costovertebral joints and posterior ribs. See the schematic illustration Figure 5–13 to assist in visualizing these structures on the radiograph. The important observations are:

1. The alignment of the vertebral bodies forms a vertical column with well-preserved intervertebral disc spaces noted.
2. Rotation present in the thoracic column is identified by the rotation of the pedicles toward midline. Note slight rotation in the lower thoracic bodies.
3. The pedicles are spaced equidistantly from the midline spinous processes. Misalignment in the relationship of these structures may be an indication of fracture-dislocation. Remember that the distance between a pair of pedicles represents the transverse diameter of the spinal canal. Compromise of this space is a threat to the spinal cord.
4. Intervals between each spinous process and, similarly, between each paired set of laminae, are compared for consistency. An increased interval at one level may indicate a torn posterior ligament complex.
5. The articular processes cast a butterfly-like shadow over the vertebral body. While the plane of the facet joints is not visible, the alignment of the articular processes is evident. Misalignment is an indication of fracture-dislocation or subluxation.
6. The costocentral and costotransverse joints are cor-

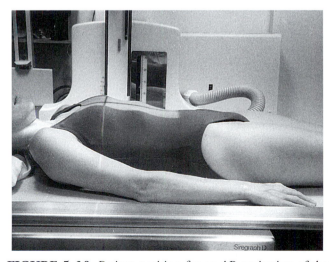

FIGURE 5–10. Patient position for an AP projection of the thoracic spine.

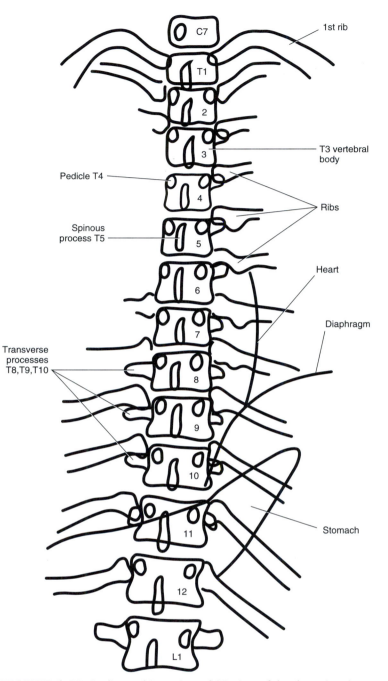

FIGURE 5–11. Radiographic tracing of AP view of the thoracic spine.

rectly articulated, and the ribs form smooth curving margins.

CLINICAL OBJECTIVES

1. Trace the thoracic vertebral bodies.
2. Trace the spinous processes.
3. Trace the pedicles.
4. Trace the transverse processes. Note the size distortion of the transverse processes of T8–T10 due to slight rotation of the bodies.
5. Trace the superior and inferior articular processes.
6. Trace the ribs and their vertebral articulations.

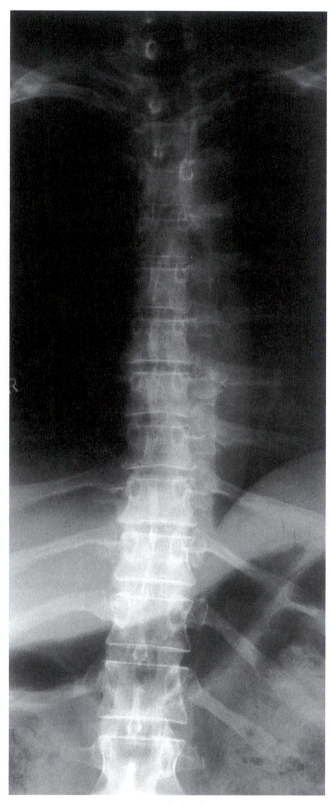

FIGURE 5–12.

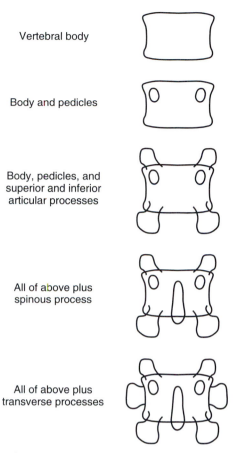

Vertebral body

Body and pedicles

Body, pedicles, and superior and inferior articular processes

All of above plus spinous process

All of above plus transverse processes

FIGURE 5–13. Schematic to distinguish vertebral structures on an AP radiograph. (Adapted from Squires, LF, and Novelline, RA: Fundamentals of Radiology, ed 4. Harvard University Press, Cambridge, MA, 1988, p 169.)

LATERAL (FIGS. 5–14, 5–15, 5–16)

This view demonstrates the thoracic vertebral bodies, intervertebral disc spaces, and intervertebral foramina. The uppermost two or three thoracic vertebrae are not well visualized because of superimposition of

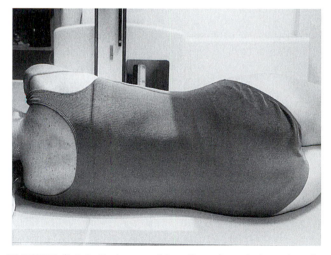

FIGURE 5–14. Patient position for a lateral thoracic spine projection.

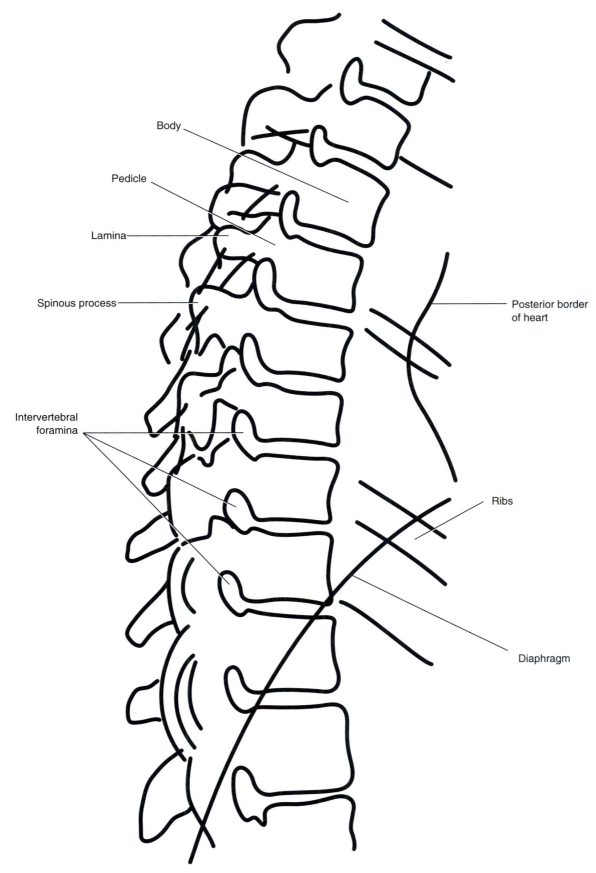

Body

Pedicle

Lamina

Spinous process

Posterior border
of heart

Intervertebral
foramina

Ribs

Diaphragm

FIGURE 5–15. Radiographic tracing of lateral view of the thoracic spine.

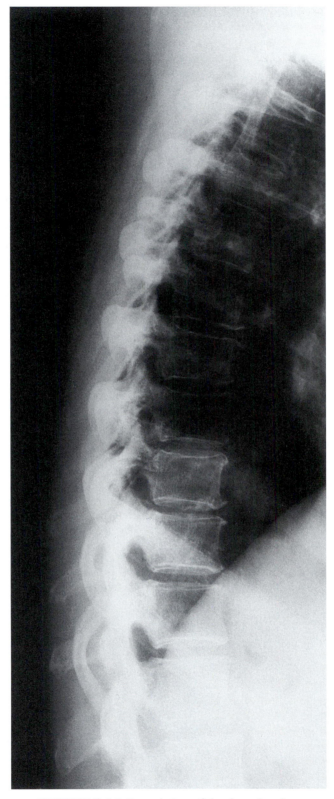

FIGURE 5–16. Lateral view of the thoracic spine.

the shoulder. If these vertebrae are of special interest, a *swimmer's lateral projection* is done with the arm positioned overhead to remove the obstruction of the shoulder. The important observations on the lateral view are:

1. As observed in the cervical spine, normal alignment of the thoracic vertebrae is similarly verified by identifying three roughly parallel lines (Fig. 5–17).

   Line 1: the *anterior vertebral body line*, representing the connected anterior borders of the vertebral bodies, forms a smooth, continuous curve.

   Line 2: the *posterior vertebral body line*, representing the connected posterior borders of the vertebral bodies, forms a continuous curve parallel to line 1.

   Line 3: the *spinolaminar line*, representing the junctions of the laminae at the spinous processes, forms a continuous curve parallel to lines 2 and 3. Because of overlapping laminae and long, downwardly inclined spinous processes, the spinolaminar line in the thoracic region exhibits a shingle effect.

   The spatial relationship of these three lines will normally remain constant during any amount of thoracic flexion or extension. Disruptions in these parallel lines may indicate fracture or dislocation. Remember that the spinal canal lies between lines 2 and 3, and compromise of this space seriously threatens the integrity of the spinal cord. In the presence of a fracture or dislocation, this space may show an increase or decrease in diameter, relative to adjacent levels.[18,19]

2. The vertebral bodies are boxlike in appearance with distinct, smoothly curved osseous margins.

3. The intervertebral foramina, through which the spinal nerves exit, are normally imaged as radiolucent ovals. Narrowed, ragged margins of the ovals indicate bony encroachment upon the spinal nerves or the spinal canal.

4. The intervertebral disc spaces normally exhibit well-preserved potential space. Note any osteo-

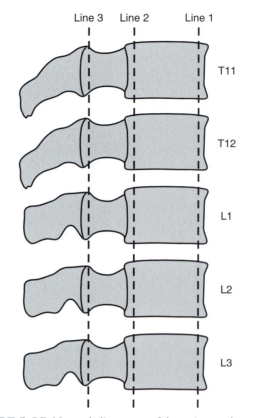

FIGURE 5–17. Normal alignment of thoracic vertebrae on the lateral view is verified by identifying three approximately parallel lines. Line 1 = anterior vertebral body line. Line 2 = posterior vertebral body line. Line 3 = spinolaminar line. This spatial relationship will normally hold true in any degree of flexion or extension.

phyte formation at the joint margins indicating degenerative changes.

5. The pedicles are superimposed as a pair at each level.

6. The axillary portions of the ribs overlay the thoracic spine but are easily projected through as they are less dense than the vertebrae. The posterior rib cage

is projected tangentially, and images as a dense border posterior to the vertebrae.

7. Facet joint articulations are partially seen at some levels.
8. The soft tissue density representing the diaphragm may be seen as a shadow superimposed over the lower thoracic vertebrae.

CLINICAL OBJECTIVES

1. Trace each **vertebral body**.
2. Trace the **pedicle, lamina**, and **spinous processes**.
3. Trace the **intervertebral foramina**.
4. Trace the **facet joints** that are visible.
5. Trace the **axillary portion of the ribs**.
6. Trace the **diaphragm**.

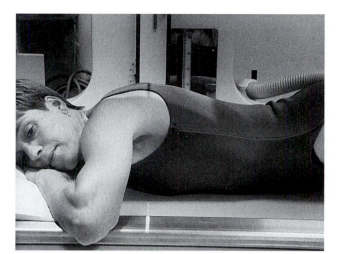

FIGURE 5–18. Patient position for RAO projection of the sternum.

Sternum[20] (Figs. 5–18 through 5–22)

Basic: Right Anterior Oblique (RAO)
Lateral

The sternum is almost impossible to see on an anteroposterior projection because of the superimposition of the denser thoracic spine. Therefore, a frontal view of the sternum is obtained by rotating the body just enough to bring the sternum out of the shadow of the spine. An RAO projection is most commonly used as this will project the sternum over the homogeneous density of the heart, allowing for contrast to delineate the image. Some distortion of the sternum occurs due to the obliquity of the projection.

The lateral view of the sternum is easily visualized as the sternum is the most anterior structure in the thorax and there is a minimum of overlying tissue.

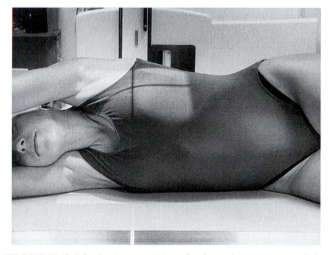

FIGURE 5–19. Patient position for lateral projection of the sternum.

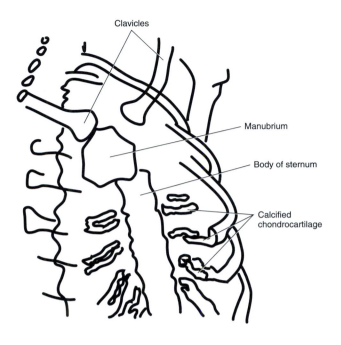

A

B

FIGURE 5–20. (A) Radiographic tracing of RAO view of the sternum. (B) Radiographic tracing of lateral view of the sternum.

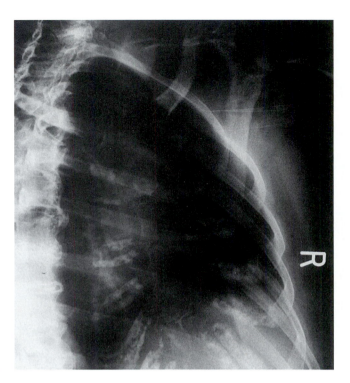

FIGURE 5–21. RAO view of sternum.

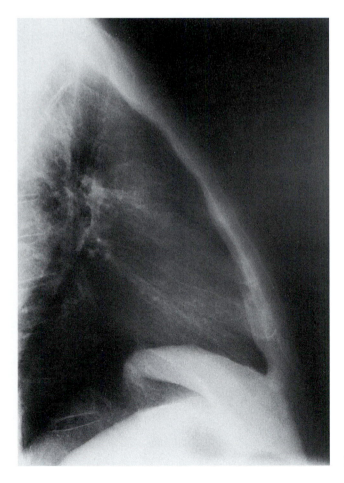

FIGURE 5–22. Lateral view of sternum.

Ribs[21] (Figs. 5–23 through 5–28)

Basic: Anteroposterior (AP) or Posteroanterior (PA)
Anterior Oblique (AO) or Posterior Oblique
(PO)
PA Chest Film

The great expanse of bone, multiplanar curves, and
superimposition of the muscular diaphragm necessitates the radiographic evaluation of the rib cage to be
done in sections. These sections include the anterior
ribs, the posterior ribs, and the axillary ribs. These sections of the ribs are again divided into the upper ribs,
which can be visualized above the density of the diaphragm, and the lower ribs, which can be imaged with
altered exposure below the level of the diaphragm. The
entire rib cage is not often radiographed in an evaluation. Rather the clinical history and symptoms define
a region of interest, and only those segments are
radiographed.

The AP projection provides an image of the posterior
ribs, which are closest to the film plate. An AP projection done above the level of the diaphragm images the
first through the eighth or ninth posterior ribs. The AP
projection done below the level of the diaphragm images the eighth through twelfth posterior ribs. Below-
diaphragm injuries are more frequently seen at the
posterior ribs.

The PA projection provides an image of the anterior
ribs, which are closest to the film plate. Above- or be-
low-diaphragm projections are defined like the AP.

The oblique projections provide an image of the axillary portions of the ribs. The axillary portions are divided into left or right sides of the body, and again
divided into anterolateral or posterolateral segments.
Similar to positioning in the spine, these obliques will
be identified as RAO, RPO, LAO, or LPO.

A PA chest film is often included in a trauma rib
series to rule out possible pneumothorax or hemotho-

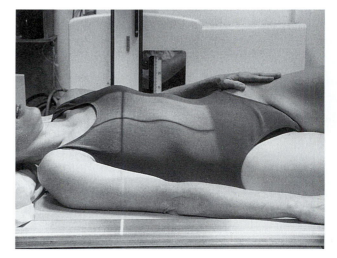

FIGURE 5–24. Patient position for PO projection of the right
posterolateral axillary ribs.

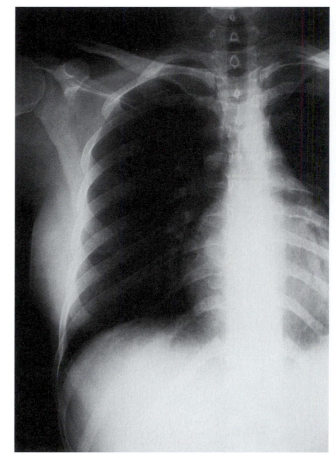

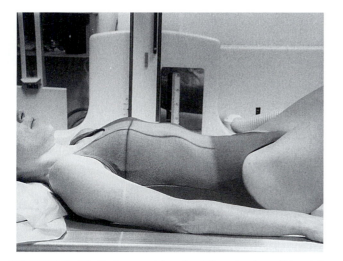

FIGURE 5–23. Patient position for AP projection of the right
posterior ribs.

FIGURE 5–25. AP view of the right posterior ribs, above
diaphragm.

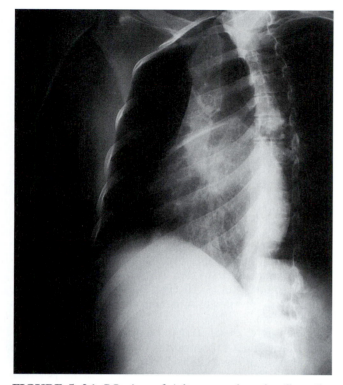

FIGURE 5–26. PO view of right posterolateral axillary ribs, above diaphragm.

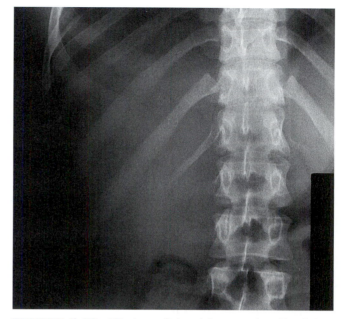

FIGURE 5–28. AP view of the right posterior ribs, below diaphragm.

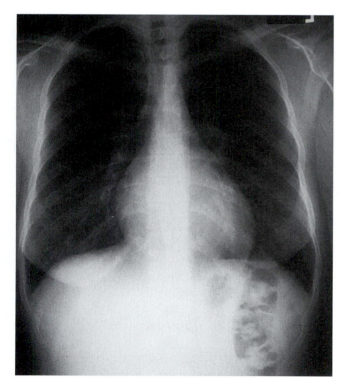

FIGURE 5–27. PA chest film radiograph. Compare with Figure 5–25 to note the altered exposure between radiographs. This radiograph was made specifically to visualize the lungs, heart, and great vessels.

rax. A PA chest film and PA rib film cover the same anatomic location of the thorax, but the radiographic exposure is different in each film. The PA chest film is made specifically to bring out the soft tissue and water densities of the lungs, heart, and great vessels.

THORACIC TRAUMA[22–24]

The thoracic spine is most commonly injured due to flexion forces. The vertebrae most commonly injured are the transitional vertebrae of the cervicothoracic and thoracolumbar regions. These regions are predisposed to injury as they are the junctions between the relatively immobile thoracic spine and the more flexible cervical and lumbar spines. The incidence of acute injury is highest in the thoracolumbar vertebrae. The 12th thoracic and first lumbar vertebrae are most frequently involved, and less often the 11th thoracic and second lumbar vertebrae. Compression fractures and fracture dislocations commonly occur in this region.

A three-column concept in viewing the thoracolumbar spine was developed to aid in determining the stability of various vertebral injuries (Fig. 5–29). The *anterior column* consists of the anterior longitudinal ligament and the anterior two-thirds of the vertebral body and annulus fibrosus. The *middle column* consists of the posterior third of the body and annulus and the posterior longitudinal ligament. The *posterior column* consists of the posterior ligament complex and the vertebral arch structures. Fractures involving only one column are considered stable injuries, and fractures involving all three columns are considered unstable in-

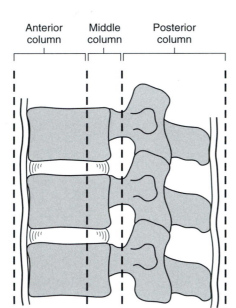

FIGURE 5–29. The three-column concept in viewing the thoracolumbar spine aids in determining the stability of various vertebral injuries.

juries. Involvement of two columns may or may not be stable, depending on the degree of injury.[25,26]

Anterior Compression Fractures[27–32]

Anterior compression fractures are caused by flexion forces that fracture and deform the anterior vertebral body while the posterior body, vertebral arches, and posterior ligaments remain intact (Fig. 5–30). The loss of anterior vertebral body height may range in severity from barely perceptible to complete collapse with comminution. Anterior compression fractures are considered stable fractures as only the anterior column is involved. However, if the force incurred

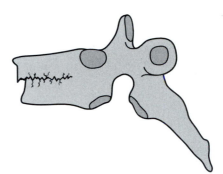

FIGURE 5–30. Anterior vertebral body compression fracture.

exceeds that which collapsed the anterior body, a distractive disruption of the posterior bony structures and ligaments can occur (Fig. 5–31). In this instance, more than one column is involved and stability is questionable.

The intervertebral disc is commonly injured in association with compression fractures. The distinction in thickness of the discs in the upper versus the lower thoracic spine alters the nature of both the injury to the disc and the deformity sustained by the vertebral bodies. In the upper thoracic spine, discs are thinner and less shock absorbing, so forces are readily transmitted to the vertebral body. The collapse of the body thus results in a true wedge-shaped deformity. In the lower thoracic and lumbar spine, discs are thicker and better shock absorbers, so forces are dispersed more readily to the disc itself and the vertebral endplates encasing it. The result is a greater occurrence of associated anterior or intervertebral disc herniations and vertebral endplate fractures and less of a vertebral body wedge deformity in this region (Figs. 5–32, 5–33). Additionally, the thickness of the discs in the lower thoracic spine also allows for greater distance between the vertebral bodies, and, in turn, greater facet joint translation is possible. A flexion force thus has the potential to translate into an anterior shearing force, tearing the

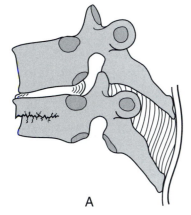

A

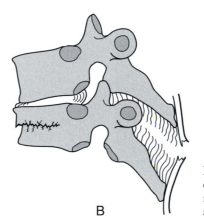

B

FIGURE 5–31. Anterior vertebral body compression fracture (*A*) with wedge deformity and intact posterior ligament complex and (*B*) with torn posterior ligament complex.

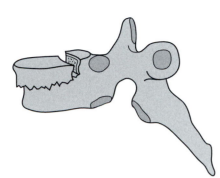

FIGURE 5–32. Anterior vertebral body compression fracture resulting in disruption of vertebral endplate.

outermost annular fibers that attach to the vertebral endplates (Sharpey's fibers) or avulsing the bony rims of the endplates (Fig. 5–34).

MECHANISM

Compression fractures are common in the thoracic and thoracolumbar spines due to multiple factors. The vertebral bodies are composed of compressible spongy cancellous bone while the vertebral arches are composed of less compressible dense cortical bone. An axial compressive force applied through the spinal column will result in a collapse of the anterior vertebral structures with relative sparing of the posterior structures. Thus, an axial force is often converted into a flexion force. A flexion force itself will load the anterior vertebral bodies first, and these areas will collapse when their weight-bearing threshold has been reached.

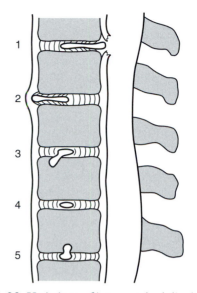

FIGURE 5–33. Variations of intervertebral disc herniations. 1 = posterior herniation through the posterior longitudinal ligament; 2 = anterior herniation; 3 = inferior intervertebral herniation; 4 = normal position of nucleus pulposus; 5 = superior intervertebral herniation.

The normal thoracic kyphosis predisposes the thoracic spine toward flexion. Additionally, humans move reflexively into flexion as a protective response; thus, anticipated trauma is often sustained in a position of truncal flexion. External factors, such as falls on the buttocks, items falling from above onto the back, or the sitting position in motor vehicles, place the spine in flexion at or prior to sustaining a compressive force.

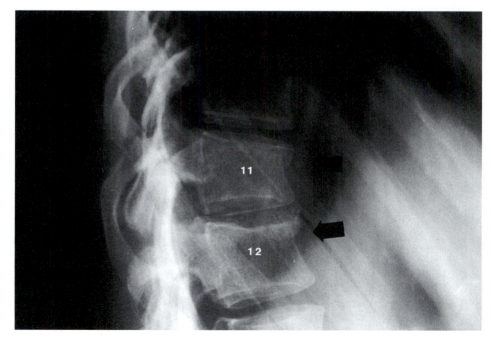

FIGURE 5–34. Traumatic compression fracture of the 11th and 12th thoracic vertebrae. This 40-year-old woman was operating a weed-whacker on a grassy slope when she slipped, sustaining these fractures as she landed on her buttocks. As is characteristic of compression fractures in the lower thoracic vertebrae, the flexion force has damaged the vertebral endplates by converting into anterior shear force, in addition to causing a compressive deformity.

ANTERIOR COMPRESSION FRACTURES IN OLDER ADULTS

Anterior compression fractures of the vertebral bodies are the most common spinal injury in all age groups detectable on radiographs (Figs. 5–35, 5–36). Over age 60, compression fractures compose the majority of all vertebral injuries. Compression fractures increase in incidence with age owing in part to degenerative changes in the vertebrae and intervertebral discs. Demineralization of bone renders the vertebrae less elastic, more brittle, and prone to fracture; dehydration of the nucleus pulposus renders the discs less resilient to compression. These decreases in shock-absorbing qualities increase the degree of trauma suffered at the vertebrae.

RADIOGRAPHIC APPEARANCE

Radiographically, compression fractures will reflect the mechanical changes described earlier. The radiographic signs of compression fracture include:

- A step defect
- A wedge deformity
- A linear zone of impaction

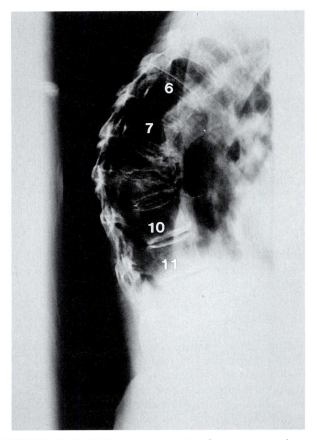

FIGURE 5–36. Multiple compression fractures secondary to osteoporosis in a 95-year-old female. Note the collapse of T8 and T9. The severity of the deformity coincides with the severity of the postural thoracic kyphosis as evident on this lateral view. Note the linear zone of impaction in both vertebral bodies representing the enmeshed trabeculae of the compressed fracture fragments.

- Displaced endplates
- Loss of intervertebral disc height
- Paraspinal edema
- Abdominal ileus[33]

1. **The step defect:** The anterior cortex of the vertebral body is the first structure to undergo strain and will suffer the greatest stress. The superior endplate is often displaced anteriorly, causing a buckling or step-off of the normally smooth concave anterior margin. This sign is best seen on the lateral view and is sometimes the only radiographic clue to a subtle compression fracture.
2. **The wedge deformity:** The collapse of the anterior vertebral body creates a triangular or trapezoidal body, apparent on the lateral view. This may result in increased kyphosis. Lateral wedging may also occur, resulting in a scoliosis, apparent on the AP view. It is estimated that at least a 30 percent loss of vertebral body height is required for the wedge deformity to be present on radiograph.
3. **Linear zone of impaction (white band of condensation):** A linear band of increased density is ap-

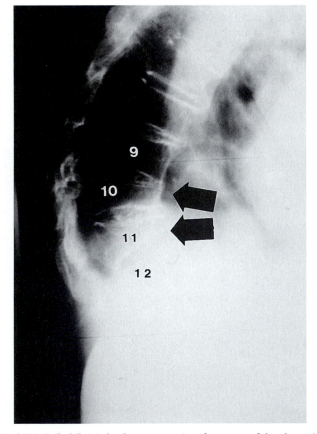

FIGURE 5–35. Multiple compression fractures of the thoracic spine secondary to osteoporosis. Note the characteristic wedge deformity of T10 and T11 caused by collapse of the cancellous bone of the anterior vertebral bodies in this 85-year-old female.

parent beneath the involved endplate. Acutely, this represents the enmeshed trabeculae of the compression fracture. Later, this same appearance represents callus formation in the healing fracture. It is best seen on the lateral view.

4. **Displaced endplates:** The anterior shearing of the intervertebral disc may avulse the bony rim of an endplate, or displace it anteriorly. The appearance on the lateral view will be a greater AP diameter of the vertebral body at the involved endplate.
5. **Loss of intervertebral disc height:** The intact disc is inferred by the well-preserved potential space between the vertebrae and the proper alignment of the vertebrae. Herniation of the disc will cause a decrease in the potential space and possibly a misalignment of adjacent vertebrae.
6. **Paraspinal edema:** Paraspinal soft tissue edema or hematoma is often associated with compression fractures. These are best seen on the AP view as increased areas of density adjacent to either side of the spine.
7. **Abdominal ileus:** Disturbance to the visceral autonomic nerves or ganglia may occur with paraspinal soft tissue trauma. The result will be excessive amounts of small or large bowel gas best seen on the AP view. The significance of this sign is that it is an indicator of underlying severe trauma, and the likelihood of fracture is great.

HEALING

Anterior compression fractures are acutely painful, and the most severe symptoms resolve in 10 to 14 days. Bracing the trunk in extension relieves much pain by unloading the anterior vertebral bodies from a certain amount of weight bearing. Bracing may not be effective or appropriate in the elderly because of pre-existing kyphotic deformities, loss of extension mobility, or intolerance to confinement of the thorax.

Vertebral body fractures heal by both endosteal and periosteal callus formation. Union occurs in 3 to 6 months. Delayed union may be due to extensive disc herniation into the fracture site, interrupted nutrient vessels, or general poor health and old age. The anterior height of the vertebral body rarely returns to normal, and the wedge deformity persists after healing. Excessive cortical thickening at the anterior vertebral margin and excessive callus formation, even extending to the anterior longitudinal ligament, are not uncommon and may persist for years. Mildly damaged discs may revascularize and function normally. Severely torn discs may calcify and form a bony ankylosis at that segment.

DETERMINING THE AGE OF A COMPRESSION FRACTURE (TABLE 5–1)

The age of a compression fracture is determined radiographically by the presence or absence of the foregoing radiographic signs. The acute compression frac-

TABLE 5–1 Age Determination of Compression Fracture

	New (<2 Mo Postfracture)	Old
Step defect	+	—
Wedge deformity	+	+
Linear zone of impaction	+	—

ture will exhibit most of the indicators, although the less severe cases will not involve the soft tissue signs. The step defect and the linear zone of impaction are the most reliable signs of a recent or healing fracture, less than 2 months old. These two radiographic signs will disappear when union is complete, usually by 3 months postinjury. Bone scans may be helpful if the age of a compression fracture is in question, as active healing will be evident. Bone scans are not precise, however, as scans may stay positive for as long as 2 years postinjury.

Fracture Dislocation[34–39]

Generally, fractures of the anterior column are considered stable injuries, and fractures or dislocations of the middle and posterior columns have the potential to be unstable injuries. The risk factors of these injuries involve the migration of a fracture fragment into the spinal canal, or a compromise of the available space for the spinal cord in the canal.

Fractures combined with dislocations are common injuries in the thoracic spine. Pure dislocations of the facet joints in the thoracic spine are rare owing to the structural stability of these joints, in comparison to the more mobile and dislocatable cervical facet joints. To dislocate a thoracic facet joint would require great force, and fractures are more likely to happen prior to a dislocation. Likewise, isolated fractures of the vertebral arch complex caused by acute trauma are also rare. To fracture the dense cortical bone of an isolated articular pillar, transverse process, or spinous process would require great force, and thus associated fractures and ligamentous damage are likely.

An exception to the rarity of isolated posterior column fractures is the avulsion fracture of spinous process commonly seen in the cervicothoracic region. This fracture is well known by the eponym "clay shoveler's fracture." The first thoracic vertebra, followed by the seventh cervical vertebra, followed by the second thoracic vertebra, is most frequently involved in this type of injury.

The majority of fracture-dislocations in the thoracic spine are the result of violent hyperflexion forces. Rotary, shear, compressive, or distractive tension forces often combine with flexion to cause characteristic patterns of injury. A summary of some fracture-dislocation injuries commonly seen in the thoracic and thoracolumbar spines is provided in Table 5–2.

TABLE 5–2 Fracture-Dislocation Patterns in Thoracolumbar Space

Mechanism	Injury	Appearance
A. Hyperflexion	Ant. Col: Vertebral body compression fracture Mid. Col: Tear of posterior longitudinal ligament Post. Col: Tear of posterior ligament complex, dislocation of facet joints	
B. Hyperflexion plus rotation	Ant. Col: Vertebral endplate fracture, disc rupture Mid. Col: Tear of posterior longitudinal ligament (PLL) Post. Col: Tear of posterior ligament complex (PLC); dislocation or fracture at facet joints	
C. Hyperflexion plus shear "traumatic spondylolisthesis"	Ant. Col: Shear fracture through vertebral body or disc Mid. Col: Body fracture and PLL tear Post. Col: Fracture of pedicles and PLC tear	
D. Hyperflexion over fixed horizontal restraint "seatbelt injury"	Ant. Col: Horizontal body fracture Mid. Col: Horizontal body fracture Post. Col: Fissuring of laminae, pedicles, and transverse processes	
E. Hyperextension	Ant. Col: Rupture of anterior longitudinal ligament and IV disc Mid. Col: Compression of posterior disc Post. Col: Compression fracture of vertebral arches or dislocation of facet joints	

Rib and Sternal Fractures

Ribs are composed of cancellous bone in thin cortical casings. Ribs are well vascularized, and fractures occurring here heal readily despite the continued movement of respiration. Nonunion of rib fractures is almost unknown. The mechanism of injury is direct blow to the ribs; occasionally in frail patients a severe coughing fit may fracture the lower ribs. Ribs are seldom dislocated due to the stability provided by the intercostal muscles. Clinically, rib fractures announce themselves by history, localized tenderness, and pain on deep inspiration. Manual compression of the rib cage in an anteroposterior direction will flair the rib cage and reproduce painful symptoms. Radiographically, rib fractures are difficult to assess due to the numerous planes of the ribs (Fig. 5–37). Often the callus formation of a healing rib fracture is the first noticeable radiographic indication that a fracture had indeed occurred. Complications of rib fractures include puncturing of the pleura causing a hemothorax, puncturing of the lung causing a pneumothorax, or contusion to the underlying lung.

Fractures of the sternum are caused by blunt force trauma and are relatively uncommon. Fractures of the xiphoid process, however, are common, because of its exposed position and brittleness after ossification. Note that the sternum is cut vertically to gain access to the heart and lungs for surgical intervention and is fixated with wire reduction postoperatively.

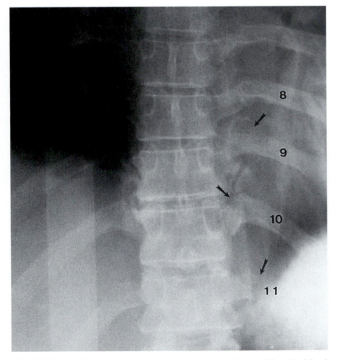

FIGURE 5–37. Multiple rib fractures are indicated by the black arrows to the left side ribs #10, and 11.

OSTEOPOROSIS[40–44]

Osteoporosis is a metabolic disease of bone, characterized by a decrease in the quantity of bone mass (see Chapter 2). The early consequences and symptomatology of generalized osteoporosis may be nonexistent. The devastating later effects include predisposition to fracture, complications in fracture healing, and, in the spine, painful, progressive deformities. Vertebral compression fractures are a common sequela of osteoporosis and can occur at multiple levels, often recurring with some frequency over successive years. Resultant increases in the kyphosis of the thoracic spine are usually quite pronounced and deforming (see Figs. 5–35, 5–36). Functional abilities are compromised as the spine and thorax lose flexibility. Ambulation is often impaired because of pain, compromised heart and lung volume, and the stressful compensatory cervical hyperextension required to bring the eyes to horizontal.

Radiographic Assessment

Osteoporosis affecting the spine demonstrates all of the general radiographic features seen elsewhere in the skeleton including:

- Increased radiolucency of vertebrae
- Thinning of cortical margins
- Alterations in trabecular patterns
- Wedge deformity
- Other deformities of vertebral body
- Endplate deformities
- Schmorl's nodes

Specific to the vertebrae, increased radiolucency is first evidenced at the cancellous vertebral bodies. Thinning of the cortices is first noted at vertebral body margins, especially at the endplates, where the cortical outline is normally relatively thick. The cortical margins of the vertebral arches also become thinned. Trabecular changes within the vertebral bodies often leave distinct vertical striations. The structurally weakened vertebral bodies often collapse under flexion or axial compressive forces (Fig. 5–38A). In severe osteoporosis these vertebral compression fractures may happen with relatively minor or normal everyday forces. The preponderance toward fracture is directly related to the severity of the osteoporosis. A summary of the various configurations of vertebral body collapse is presented in Figure 5–38B.

As discussed earlier, osteoporosis is a clinical diagnosis and therefore is not used as a descriptive term in the radiographic assessment. Osteoporotic bone is described on radiographs by the pathologic changes in the cortex and trabeculae and the presence of old or new compression fractures or deformities. The increased radiolucency of bone is described as *diffuse demineralization* or *osteopenia*.

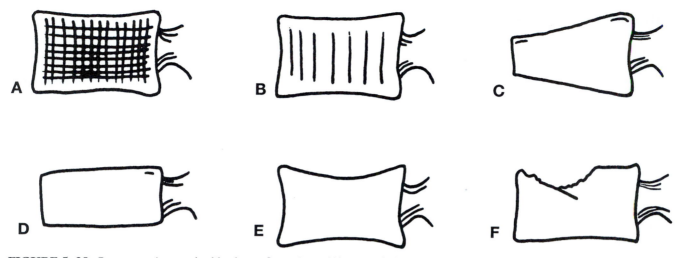

FIGURE 5–38. Osteoporosis: vertebral body configurations. (A) Normal. (B) Normal shape, with pencil-thin cortices. (C) Wedge shape due to anterior loss of height. (D) Plana with both anterior and posterior collapse. (E) Biconcave ("fish" vertebra) due to gradual end plate depression. (F) Angular end plate depressions from acute fractures.

SCOLIOSIS[45–48]

Pathogenesis

Scoliosis is a lateral deviation of the spine from the midsagittal plane combined with rotational deformities of the vertebrae and ribs. Pathologic changes due to compressive forces on the concave side of a curvature include narrowed disc spaces, wedge-shaped vertebral bodies, shorter and thinner pedicles and laminae, and narrowed intervertebral foraminal and spinal canal spaces. Pathologic changes on the convex side of a curvature include widened rib spaces and a posteriorly positioned rib cage, resulting in the deforming "rib hump" (Fig. 5–39).

Classification

Scoliosis is broadly classified into *structural* and *nonstructural scoliosis*. Nonstructural scoliosis designates a curvature that retains flexibility and will reverse or straighten on lateral flexion toward the convex side. Structural scoliosis designates an inflexible curvature that remains unchanged during lateral flexion to the convex site.

Idiopathic Scoliosis

The majority of structural scoliotic cases are termed *idiopathic scoliosis*, as the etiology remains unknown.

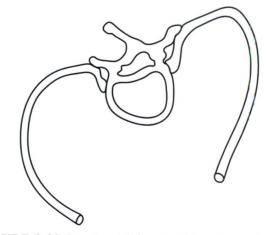

FIGURE 5–39. Rotational deformity of thoracic vertebrae and ribs in scoliosis, top view.

Although various factors are implicated, genetics appears to play a significant role.

Idiopathic scoliosis appears at any age during the skeletal growth period but primarily develops in adolescence, from 12 to 16 years of age. Females outrank males in incidence by 9 to 1. Skeletal maturity usually arrests the progressive development of a curve and also halts the treatment effectiveness.

Curve Patterns

Four distinct patterns of curvature are common (Fig. 5–40). Curves are named by the side of the convexity.

1. **Right thoracic curve:** The most frequently seen curve is the right convex thoracic curve. This major curve extends from T4, 5, or 6 to T11 or 12 or L1. Often, secondary or minor curves are seen above and below the major curve. These are compensatory and initially nonstructural curves that aid in balancing the spine and keeping the eyes oriented to the horizontal. Secondary curves may also be present in any of the following curve patterns.
2. **Right thoracolumbar curve:** This major curve is longer, extending from T4, 5, or 6 to L2, 3, or 4. It can appear to either side, but right is most common.
3. **Left lumbar curve:** This curve extends from T11 or T12 to L5. It also can appear to either side, but left is most common.
4. **Left lumbar—right thoracic curve:** This double major curve consists of two structural curves of equal prominence. This pattern may be the end result of what began as a major thoracic curve with a compensatory secondary lumbar curve, but progressed into two structural curves.

Treatment

Treatment choices fall into three groups: (1) no active treatment but close observation for months or years to determine if a curve is progressing; (2) spinal bracing combined with exercise, for several months or years until skeletal maturity is reached; and (3) surgical fixation.

Treatment choice is predicated on the amount of curvature present, how fast the curve is progressing, how flexible the curve is, and the level of skeletal maturity present. Bracing is not usually prescribed for curves less than 20 degrees. However, during the rapid growth period (10–15 years of age), radiographic re-evaluation is necessary every 3 months, and subsequent increases in curvature greater than 5 degrees may indicate the need for bracing. In general, bracing is effective in immature spines with flexible curves in the 20- to 40-degree range. Surgery may be indicated in rapidly progressing curves, in curves greater than 40 degrees, or if an underlying abnormality can be treated. These criteria are not definitive, however.

Radiographic Assessment

Radiographs are the most definitive and diagnostic modality in the management of the patient with scoliosis. Radiographs serve these purposes:

1. Determine or rule out the various etiologies of the scoliosis
2. Evaluate the curvature size, site, and flexibility
3. Assess the skeletal maturity or bone age
4. Monitor the curvature progression or regression

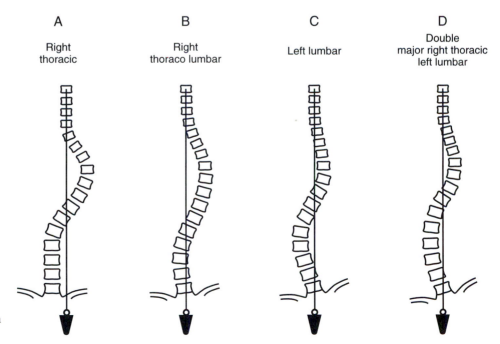

A	B	C	D
Right thoracic	Right thoraco lumbar	Left lumbar	Double major right thoracic left lumbar

FIGURE 5–40. Four common curve patterns seen in scoliosis.

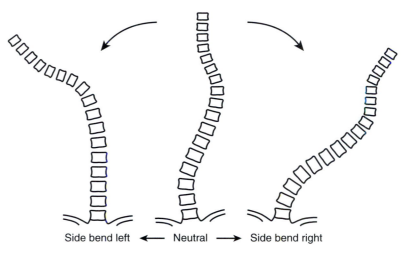

FIGURE 5–41. Schematic of AP side-bending radiographs done to evaluate the amount of flexibility present in a double major spinal curve. *Side bending left*: Shows a correction or reversal of the lumbar curvature, indicating a flexible, nonstructural curve in the lumbar spine. *Side bending right*: Shows no correction of the thoracic curvature, indicating a rigid, structural curve in the thoracic spine.

Side bend left ◄— Neutral —► Side bend right

All of the foregoing influence the choice of treatment plan, modifications of the treatment plan, and the determination of when to discontinue treatment.

The routine radiographic scoliosis evaluation consists of (1) erect anteroposterior, (2) erect lateral, and (3) erect anteroposterior lateral flexion views of the spinal column. The AP lateral flexion views are taken at the end ranges of sidebending right and sidebending left. This will expose the amount of flexibility or rigidity in a curve. Flexible nonstructural curves will reverse or straighten upon sidebend to the convexity. Rigid, structural curves will not be altered during sidebending (Fig. 5–41).

In addition to the spinal films a "spot film," or one-view, AP radiograph of the left hand and wrist is made. This film is compared to standardized films in the Greulich and Pyle Atlas[49] to provide an accurate assessment of bone age. Bone age refers to the physiologic stage of skeletal maturity and is often different from the chronologic age. Thus, a 16-year-old girl may have an immature bone age of 14, and so corrective treatment is still possible. Two other indicators of skeletal maturity are seen on the spinal films. As discussed earlier, fusion of the vertebral ring apophyses closely parallels the end stages of skeletal maturity. Additionally, the process of skeletal maturity is reflected in the appearance of the apophyses of the iliac crests. Referred to as Risser's sign, the apophyses first appear at the anterior superior iliac spines and progress over a year's time posteromedially to the posterior superior iliac spines and then complete fusion in an additional 2- to 3-year period (Fig. 5–42). The formation of the apophyses is graded in quarters relative to the excursion of the apophysis over the extent of the crest. A 1+ Risser's sign indicates an excursion of the apophysis over 25 percent of the crest, 2+ means 50 percent of the crest is "capped," 3+ is 75 percent capped, and 4+ is 100 percent capped. A 5+ indicates osseous fusion is complete. Skeletal spinal maturity is thought to be complete when a 5+ Risser's sign is present and the

vertebral ring apophyses complete fusion. Progression of a scoliotic curve is strongly inhibited after this point. Bracing is gradually weaned as significant further corrective treatment is also inhibited.

Measurements of scoliotic curves are done on the erect AP radiograph. The Cobb method is the widely

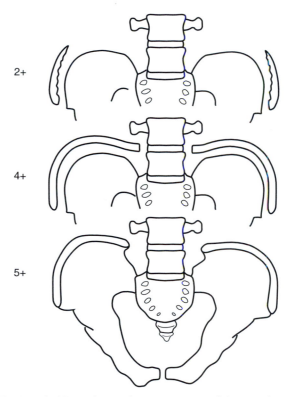

2+

4+

5+

FIGURE 5–42. Radiographic appearance of the apophyses at the iliac crests at different stages of skeletal maturity. Referred to as Risser's sign, formation of the apophyses is graded by the percentage of bone covering the crests. Complete fusion is graded as 5+.

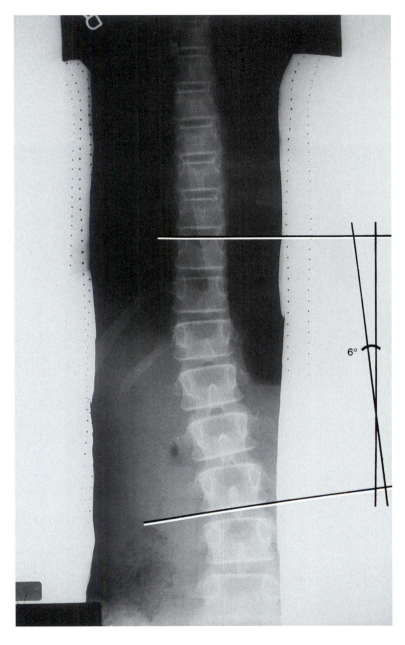

6°

FIGURE 5–43. Mild scoliosis of the thoracic spine, measured by the Cobb method to be a 6 degree curve.

accepted form of measurement and provides a value for the amount of curvature in the frontal plane (Fig. 5–43, 5–44). In addition, the pedicle method provides a value for the amount of axial rotation that has occurred in combination with the lateral curve.

The Cobb method is done by (Fig. 5–45):

1. Identifying the uppermost involved vertebra of the curve that tilts significantly toward the concavity and drawing a line through its superior endplate
2. Identifying the lowest involved vertebra of the curve that tilts significantly toward the concavity and drawing a line through its inferior endplate
3. Drawing perpendicular lines through those two

lines and measuring the resulting intersecting angle. This angle represents the value assigned to the scoliotic curve

The pedicle method of measuring rotation is done by identifying how far the convex side pedicle has rotated toward midline (Fig. 5–46). A 0 to 4+ grading system is used. A 0 indicates normal position. A 1+ indicates the pedicle has moved a third of the way toward midline from its normal position, 2+ indicates the pedicle has moved two-thirds of the way, 3+ indicates that the pedicle is in the midline of the image of the vertebral body, and 4+ indicates that the pedicle has rotated beyond midline.

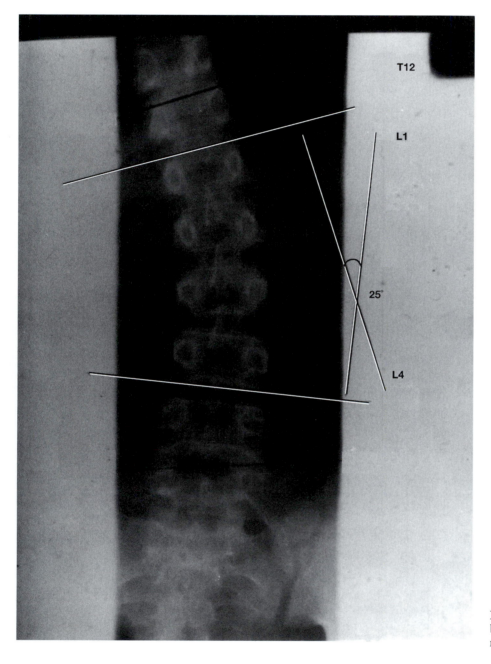

FIGURE 5–44. Scoliosis of the lumbar spine measured by the Cobb method to be a 25 degree curve.

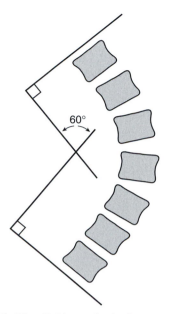

FIGURE 5–45. The Cobb method of measuring spinal curvatures on the AP radiograph.

THORACIC, RIB, AND STERNAL ANOMALIES[54–57]

Congenital or developmental anomalies occur with frequency at the junctions of the spinal curvatures. The thoracolumbar junction is often the site of vertebral anomalies. As stated in the cervical spine chapter, spinal anomalies are related to a structure's (1) failure to develop, (2) arrested development, or (3) development of accessory bones. Spinal anomalies may occur in isolation or in combination with other spinal, visceral, or soft tissue malformations.

Rib and anterior chest anomalies are not uncommon and are usually clinically insignificant.

Examples of anomalies of the thoracic spine and thorax, their clinical significance, radiographic features, and appearances are presented in Table 5–3. (See Figures 5–47 and 5–48 for radiographs of anomalies.)

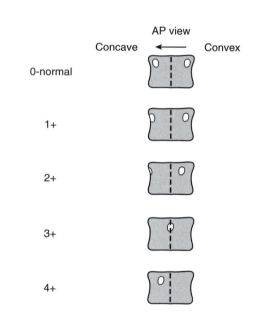

FIGURE 5–46. The pedicle method of measuring vertebral rotation in scoliosis.

TABLE 5–3 Anomalies of the Vertebrae, Ribs, and Sternum

Anomaly	Clinical Considerations	Radiographic Features	Appearance
Block Vertebrae: Two adjacent vertebrae fused at birth. Partial or complete fusion of bodies, facets, spinous processes may be present.	No motion at fused segment. Excessive compensatory motion at adjacent freely moving joints with resultant accelerated degenerative changes. Common in both the thoracic and lumbar spines.	**Lateral film:** Small AP diameter of bodies with indented "wasp-waist" appearance of the fused intervertebral disc space. Facets fused in half the cases. Spinous processes may be fused or malformed.	
Butterfly Vertebrae: The endplates are indented toward the center of the body and filled with continuous disc material from adjacent superior and inferior disc spaces.	Usually clinically insignificant. The divided body halves are approximately symmetrical and maintain axial alignment of the vertebrae. Common in both the thoracic and lumbar spines.	**AP film:** The lucency of the invaginating disc material creates the appearance of the vertebral body as a pair of butterfly wings.	
Hemivertebrae: Failure of one half of the vertebral body to grow.	Often associated with other vertebral anomalies. In isolation a hemivertebra will become the apex of a structural scoliosis. Common in lower thoracic and upper lumbar spines.	**AP film:** The involved vertebral body presents a triangular appearance. Adjacent disc spaces are of normal height but adjacent vertebral endplates may be deformed, slightly altering the shape of the bodies.	
Schmorl's Nodes: Weakening of the cartilaginous endplates that permit herniation of disc material through the plates and into the vertebral body.	Associated with developmental weakness of the endplates, trauma, or various pathologic conditions that weaken bone, such as osteoporosis, Paget's disease, DJD, sickle cell anemia, and malignancies. Common in thoracic and lumbar spines.	**Lateral film:** Protrusions of disc material into the body create cavities that eventually ossify. These cavities then radiograph as distinct squared-off sclerotic nodes. More nodes may be present but not seen on radiograph if the cavities have not ossified yet.	

Rudimentary 12th rib: Arrested development of the 12th pair of ribs.	Clinically insignificant.	**AP film:** Small irregularly shaped stubs of bone present instead of well-formed ribs
Lumbar Ribs: Accessory ribs seen most often at L1. These ribs may have all the characteristics of a thoracic pair of ribs, or may present only as rudimentary stubs of bone.	Clinically insignificant. Important in the differential diagnosis of transverse process fractures of the lumbar spine.	**AP film:** Note either well-developed thoracic-like rib pairs present at L1, or small irregularly shaped stubs of bone that are distinct from the transverse processes.
Srb's anomaly: Diminished size or incomplete fusion of one or both first ribs.	Clinically insignificant.	**AP or PA film:** Note malformation of first ribs. May see congenital synostosis of the first rib to the second rib.
Rib foramen: Formation of an opening within the shaft of the rib	Clinically insignificant.	**AP or PA film:** Note radiolucent oval within the shaft of the rib.
Luschka's bifurcated rib: A split at the anterior end of an upper rib.	Clinically insignificant. To be differentiated from a cavity within the lung.	**AP or PA film:** Note bifurcation of rib creating radiolucent area.
Congenital synostosis: Developmental fusion of adjacent ribs.	Clinically insignificant.	**AP or PA film:** Note fusion of adjacent ribs.

Chest Anomalies

Pectus excavatum: Congenital condition in which the sternum is abnormally depressed. Commonly termed "funnel chest."	Severe cases may compromise functioning of the heart and lungs and require surgical intervention.	**Lateral film:** Note posterior position of sternum.
Pectus carinatum: Congenital abnormal prominence of the sternum. Commonly termed "pigeon breast."	Severe cases increase the AP diameter of the thorax enough to impair coughing and restrict the volume of ventilation. Surgery may be warranted to place the sternum in a more normal position via resection of the costal cartilages.	**Lateral film:** Note anterior position of sternum.

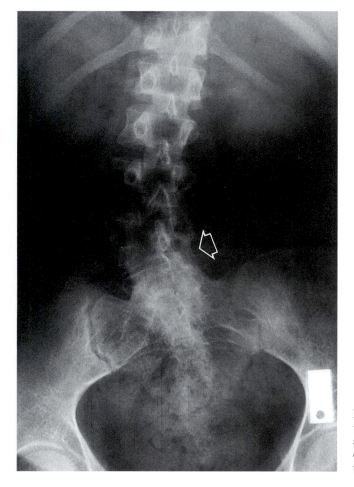

FIGURE 5–47. Lumbar scoliosis. This anteroposterior view of the lumbar spine of a 28-year-old female shows a congenital anomaly of block vertebrae or synostosis of the left-side portions of L5 and S1. The asymmetry of this anomaly has contributed to the development of scoliosis.

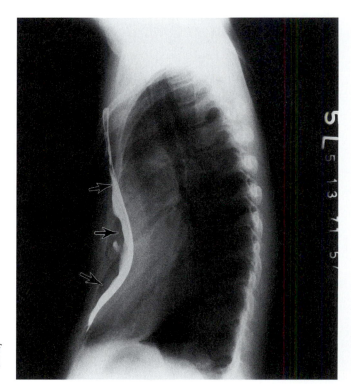

FIGURE 5–48. Pectus excavatum. This congenital anomaly of a posteriorly positioned sternum is demonstrated on this lateral film of a 9-year-old girl.

SUMMARY OF KEY POINTS

1. The routine radiographic evaluation of the thoracic spine includes two projections:
   - **Anteroposterior:** Demonstrates all 12 vertebrae
   - **Lateral:** Demonstrates all vertebrae except the upper two or three, which are obscured by the shoulder; a swimmer's lateral, which positions the arm overhead, may be done for the purpose of evaluating these upper vertebrae
2. The routine radiographic evaluation of the sternum includes the oblique and lateral projections.
3. The routine radiographic evaluation of the ribs includes the oblique and lateral projections, directed to specific regions of the rib cage as indicated by clinical history. In trauma cases, a posteroanterior chest film is included in the routine evaluation to determine if a rib fracture has punctured the pleura.
4. Normal vertebral alignment in the thoracic spine is demonstrated on the lateral projection via three parallel line images construed at (a) the borders of the anterior vertebral bodies, (b) the borders of the posterior vertebral bodies, and (c) the junctions of the laminae to the spinous processes (the spinolaminar line). Discontinuity in the spatial relationships of these line images may indicate the presence of fracture or dislocation.
5. The thoracic spine is most frequently injured due to flexion forces. The incidence of acute injury is highest in the thoracolumbar spine (T11, T12, L1, L2).
6. Anterior compression fractures of the vertebral bodies are the most common spinal injuries in all age groups detectable on radiographs. Compression fractures increase in incidence with age owing to degenerative changes in the vertebrae and the intervertebral discs.
7. Osteoporosis is a metabolic disease of bone characterized by a decrease in the quantity of bone mass. Vertebral compression fractures are a common sequela of osteoporosis and can result in progressive kyphotic deformities of the spine.
8. Scoliosis is a lateral deviation of the spine from the midsagittal plane combined with rotational deformities of the vertebrae and ribs. Radiographs are the most definitive and diagnostic modality in the management of the patient with scoliosis.

REFERENCES

1. Rockwood, CA and Green, DP (eds): Fractures in Adults, Vol 2. JB Lippincott, Philadelphia, 1984, p 1036.
2. Netter, FH: The Ciba Collection of Medical Illustrations, Vol 8, Part I, Musculoskeletal System. Ciba-Geigy Corporation, Summit, NJ, 1978, pp 9–15, 33.
3. Basmajian, TH: Imaging of Orthopedic Trauma, ed 2. Raven Press, New York, 1993, pp 391–397.
4. Magee, DJ: Orthopedic Physical Assessment, ed 2. WB Saunders, Philadelphia, 1992, pp 15–155.
5. Gehweiler, JA, Osborne, RL, and Becker, RF: The Radiology of Vertebral Trauma. WB Saunders, Philadelphia, 1980, p 54.
6. Epstein, BS: The Spine: A Radiological Text and Atlas. Lea & Febiger, Malvern, PA, 1976, p 69.
7. Meschan, I: An Atlas of Normal Radiographic Anatomy. WB Saunders, Philadelphia, 1960, p 389.
8. Netter, pp 9, 125–131.
8a. Yochum, TR and Rowe, LJ: Essentials of Skeletal Radiology. Williams & Wilkins, Baltimore, 1987, p 238.
9. Murray, RO and Jacobson, HG: The Radiology of Skeletal Disorders, ed 2. Churchill-Livingstone, New York, 1977.
10. Grainger, RG and Allison, DJ: Diagnostic Radiology. Churchill-Livingstone, New York, 1986.
11. Greenspan, A: Orthopedic Radiology: A Practical Approach, ed 2. Raven Press, New York, 1992, pp 10.27–10.30.
12. Meschan, pp 406–415, 471–473, 482.
13. Bontrager, KL: Textbook of Radiographic Positioning and Related Anatomy, ed 3. Mosby, St Louis, 1993, pp 271–285.
14. Wicke, L: Atlas of Radiologic Anatomy, ed 5. Lea & Febiger, Malvern, PA, 1994, p 32.
15. Fischer, HW: Radiographic Anatomy: A Working Atlas. McGraw-Hill, New York, 1988, p 78.
16. Weir, J and Abrahams, P: An Atlas of Radiological Anatomy. Yearbook Medical Publishers, Chicago, 1978, p 93.
17. Yochum, pp 24–25, 217.
18. Meschan, p 409.
19. Yochum, p 290.
20. Bontrager, pp 297–311.
21. Ibid.

22. Weissman, BW and Sledge, CB: Orthopedic Radiology. WB Saunders, Philadelphia, 1986, p 325.
23. Rockwood, p 1036.
24. Gehweiler, pp 306–314.
25. Greenspan, p 10.34.
26. Weissman, p 329.
27. Rockwood, pp 1036–1085.
28. Gehweiler, pp 262–305.
29. Greenspan, p 10.36.
30. Yochum, pp 477–450, 1031–1038.
31. Netter, pp 218–221.
32. Weissman, pp 325–326.
33. Yochum, p 448.
34. Ibid, pp 447–454.
35. Schultz, pp 140–144, 245–248.
36. Weissman, pp 325–329.
37. Gehweiler, pp 306–376.
38. Rockwood, pp 1036–1092.
39. Greenspan, pp 10.34–10.55.
40. Netter, pp 216–228.
41. Yochum, pp 1031–1041.
42. Greenspan, pp 22.1–22.6.
43. Salter, RB: Textbook of Disorders of Injuries of the Musculoskeletal System, ed 2. Williams & Wilkins, Baltimore, 1984, pp 152–156.
44. Brashear, HR and Raney, RB: Shand's Handbook of Orthopedic Surgery. Mosby, St Louis, 1974, pp 101–103.
45. Yochum, pp 225–242.
46. Keim, HA: Clinical Symposia: Scoliosis, Vol 30, No 1. Ciba-Geigy Corporation, Summit, NJ, 1978.
47. Weissman, pp 288–297.
48. Bontrager, pp 266–270.
49. Greulich, WW, and Pyle, SI: Radiographic Atlas of Skeletal Development of the Hand and Wrist, ed 2, Stanford University Press, Stanford, 1959.
50. Yochum, pp 112–135.
51. Gehweiler, pp 286–289, 353.
52. Greenspan, p 26.1.
53. Brashear, p 332.
54. Yochum, pp 112–135.
55. Gehweiler, pp 286–289, 353.
56. Greenspan, p 26.1.
57. Brashear, p 332.

SELF-TEST

Chapter 5

REGARDING FILM A:

1. What section of ribs is this film evaluating? Identify AP or PA, right or left, above or below diaphragm.
2. Give the radiographic or anatomic rationale for how you determined each of the above.

REGARDING FILM B:

3. Identify this projection.
4. How many thoracic vertebrae are visible? How many lumbar vertebrae are visible?
5. Note the scoliosis. Name the curvature pattern.
6. What can or cannot be said about the lumbar spine in regard to the scoliosis?
7. What additional projections would be helpful in determining if the scoliosis is structural or nonstructural?

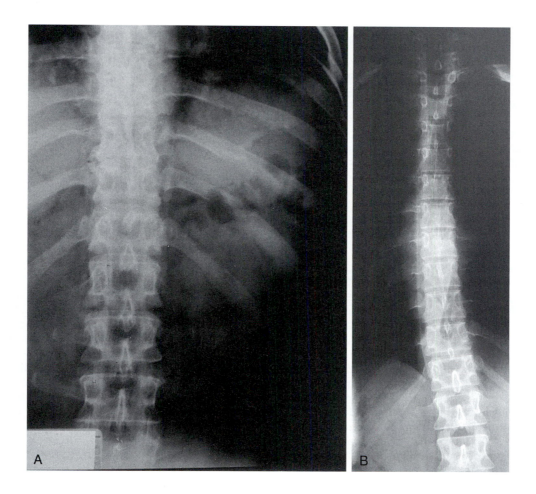

A

B

Lumbosacral Spine and Sacroiliac Joints

The lumbar spine, lumbosacral articulation, and sacroiliac joints are prone to numerous dysfunctions related to mechanical stresses and degenerative changes. Additionally, this region is vulnerable to acute trauma from falls or heavy lifting and chronic strain from repetitive movements, ligamentous laxity, and poor posture. Resultant low back and buttock pain syndromes represent one of the most frequently treated patient groups seen in the clinic. As noted in discussion of the cervical spine, it is essential that the clinical evaluation includes knowledge of the underlying degenerative changes in the spine revealed on radiographs. The degree of severity of degeneration will affect the ability of the spine to withstand trauma, assume postural changes, and make functional gains in mobility and movement patterns.

Many dysfunctions in the lumbar spine share common features with similar dysfunctions in the cervical and thoracic spines. Discussions of degenerative joint disease and degenerative disc disease, presented previously in Chapter 4, are not repeated here, as the pathologic and radiographic characteristics are grossly similar to those seen in the cervical spine. Likewise, fractures and dislocations, discussed in Chapter 5, are not repeated here as the mechanisms and appearances of lumbar spine fractures are grossly similar to those seen in the thoracic spine. Presented at this time are those dysfunctions commonly associated with the lower lumbar spine and lumbosacral junction: stenosis, spondylolysis, spondylolisthesis, posterior intervertebral disc herniations, and sacroiliac joint dysfunction.

The goals of this chapter are first to provide a review of osseous radiographic anatomy. Next, a brief review of ligamentous anatomy and lumbosacral joint mobility to assist the reader in understanding the mechanics of common dysfunctions in this region is presented. The routine radiographic examination of the lumbar spine and sacroiliac joints follows. Here the reader has an opportunity to interact and learn radiographic anatomy by tracing a radiograph with a marker on a transparency sheet, and then comparing it with the radiographic tracing. Additional goals are to present the radiographic findings characteristic of the pathologies listed above. Illustrations and films of osseous anomalies frequently appearing in this region are also presented. A summary of practical points highlighting the clinical aspects of this region follows. A self-test concludes the chapter and challenges the reader's visual interpretation skills.

RADIOGRAPHIC ANATOMY

Osseous Anatomy[1,2]

The five lowermost vertebrae of the spinal column make up the *lumbar spine* (Fig. 6–1). The fifth lumbar vertebra is joined to the sacrum via the articulation of the *inferior articular processes* of L5 to the *superior articular processes* of the *sacrum*, and additionally the L5–S1 *intervertebral disc*. These articulations define the *lum-*

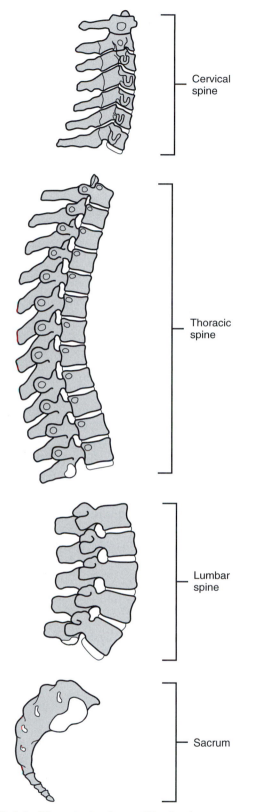

FIGURE 6–1. The spinal column. The five lowermost vertebrae make up the lumbar spine.

bosacral junction (Fig. 6–2). The transformation of the lumbar lordosis to the convexity of the sacrum at this junction defines the *lumbosacral angle*. The caudal end of the sacrum articulates with the *coccyx*.

Lumbar vertebrae are characterized by large *bodies* increasing in size from the first to the fifth lumbar vertebrae (Fig. 6–3). Short *pedicles* project posteriorly from the body and give rise to paired *superior and inferior articular processes*. Short, broad *laminae* unite in midline to form large, blunt, horizontally inclined *spinous processes*. *Transverse processes* are slender in the lumbar spine. *Spinal nerves* exit the *intervertebral foramen* bounded by co-adjacent pedicles. *Facet*, or *zygapophyseal*, *joints* articulate in a sagittally oriented plane, with the exception of the inferior articular facets of L5. The lumbosacral facet joints lie in more frontal plane orientation (Fig. 6–4). The intervertebral discs of the lower two lumbar segments and especially the lumbosacral junction possess greater anterior than posterior height and exhibit a wedgelike shape.

The *sacrum* represents the fusion of five sacral bodies into a single bone. The superior end of the sacrum is its *base*, and the inferior end is the *apex*. The large masses of bone lateral to the first sacral body segment are the *alae* or *wings* of the sacrum. The anterior surface of the sacrum is concave, smooth, and marked by four pairs of anterior *sacral foramina*. The rough, irregular, convex posterior surface is marked by a midline *sacral crest*, representing the fused spinous processes; four pairs of posterior sacral foramina, corresponding with the anterior pairs; and large auricular surfaces that articulate with surfaces on the ilium, forming the *sacroiliac joints*. The failure of the fifth sacral laminae to unite leads to the development of the *sacral hiatus*, which is sometimes used as a portal for injection into the *epidural space*.

The *sacroiliac joints* are formed primarily by the upper three sacral vertertebrae. The articular surfaces are irregularly shaped but fit snugly into corresponding irregularities on the ilia, and this contributes to the inherent stability of the joint. The joint itself lies in an oblique orientation to the frontal plane, with variations in angulation and shape.

The *coccyx* represents the fusion of three to five segments of bone into a single bone. The superior end of the coccyx is its *base*, and the inferior end is the *apex*. The coccyx articulates to the sacrum in such a way that it lies continuous with the dominant curve of the sacrum, and its tip points anteriorly toward the *symphysis pubis*.

Ligamentous Anatomy[3,4]

LUMBAR SPINE

The vertebral column ligaments (Fig. 6–5) that arise in the upper cervical region and extend downward reach their termination at the sacrum. The *anterior longitudinal ligament* extends from the atlas to the sacrum and increases in width as it descends, providing a

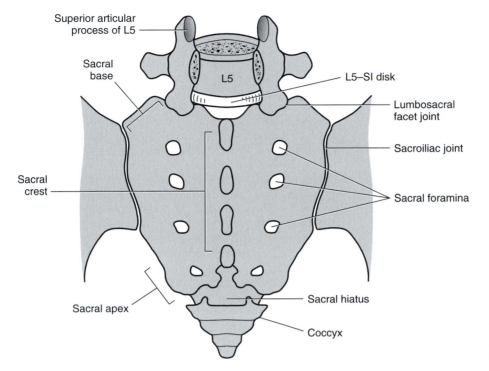

FIGURE 6–2. Posterior view of the lumbosacral articulation, sacrum, coccyx, and sacroiliac articulations.

strong anterior support in the lumbar spine. The *posterior longitudinal ligament* extends from the axis to the sacrum and decreases in width as it descends, providing less certain posterior support for the lumbar intervertebral discs. The remaining posterior ligaments, including the *ligamenta flava* and *supraspinous, interspinous, intertransverse,* and *articular facet capsules,* function similarly in the lumbar spine as in the cervical and thoracic regions, providing restraints to excessive flexion and rotation.

LUMBOSACRAL SPINE

The *iliolumbar ligament* (Fig. 6–6) extends from the transverse processes of the fifth lumbar vertebra to the posterior iliac crests, providing a major restraint against excessive shear of L5 on the sacrum. The lumbosacral joint receives additional ligamentous support, similar to any other vertebral segment, from the anterior longitudinal ligament and the posterior ligaments, as described earlier.

SACROILIAC JOINT

The primary ligamentous stabilizer of the sacroiliac joint is the *interosseous ligament,* extending between the sacrum and ilia. Posterior support is provided by the *posterior sacroiliac ligaments,* and anterior support is provided by the *anterior sacroiliac ligaments.* Additional extrinsic support is provided by the *sacrospinal ligament,* extending from the ischial spine to the lower side of the sacrum and coccyx, and the *sacrotuberous ligament,* extending from the ischial tuberosity to the back of the sacrum and the posterior superior iliac spine.

Joint Mobility[5–7]

The lumbar facet joints L1–L4 are vertically oriented in a sagittal plane. This orientation facilitates flexion and extension and somewhat limits rotation and lateral flexion. The mechanics of the lumbosacral joint, L5–S1, are unique. The change of facet orientation into

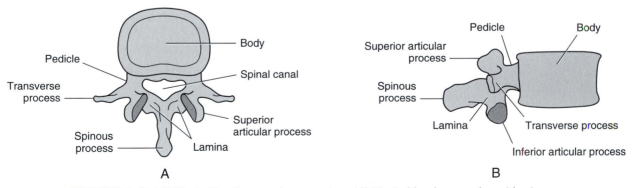

FIGURE 6–3. (*A*) Typical lumbar vertebra, top view. (*B*) Typical lumbar vertebra, side view.

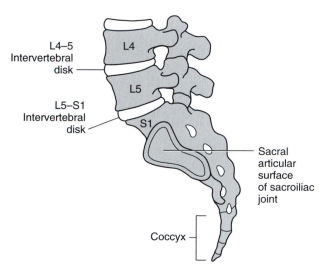

FIGURE 6–4. Lumbosacral spine, side view.

a more frontal plane, the degree of inclination of the lumbosacral angle, and the articulation of the sacroiliac joints all directly affect the amount of mobility and the resistance to shear forces at this segment. The anteriorly directed shear forces that are imposed by normal upright posture have been estimated to be at least half of the total body weight. This tremendous amount of joint stress predisposes the segment to degenerative conditions and complications when fractured.[8]

SACROILIAC JOINT[9,10]

The type and amount of movement at the sacroiliac joints are controversial, and values differ according to various researchers. Despite the differing theories on where the axes of joint motion are located, it is generally accepted that (1) movement at the sacroiliac joints

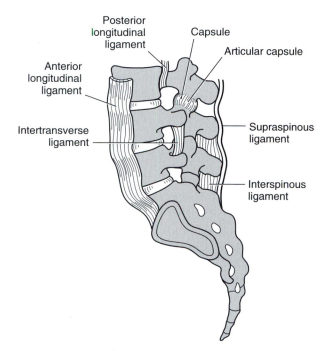

FIGURE 6–5. Ligaments of the lumbar spine.

occurs in response to movement at adjacent bones or body segments and (2) the cartilaginous, irregularly shaped articular surfaces permit adaptive deformation to a variety of imposed stresses. Thus, movement at the sacroiliac joint occurs not in isolation but in combination with and as a result of extrinsic movement. Trunk flexion, for example, incurs a reversal of lumbar lordosis, pelvic rotation about the hip joints, flaring of the posterior ilia, and a counternutation of the sacrum. These smoothly coordinated joint movements acting in concert and including sacroiliac motion are referred to in a functional sense as the *lumbopelvic rhythm.*

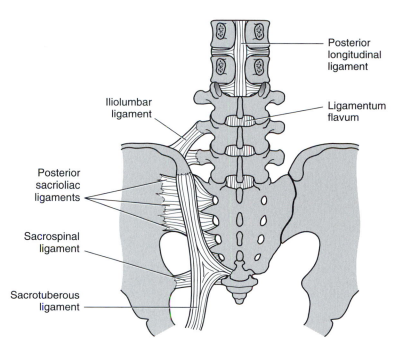

FIGURE 6–6. Lumbosacral ligaments. The first and second lumbar vertebrae are cut away through the pedicles in order to view the posterior longitudinal ligament.

GROWTH AND DEVELOPMENT[11,12]

The ossification process, newborn appearance, development, and maturity of lumbar vertebrae are similar to those of the thoracic vertebrae and are described in Chapter 5.

The sacrum of the newborn is not fused and the individual sacral bodies, separated by intervertebral disc spaces, are evident on the lateral radiograph (Fig. 6–7). The transverse processes of the sacral bodies may also be unfused. The coccyx at birth usually exhibits ossification of the first segment, and the remaining car-

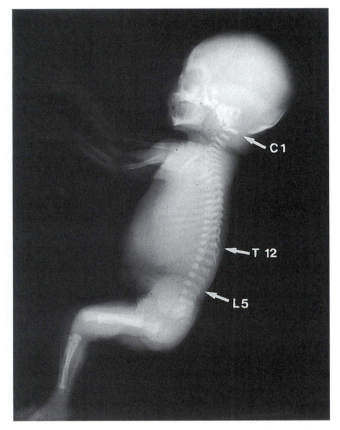

FIGURE 6–7. Normal radiographic appearance of a healthy 6-month-old infant. On this lateral view, the oval-shaped vertebral bodies and the individual sacral bodies are demonstrated.

tilaginous segments are not easily visualized on radiograph.

The dorsal convexity of the sacrum is a primary spinal curvature that is present in utero and at birth (see Fig. 4–13). The secondary spinal curve of *lumbar lordosis* begins development with the onset of active prone extension, standing, and ambulatory skills. The development of the lumbar lordosis over the base of the sacrum also develops the lumbosacral angle. The inclination of this angle affects the amount of shear force the lumbosacral joint sustains during erect postures.

The sacroiliac joint is in part a synovial joint that undergoes marked changes in adulthood. Fibrous and bony ankylosis uniting the joint surfaces are normal aging changes that begin in late middle age. Women and men differ in the amount of mobility that remains preserved in this joint, and numerous factors influence this difference, including the lumbosacral articulation, configuration of the pelvic bones, and ligamentous laxity promoted by pregnancy and childbirth.

ROUTINE RADIOGRAPHIC EVALUATION

Lumbosacral Spine[13–20]

Lumbosacral Spine
Basic: Anteroposterior (AP)
         Lateral
         Right oblique
         Left oblique
         Lateral L5–S1

The routine evaluation of the lumbar spine is similar to the cervical spine in that right and left oblique views are standard. However, whereas the oblique views of the cervical spine visualize the *intervertebral foramina*, oblique views in the lumbar spine visualize the *facet joints*. Table 1–2 gives a summary of radiographic views visualizing intervertebral foramina versus those of the facet joints in the various spinal regions.

Radiographic evaluation of the sacroiliac joint is separate from the lumbar spine evaluation. The orientation of the joint planes necessitates a separate examination. Both sacroiliac joints are viewed simultaneously on the axial AP projection, and each joint is viewed individually on the oblique projections.

The sacrum is well visualized on a basic lumbar spine series but is also radiographed as a separate examination if it is the area of interest. Specific radiographic evaluation of the sacrum includes an AP and a lateral view, extending from L5 to the coccyx. Similarly, if the coccyx is the area of interest, a basic coccyx radiographic evaluation includes an angled AP to avoid superimposition of the symphysis pubis, and a lateral view demonstrating the normal anterior curvature of the coccyx.

ANTEROPOSTERIOR (FIGS. 6–8, 6–9, 6–10)

This view demonstrates the lumbar vertebral bodies, intervertebral disc spaces, and alignment of the pedicles and spinous processes. The important observations are:

1. Depending on the facility, the patient may be positioned supine with the knees *straight*, preserving a lumbar lordosis, or with the knees *flexed*, eliminating the lordosis. The different positions produce

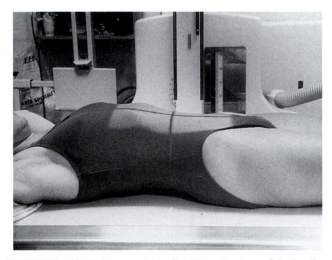

FIGURE 6–8. Patient position for AP projection of the lumbar spine.

slightly different images. In the former, the joint spaces undergo some distortion owing to the lordosis. In the latter, the joint spaces are in neutral.
2. The alignment of the vertebral bodies forms a vertical column with well-preserved intervertebral joint spaces.
3. The pedicles are oval densities on either side of teardrop-shaped spinous processes (Fig. 6–11). The pedicles are spaced equidistantly from midline spinous processes. Misalignment in the relationship of these structures may indicate a fracture-dislocation. Remember the distance between a pair of pedicles represents the transverse diameter of the spinal canal. A decrease in this space may compromise the spinal cord.
4. Intervals between each spinous process and, similarly, between each paired set of laminae are compared for consistency. An increased interval at one level may indicate a torn posterior ligament complex.
5. The articular processes cast a butterfly-like shadow over the vertebral body. Although the facet joints themselves are not visible, the alignment of the articular processes is. Misalignment is an indication of fracture-dislocation.
6. The upper margins of the proximal sacral foramina are identified as paired sharp arcuate lines in the paramedian area of the sacrum. Interruption of the smooth contour of these images could represent fracture. Absence of these images could indicate bone destruction.

CLINICAL OBJECTIVES

1. Trace the lumbar vertebral bodies.
2. Trace the spinous processes.
3. Trace the pedicles.
4. Trace the transverse processes.
5. Trace the superior and inferior articular processes.
6. Trace the sacrum.

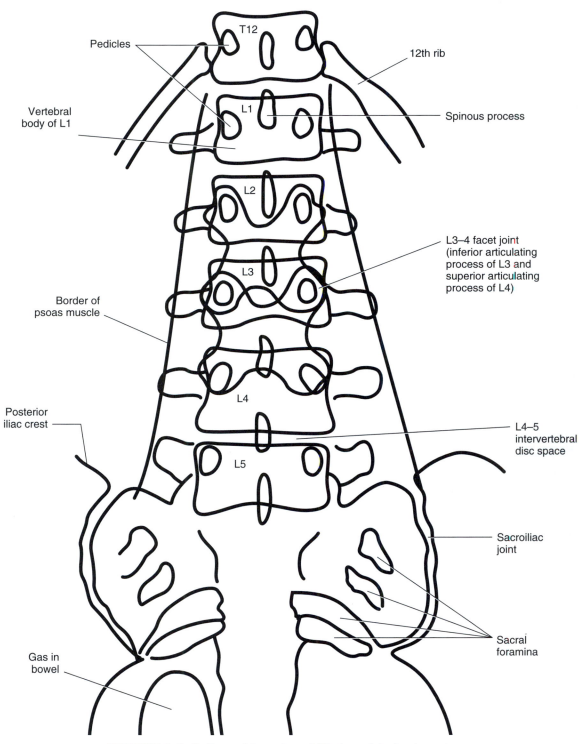

FIGURE 6–9. Radiographic tracing of AP view of the lumbar spine.

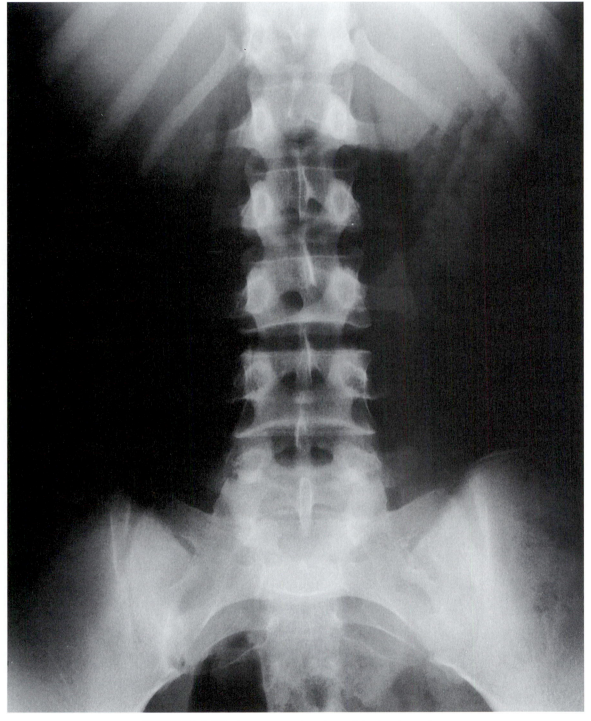

FIGURE 6–10. Anteroposterior view of the lumbar spine.

Vertebral body

Body and pedicles

Body, pedicles, and
superior and inferior
articular processes

All of above plus
spinous process

All of above plus
transverse processes

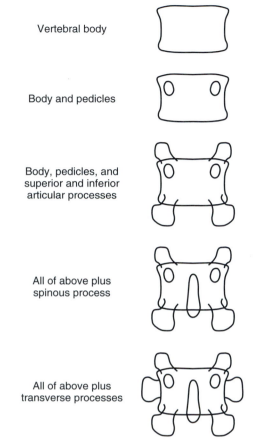

FIGURE 6–11. Schematic to distinguish vertebral structures on an AP radiograph. (Adapted from Squires, LF, and Novelline, RA: Fundamentals of Radiology, ed 4. Harvard University Press, Cambridge, MA, 1988.)

LATERAL (FIGS. 6–12, 6–13, 6–14)

This view demonstrates the lumbar vertebral bodies, intervertebral disc spaces, pedicles, spinous processes, intervertebral foramina, and the lumbosacral articulation. The important observations on the lateral view are:

1. As observed in the cervical and thoracic spines, normal alignment of the vertebrae is verified by identifying three roughly parallel lines (see Fig. 6–14B):
   - **Line 1:** The anterior vertebral body line, representing the connected anterior borders of the vertebral bodies, forms a continuous lordotic curve.
   - **Line 2:** The posterior vertebral body line, representing the connected posterior borders of the vertebral bodies, forms a continuous curve parallel to line 1.
   - **Line 3:** The spinolaminar line, representing the junctions of the laminae at the spinous processes, forms a continuous curve parallel to lines 1 and 2.

   The spatial relationship of these three lines will remain constant during any amount of lumbar flexion or extension. Disruptions in these parallel lines may indicate fracture or dislocation. Remember that the spinal canal lies between lines 2 and 3, and compromise of this space seriously threatens the integrity of the spinal cord.

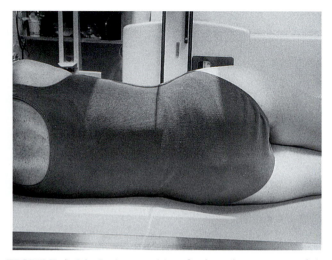

FIGURE 6–12. Patient position for lateral projection of the lumbar spine.

2. The vertebral bodies are boxlike with distinct, smoothly curved osseous margins. Note any osteophyte formation at the joint margins, indicating degenerative changes.
3. The intervertebral disc space height is largest in the lumbar spine because of the thickness of the lumbar discs. Note the normal wedge shape of the disc spaces in the lowest lumbar segments and especially L5–S1.
4. The pedicles are superimposed as a pair at each level.
5. The intervertebral foramina image as radiolucent ovals. The foramina of L1–L2 through L4–L5 are best seen. The foramina of L5–S1 are less easily visualized owing to the transitional anatomy at this level. Additionally, the L5–S1 foramina are typically smaller than the other lumbar levels, and this feature is important to recognize in order to prevent or avoid a misleading interpretation of foraminal stenosis.

CLINICAL OBJECTIVES

1. Trace the three lines of alignment just described.
2. Trace each vertebral body.
3. Trace each intervertebral foramen.
4. Trace the pedicles, laminae, and spinous processes.
5. Trace the lumbosacral articulation.
6. Trace the sacrum.

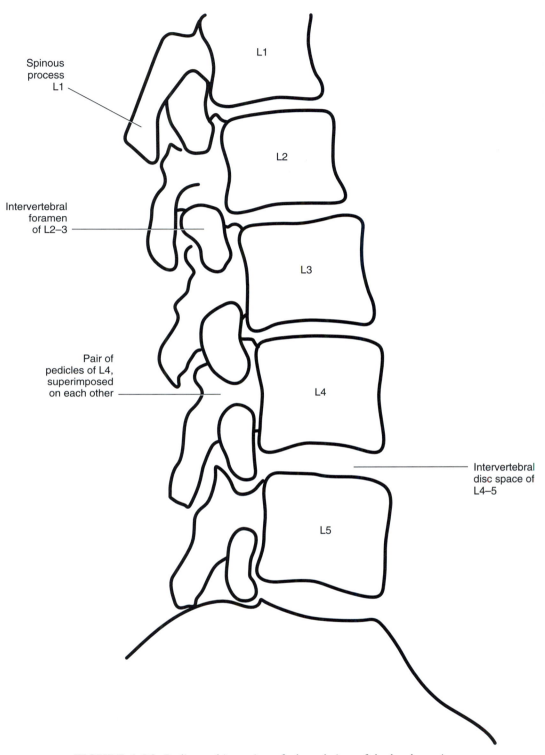

FIGURE 6–13. Radiographic tracing of a lateral view of the lumbar spine.

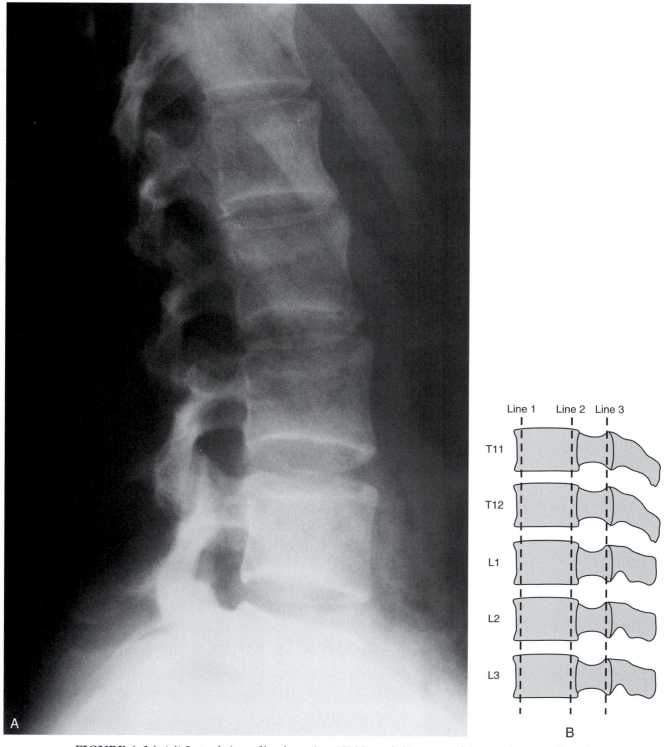

FIGURE 6–14. (*A*) Lateral view of lumbar spine. (*B*) Normal alignment of the vertebrae on a lateral radiograph is verified by identifying three roughly parallel lines. Line 1 = anterior vertebral body line. Line 2 = posterior vertebral body line. Line 3 = spinolaminar line. The *spatial* relationship of these lines will remain constant in any degree of flexion or extension, under normal conditions.

OBLIQUES, R AND L (FIGS. 6–15, 6–16, 6–17)

This view demonstrates the facet (zygapophyseal) joints, the superior and inferior articular processes, the pars interarticularis, and the pedicles. Both right and left oblique projections are included in a lumbar spine study. The right posterior oblique (RPO) demonstrates right-side structures, and the LPO demonstrates left-side structures. The important observations are:

1. The articulation of two adjacent vertebrae causes a radiographic image of a "Scottie dog." The significance of clearly realizing this image is that the viewer is assured the articulating processes and facet joints are well demonstrated, as well as the pars interarticularis.
2. The configuration of the "Scottie dog" body parts represents these anatomic landmarks (see Fig. 6–16C): the nose = transverse process; eye = pedicle; ear = superior articular process; neck = pars interarticularis; foreleg = the inferior articular process; body = lamina and spinous process; tail = superior articular process of opposite side; hindleg = inferior articular process of opposite side.[21]
3. The oblique views may be radiographed from either the anterior or posterior aspect. The posteroanterior obliques (RPO and LPO) demonstrate right and left side facets, respectively. The anteroposterior obliques (RAO and LAO) demonstrate left and right facets, respectively.

CLINICAL OBJECTIVES

1. Trace the image of the "Scottie dog" at one level.
2. Trace the pedicles.
3. Trace the superior and inferior processes.
4. Trace the facet joints.

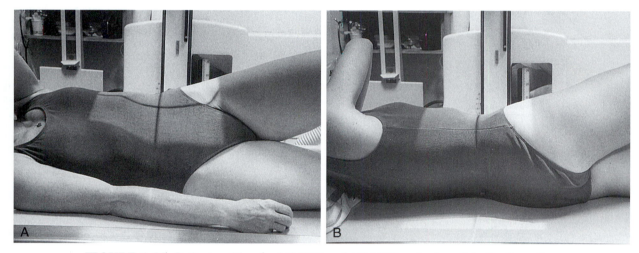

FIGURE 6–15. Patient position for (*A*) RPO and (*B*) LPO projection of the lumbar spine.

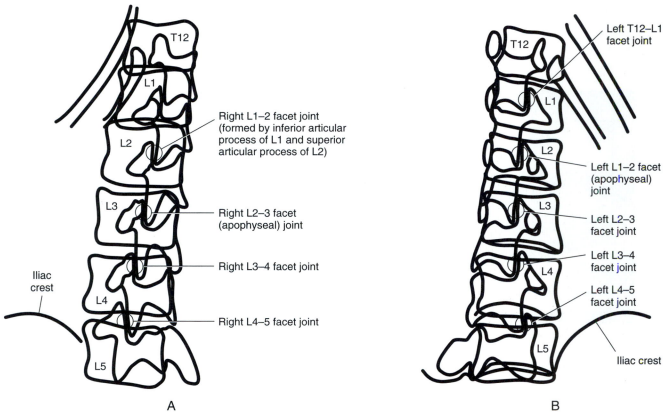

FIGURE 6–16. Radiographic tracings of (*A*) RPO and (*B*) LPO views of the lumbar spine.

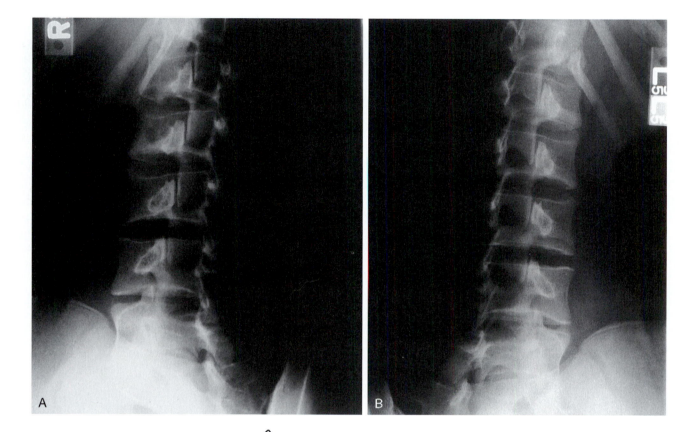

FIGURE 6–17. (*A*) Right oblique projection of lumbar spine. (*B*) Left oblique projection of lumbar spine. (*C*) the image of a "Scottie dog" as seen on an oblique radiograph of the lumbar spine.

Transverse process

Pedicle

Superior articular process

Neck–pars interarticularis

Superior articular process of opposite side

Inferior articular process

Lamina and spinous process

Inferior articular process of opposite side

C

LATERAL L5–S1 (FIGS. 6–18, 6–19, 6–20)

This view is a spot film of the lumbosacral junction. The scope of the radiograph is scaled down to image in greater detail the sole area of interest. The radiographic exposure is adjusted to view optimally L5–S1 through the superimposed density of the ilia. The important observations are:

1. The three parallel lines of vertebral body alignment, as described in the lateral lumbar spine view, continue to hold true in this spot film of the lumbosacral junction. Extensions of the lines now include the sacral body:
   • The anterior vertebral body line, extending from L4 to the anterior body of the sacrum, is normally

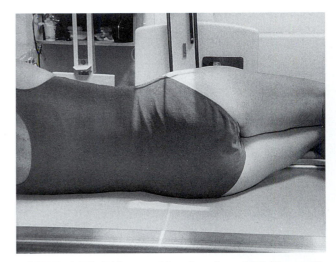

FIGURE 6–18. Patient position for a lateral L5-S1 spot film projection.

smooth and continuous, including the area of transition at the lumbosacral junction. Step-offs in this line may be an indication of fracture, subluxation, dislocation, or retro- or anterolisthesis.

- The posterior vertebral body line, extending from L4 to the posterior body of the sacrum, is likewise evaluated for abnormal step-offs.
- The spinolaminar line, extending from L4 to the sacrum, is likewise evaluated for step-offs.

2. The L4–L5 and L5–S1 intervertebral disc spaces are observed for well-preserved potential spaces. Narrowing of the joint spaces, sclerotic joint margins, osteophyte formation, or lucency indicating vacuum phenomenon are all indicators of degenerative discs.

CLINICAL OBJECTIVES

1. Trace the lumbar vertebral bodies.
2. Trace the pedicles, laminae, and spinous processes.
3. Trace the intervertebral discs: L4–L5, L5–S1.
4. Trace the sacrum.

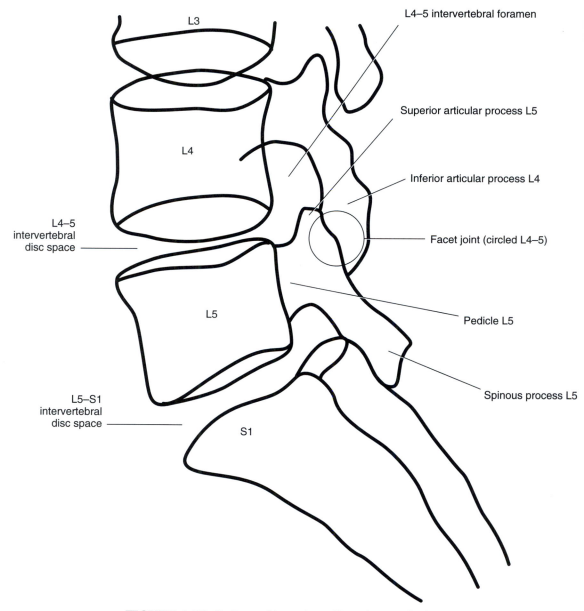

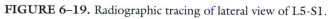

FIGURE 6–19. Radiographic tracing of lateral view of L5-S1.

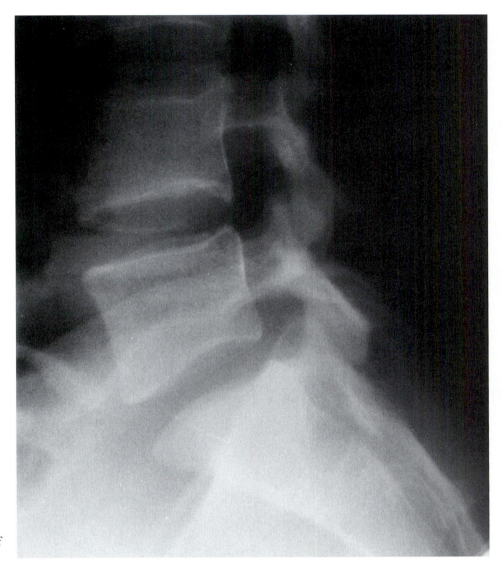

FIGURE 6–20. Lateral view of L5-S1.

Sacroiliac Joint

AP AXIAL (FIGS. 6–21, 6–22, 6–23)

Sacroiliac Joints
Basic: AP axial
R and L obliques

This view demonstrates the bilateral sacroiliac joints (SIJ). It is projected anteroposteriorly and angled in an inferior to superior direction so that the greatest surface area of the joints is exposed. Due to the irregular topography and multiplanes of the joint surfaces, the entire SIJ cannot be visualized on a single view. The important observations are:

1. The articular surfaces are superimposed on each other, so each sacroiliac joint images as two radiolucent joint lines.

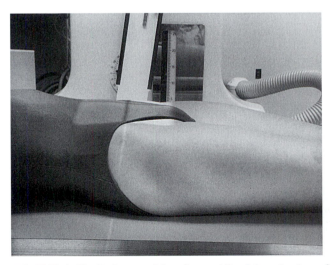

FIGURE 6–21. Patient position for an AP axial projection of the bilateral sacroiliac joints.

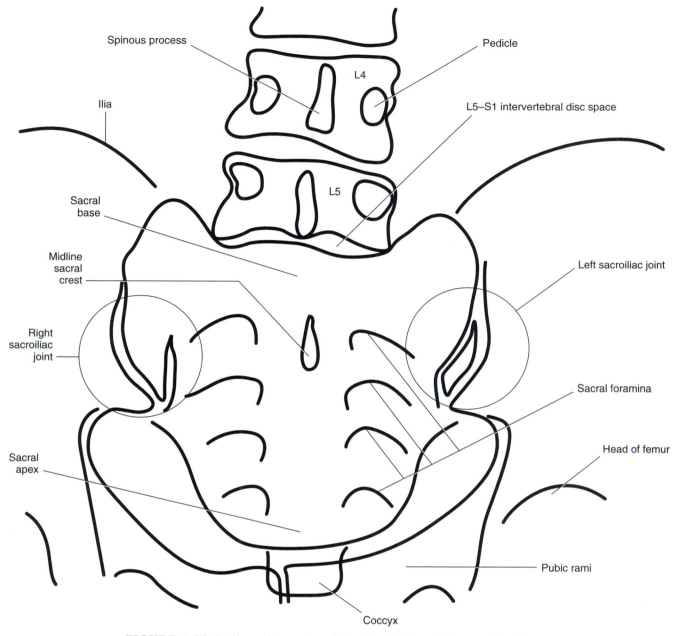

FIGURE 6–22. Radiographic tracing of the AP axial view of the sacroiliac joints.

2. The articular surfaces are evaluated for smooth osseous margins.
3. The bilateral sacroiliac joints are evaluated for symmetry.
4. The L5–S1 articulation is not well demonstrated in this view because of the angled projection.

CLINICAL OBJECTIVES

1. Trace the body of l5.
2. Trace the body of sacrum, including the sacral spinous tubercles and foramina.
3. Trace the sacroiliac joints.
4. Trace the coccyx.

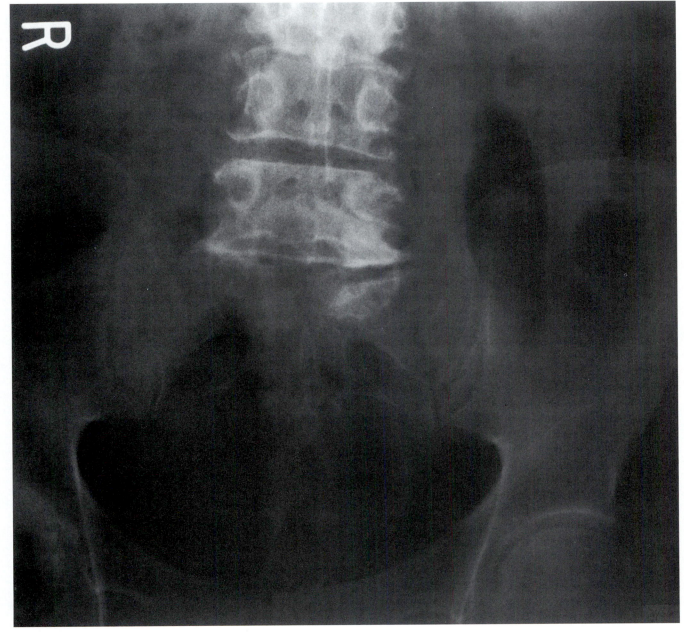

FIGURE 6–23. AP axial view of the sacroiliac joints.

R AND L OBLIQUES (FIGS. 6–24, 6–25, 6–26)

Each oblique demonstrates an individual sacroiliac joint. These views are projected anteroposteriorly, with the pelvis rotated enough to prevent superimposition of the ilia over the sacroiliac joint. Both right and left posterior obliques are done for comparison purposes. The important observations are:

1. The obliquity of the projection permits visualization of the margins of the joint space along its entirety.
2. The joint spaces are evaluated for preserved joint space.
3. The joint spaces are evaluated for degenerative changes, normally evident beginning in late middle age. Degenerative changes prominent in males include fibrosus and bony ankylosis across the joint space.

CLINICAL OBJECTIVES

1. Trace the ilium.
2. Trace the wing of the sacrum.
3. Trace the sacroiliac joint.

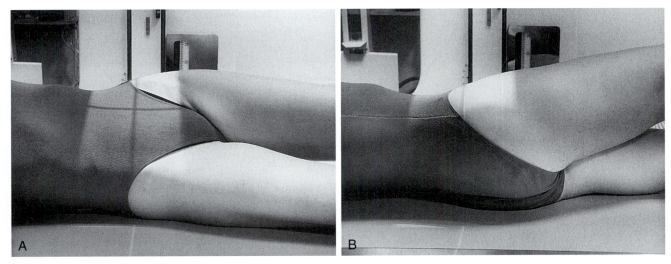

FIGURE 6–24. Patient position for (*A*) RPO projection of the right SIJ and (*B*) LPO projection of the left SIJ.

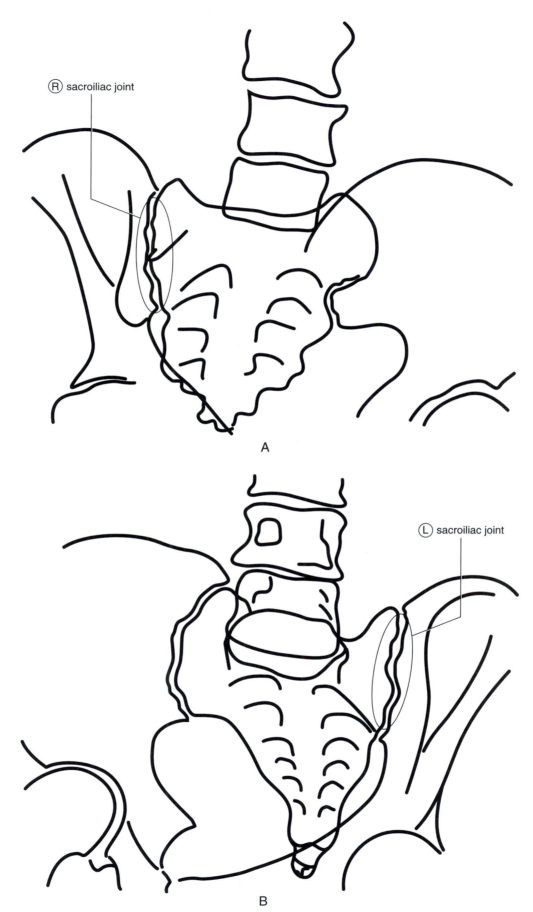

FIGURE 6–25. Radiographic tracing of an oblique view of the (A) right sacroiliac joint and (B) the left sacroiliac joint.

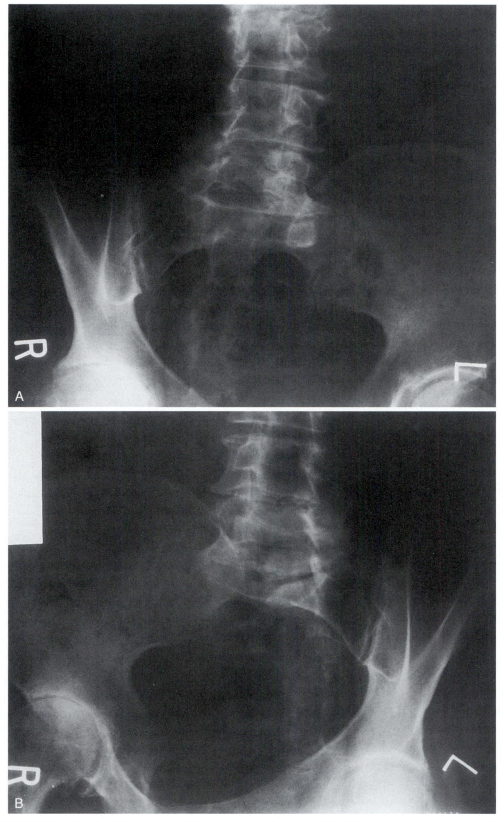

FIGURE 6–26. (*A*) Oblique view of the right sacroiliac joint. (*B*) Oblique view at the left sacroiliac joint.

LUMBAR TRAUMA

Fractures and Dislocations[22–28]

Compression fractures and fracture-dislocations in the lumbar spine share similar mechanisms of injury and similar radiographic appearances as the same injuries located in the thoracic spine. See Chapter 5 for detailed description of compression fractures and refer to Tables 5–1 and 5–2 regarding these and other fractions and dislocations of the thoracolumbar region. See Figures 6–27 and 6–28 for specific examples of plain film and magnetic resonance imagery (MRI) studies of lumbar fractures.

SPONDYLOLYSIS AND SPONDYLOLISTHESIS[29–38]

Spondylolysis is a defect at the pars interarticularis. The defect may be secondary to acute fracture or, more

commonly, a stress fracture due to chronic strain. Spondylolysis may occur bilaterally or unilaterally (Fig. 6–29). A potential consequence of spondylolysis is *spondylolisthesis* (Figs. 6–30, 6–31). Spondylolisthesis defines the forward slippage of one vertebra upon the stationary vertebra beneath it. Due to the location of the fracture, only the vertebral body, pedicle, and superior articular process actually slip forward. The spinous process, lamina, and inferior articular process remain in a relatively normal position. Although traditionally the term "spondylolisthesis" has been synonymous with *forward displacement*, a more precise term for this is *anterolisthesis*. Additionally, the term *retrolisthesis* defines the posterior displacement of a vertebra. All of these terms are in current usage in the medical literature.

Spondylolisthesis may also occur in the absence of fracture, due instead to degenerative changes in the intervertebral disc and facet joints. Loss of optimal articulation from decrease in disc height and overstretched capsules and ligaments may lead to subluxation at these joints. In this case the forward slippage of the involved vertebra is sometimes referred to as pseudospondylolisthesis or degenerative spondylolisthesis. The vertebra itself remains intact and slips forward as a complete unit (Fig. 6–32).

The anatomic differences in fracture spondylolisthesis versus degenerative spondylolisthesis can be discerned both clinically and radiographically by the spinous process sign (Fig. 6–33). In fracture spondylolisthesis, the forward slippage of only the anterior portion of the vertebra creates a palpable step-off of the spinous process at the interspace above the level of the slip. In degenerative spondylolisthesis the forward slippage of the entire vertebra creates a palpable step-off of the spinous process at the interspace below the level of the slip.

Radiographically, spondylolysis is diagnosed on the oblique projection. The "neck" of the Scottie dog image represents the area of the pars interarticularis. A fracture of the pars will appear as a radiolucent streak across the neck, sometimes referred to as the image of a collar on the Scottie dog (see Fig. 6–29). Spondylolisthesis is evaluated on the lateral view. The amount of forward slippage is graded in quarters, in reference to the extent the vertebral body surpasses the normal anterior vertebral body line (Fig. 6–34). For example, if 25 percent of the involved vertebral body overhangs the subjacent vertebra, a grade 1 spondylolisthesis is diagnosed; 50 percent of the vertebral body = grade 2; 75 percent = grade 3; 100 percent or complete dislocation = grade 4. In degenerative spondylolisthesis, the amount of displacement may not be obvious on routine films, and lateral flexion and extension films are then done to reveal the actual stability or instability of the involved segment. As described in Chapter 4 regarding the cervical spine, lateral flexion and extension radiographs are taken at the end ranges of each of these movements to stress the supporting ligaments and evaluate their ability to check excessive joint motion.

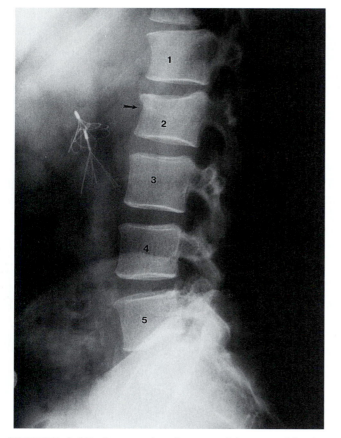

FIGURE 6–27. Compression fracture of the second lumbar vertebra, 5 months after injury. This 38-year-old man had injured his back as he fell off a horse during a rodeo competition. This follow-up film shows good healing of the fracture and the residual deformity of the compressed anterior superior end plate (arrow). This deformity will remain unchanged over time.

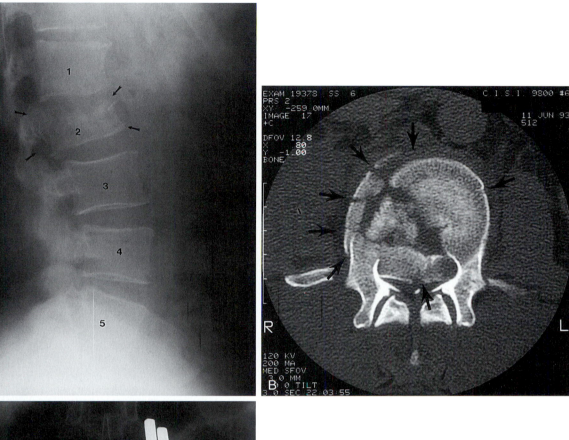

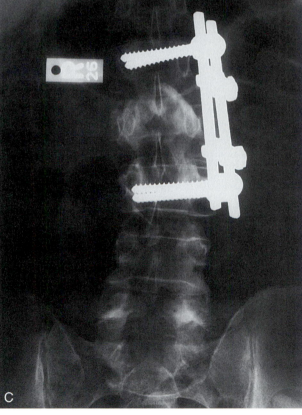

FIGURE 6–28. Burst fracture of L2. This 46-year-old man fractured his second lumbar vertebra when he fell 20 feet out of a tree as he was hanging Christmas lights (see Figs. 5–37 and 9–38 for additional fractures sustained from this fall). (*A*) Lateral plain film shows the compression deformity of the second lumbar vertebra (arrows). (*B*) Transverse axial MR image of L2 demonstrates a comminuted burst fracture of the body (arrows indicate multiple fracture sites). (*C*) Anteroposterior plain film made postoperatively demonstrates internal fixation.

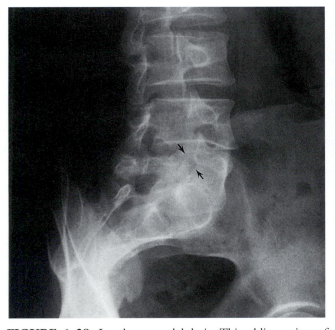

FIGURE 6–29. Lumbar spondylolysis. This oblique view of the lumbar spine demonstrates spondylolysis, a defect in the pars interarticularis. The arrows bracket the extent of the defect. The radiolucent line image caused by the defect has been referred to as "a collar on the Scottie dog." No associated spondylolisthesis is apparent on this view.

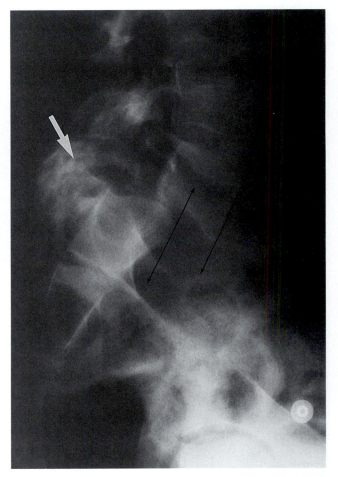

FIGURE 6–30. Lumbar spondylolisthesis. This 15-year-old boy underwent a bone graft procedure several months earlier in order to correct the anterolisthesis of L5. The grafting (arrow) was unsuccessful. Over 50% of the body of L5 has slipped forward past the anterior border of the body of S1 (see line arrows), thus this is described as a *grade 2–3 spondylolisthesis* or *anterolisthesis.*

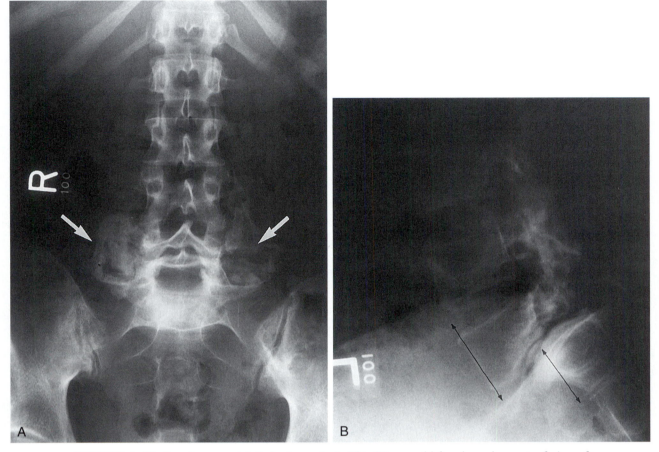

FIGURE 6–31. Lumbar spondylolisthesis, grade 3. This 32-year-old female underwent a fusion of L4 to L5 in order to correct a severe anterolisthesis. The procedure failed over time. (*A*) Bone grafts are noted on the anteroposterior film (white arrows). (*B*) Lateral spot film of the lumbosacral junction shows a grade 3 spondylolisthesis of L5–S1 (line arrows).

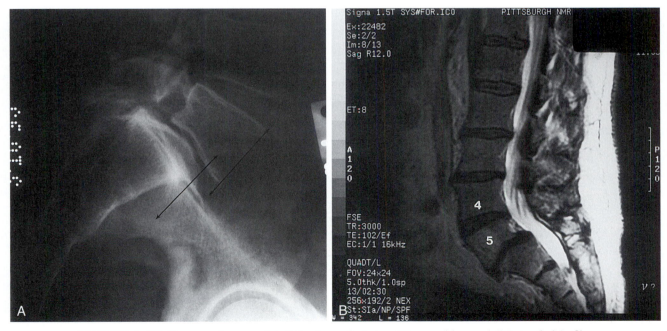

FIGURE 6–32. Degenerative spondylolisthesis, grade 1, in a 60-year-old man. (*A*) Lateral plain film of the lumbosacral junction. Line arrows mark the forward displacement of L5. (*B*) Sagittal MR image of the lumbar spine demonstrating the grade 1 degenerative spondylolisthesis.

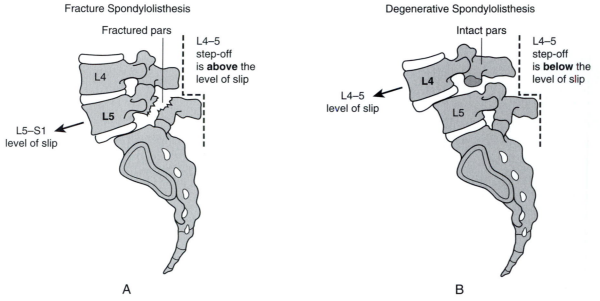

Fracture Spondylolisthesis

Fractured pars

L4

L5

L5–S1
level of slip

L4–5
step-off
is **above** the
level of slip

A

Degenerative Spondylolisthesis

Intact pars

L4

L5

L4–5
level of slip

L4–5
step-off
is **below** the
level of slip

B

FIGURE 6–33. (*A*) Fracture spondylolisthesis can be differentiated from (*B*) degenerative spondylolisthesis by the "spinous process sign." In (*A*), the forward slippage of the anterior portion of the vertebra creates a palpable step-off of the spinous processes at the interspace *above* the level of the slip. In (*B*), the intact vertebra slips forward as a unit, creating a step-off at the interspace *below* the level of the slip. (Adapted from Greenspan,[20] pp 10–42.)

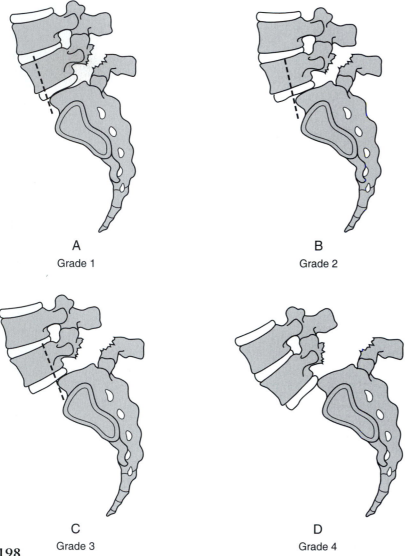

A
Grade 1

B
Grade 2

C
Grade 3

D
Grade 4

FIGURE 6–34. Grades of spondylolisthesis, based on the amount of vertebral body surpassing the normal anterior vertebral border line. (*A*) In grade 1, 25% of the vertebral body has subluxed forward; (*B*) grade 2, 50%; (*C*) grade 3, 75%; (*D*) grade 4, 100% of the vertebral body has surpassed the normal anterior vertebral body line. (Adapted from Greenspan,[20] pp 10–45.)

LUMBAR STENOSIS[39–43]

The lumbar spine is often the site of degenerative disc disease and degenerative joint disease related to aging and various other factors. See Chapter 4 for the radiographic descriptions of these processes. *Spinal stenosis* can be considered a complication or advanced stage of both these degenerative conditions.

Spinal stenosis defines a narrowing or constriction of the spinal canal (Fig. 6–35). Numerous structures altered by degenerative changes may contribute to the constriction: osteophytes at joint margins, bony hypertrophy of the pedicles, laminae, and facet joints, thickening of the ligamenta flava, intervertebral disc bulging, or displacement of the entire vertebra itself in the case of degenerative spondylolisthesis. The location of lumbar stenosis is divided into three anatomic regions: (1) stenosis of the central spinal canal, (2) stenosis of the intervertebral foramina, and (3) stenosis of the subarticular or lateral recesses. More than one region may be involved at the same segment.

Clinically, the signs and symptoms of stenosis are related to vascular and neurogenic compression resulting in diffuse unilateral or bilateral low back and/ or lower extremity pain, numbness, and weakness. Symptoms are often aggravated with standing and walking and relieved with sitting. Lumbar extension in general will narrow the canals and exacerbate the symptoms while lumbar flexion opens the available space and provides some relief.

Radiographically, stenosis is suggested by the location of severe degenerative changes in the structures just listed. Additional imaging studies are done to diagnose and define the extent of the disease. Myelography will show the amount of actual constriction of the thecal sac (Fig. 6–36). Computed tomography will show in an axial view the amount of bony encroachment narrowing the spinal canal (Fig. 6–37). Magnetic resonance imaging will define the anatomic compromises of stenosis in multiple planes.

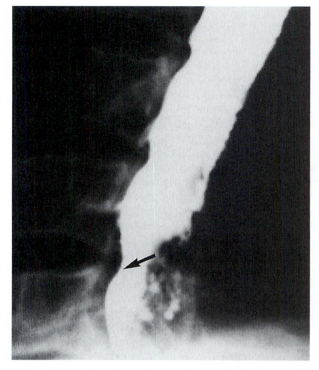

FIGURE 6–36. Lumbar spine myelogram. Indentation of the opacified thecal sac is noted at the stenotic interspace (arrow). Lesser indentations at the posterior aspect of other interspaces are not significant. (From Yochum and Rowe,[22] p 306, with permission.)

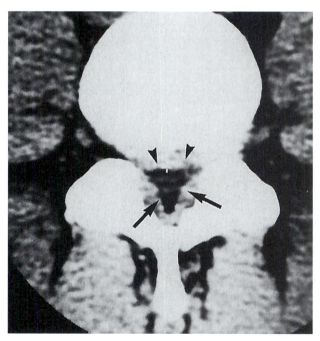

FIGURE 6–37. Transverse axial CT image of stenosis. The thickened ligamentum flavum (arrows) narrows the spinal canal significantly. There is also a posterior disc bulge (arrowheads). The dorsal sac is compromised of *stenosis* from both of these abnormalities. (From Yochum and Rowe,[22] p 308, with permission.)

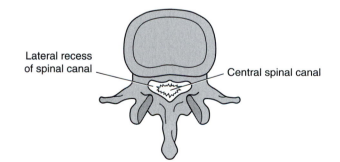

FIGURE 6–35. Spinal stenosis is a constriction of the spinal canal. The location of lumbar stenosis is divided into three anatomic locations: (1) stenosis of the central spinal canal, (2) stenosis of the intervertebral foramina, and (3) stenosis of the lateral recesses.

INTERVERTEBRAL DISC HERNIATIONS[44-50]

Intervertebral disc herniations are one of the most frequent pathologies affecting the discovertebral junction. Herniations of nuclear material through the confines of the annulus fibrosus may occur *anteriorly*, *intravertebrally*, or *intraspinally* (Fig. 6–38).

Anterior disc herniations may be due to acute compression injuries (see Chapter 5) or to a weakness in the attachment of the annulus to the vertebral rim via Sharpey's fibers. Protrusion of the nucleus may elevate the anterior longitudinal ligament and lead to osteophyte formation at the anterior and lateral vertebral joint margins (Fig. 6–39). This condition is known as *spondylosis deformans*.[51]

Intravertebral disc herniations may be due to acute trauma or, more commonly, due to a weakening of the vertebral end plate, as in osteoporosis (see Chapter 5). Protrusion of nuclear material into the vertebral body may lead to the formation of small osseous cavities known as *Schmorl's nodes*.[52,53] Protrusion of nuclear material at the anterior edge of the vertebral body that causes a triangular fragment of bone to be separated from the body is called a *limbus vertebra*.[54] Anterior and intravertebral disc herniations, by themselves and excluding associated trauma, are usually devoid of clinical symptomatology.

Intraspinal disc herniations are posterior or posterolateral protrusions of nuclear material that have the potential to compromise the spinal canal and neural elements, presenting significant symptomology often requiring therapeutic or medical intervention. Intraspinal herniations may result from acute trauma such as falls or heavy lifting, or from pre-existing degener-

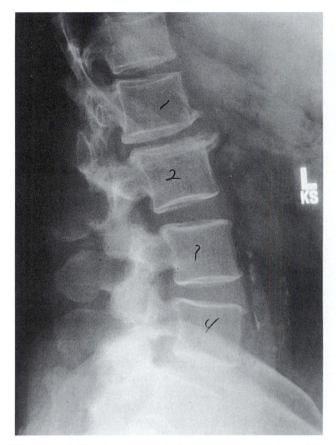

FIGURE 6–39. Spondylosis deformans. Degeneration of the annulus fibrosus may result in osteophytic build-up along the margins of the vertebral end plate. These osteophytes occur predominantly at the sites of attachment of the anterior longitudinal ligament along the anterior and anterolateral aspects of the vertebral bodies. In this lateral plain film of the lumbar spine, large osteophytes are present at L1 and L2. When the osteophytes occur along the margins of the vertebrae, they are sometimes referred to as *claw spurs*; when they are nonmarginal, they are sometimes referred to as *traction spurs*.

ative conditions that weaken the elasticity and resiliency of the annulus and the posterior ligaments, rendering the disc unable to withstand normal stresses. The physical characteristics of an intraspinal herniation are variable, as is the degree of symptoms that may appear. Terminology to describe the various degrees of disc herniations has not been standardized within the literature. Some more commonly used descriptions are (Fig. 6–40):

Posterior prolapse: The nucleus pulposus is displaced posteriorly within the confines of the annulus fibrosus, causing a distortion of the posterior boundaries of the annular ring. The annulus may or may not protrude into the spinal canal.

Contained disc herniation: Radial tears extend to the posterolateral corner of the annulus and a portion of the nucleus displaces to the extent of the tear, but remains contained under the posterior longitudinal ligament.

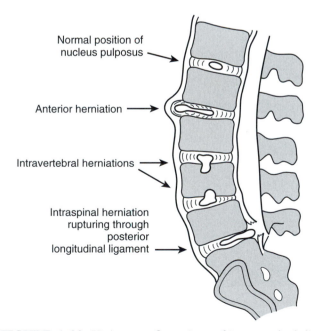

FIGURE 6–38. Various configurations of intervertebral disc herniations.

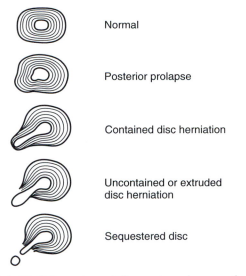

Normal

Posterior prolapse

Contained disc herniation

Uncontained or extruded disc herniation

Sequestered disc

FIGURE 6–40. Schematic to define various degrees of posterior disc herniations, as viewed in cross section.

FIGURE 6–41. Degenerative disc disease of the lumbar spine in a 66-year-old female. (*A*) Lateral film demonstrates decreased disc space height at all lumbar segments and lower thoracic segments. Spondylosis deformans (osteophyte formation in response to degenerative disc disease) is evident at all vertebral margins both anteriorly and posteriorly (see all arrows). The L4–5 disc space is greatly diminished, and a radiolucency is seen paralleling the end plate. This is known as the *vacuum sign* and is thought to represent a collection of nitrogen gas from adjacent extracellular fluid that has seeped into the discal fissures. In movements of the spine that produce a decrease of pressure in the disc, such as extension, nitrogen is released from the adjacent extracellular fluid and, because of the pressure gradient, accumulates in the fissures of the disc. This collection of gas can be made to disappear with spinal flexion and reappear with extension. Studies have shown this vacuum sign to be a common sign of disc aging and degeneration with an incidence of 2 to 3% in the general population. The large arrow indicates the vacuum sign. (*B*) An anteroposterior view of the spine demonstrates marginal spurs, a scoliosis, and, again, the radiolucency in the L4–5 interspace, which is referred to as the vacuum sign.

Uncontained or extruded disc herniation: Pressure of the herniation forces the nucleus through the annulus and causes the posterior longitudinal ligament to protrude into the spinal canal.

Sequestered disc: A portion of the nucleus has separated and migrated into the spinal canal.

Standard radiographic evaluation for disc herniation is of little value and will read normal except for pre-existing degenerative changes (Fig. 6–41). Ancillary imaging techniques, including myelography, discography, computed tomography (CT), and MRI, are used alone or as complementary investigative studies to diagnose and determine a treatment plan. See Figure 1–26 for a myelogram study of a posterior disc herniation in the lumbar spine. See Figure 4–36 for an MRI study of a disc herniation in the cervical spine.

SACROILIAC PATHOLOGY[55,56]

Ligamentous Injury

As the characteristics of motion at the sacroiliac joints remain controversial, so it follows that the characteristics of injury patterns sustained by the joints are also controversial. Subluxation hypotheses and various types of strain and sprain attributed to the sacro-

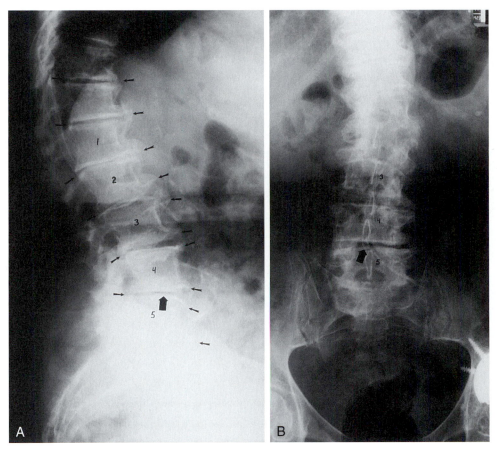

A   B

iliac joints are debated for their role in low back pain syndromes. The extreme stability of the joints afforded by the topographical anatomy discourages hypermobility theories, while the fact that the joints are synovial and innervated strongly supports joint susceptibility to painful ligamentous strain, inflammation, hypo- or hypermobility, and degenerative changes.

Radiographic examination of the sacroiliac joints is not able to evaluate sacroiliac joint stability or instabilities. The presence of acute inflammation and degenerative changes is discussed next.

Degenerative Joint Disease

Degenerative changes in the sacroiliac joints manifest the same hallmarks as seen radiographically in any synovial joint: decreased joint space, subchondral sclerosis, and osteophyte formation at joint margins.

Radiographically, only the lower halves of the joint space image represent the synovial portion of the joints. The upper portions of the joints are syndesmotic. Thus, evaluation of degenerative joint disease is confined to the lower half of the radiographic joint space.

Sacroiliitis

Sacroiliitis is inflammation of the synovial portions of the sacroiliac joints. Etiology may be an inflam-

matory disorder, infection, or early degenerative processes.

Radiographically, the lower half of the joint space will appear wide secondary to progressive inflammatory erosions. In later subacute stages the joint spaces will be narrowed and exhibit other changes typical of degenerative joint disease (Fig. 6–42).

Ankylosing Spondylitis[57–60]

Ankylosing spondylitis is a chronic, progressive, inflammatory arthritis characterized by joint sclerosis and ligamentous ossification. The disease usually manifests first in stiffness of the sacroiliac joints and later extends to the lumbar and thoracic spines. Numerous extra-articular features including pulmonary fibrosis and cardiac insufficiencies may complicate the disease. Men are affected with seven times greater incidence than women, with onset predominantly in the 20s. Early diagnosis is confirmed by laboratory studies.

Radiographic evidence of the disease often appears first in abnormal narrowing of the upper half of the sacroiliac joints. Fusion of the joint spaces eventually occurs (Fig. 6–43). Squaring-off of the anterior borders of the vertebral bodies is another early radiographic indicator of the disease. In later stages, syndesmophytes form, bridging the vertebral bodies. Additionally, facet joints and intervertebral joints fuse, and the entire spine then exhibits the hallmark radiographic image of the disease known as the "bamboo spine."

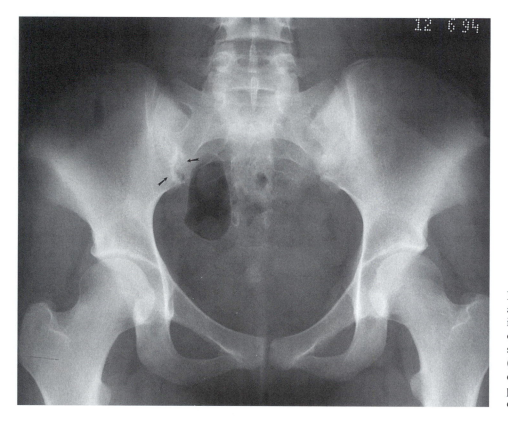

FIGURE 6–42. Sacroiliitis. This anteroposterior view of the sacroiliac joints demonstrates narrowing of the right sacroiliac joint with sclerosis of the subchondral bone (arrows). The possible differential diagnosis for this patient included psoriatic arthritis, Reiter's syndrome, and infection.

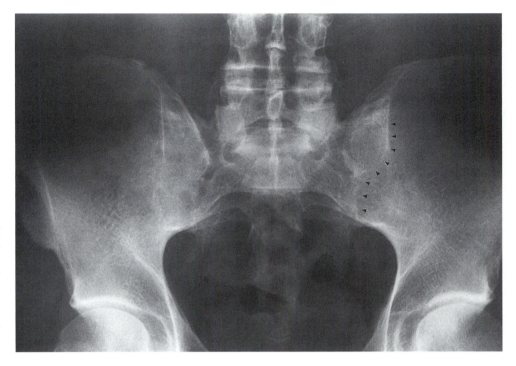

FIGURE 6–43. Ankylosing spondylitis. This 54-year-old man was diagnosed with ankylosing spondylitis several years ago. The location of the left sacroiliac joint is barely discernible (arrowheads). Much of the right sacroiliac joint has been totally obliterated by bony fusion across the joint space.

LUMBOSACRAL ANOMALIES[60–65]

As noted previously, congenital or developmental anomalies occur with frequency at the junctions of the spinal curvatures. The lumbosacral junction, similar to the thoracolumbar junction, is often the site of vertebral anomalies. Anomalies are generally related to a structure's (1) failure to develop, (2) arrested development, or (3) development of accessory bones. Spinal anomalies may occur in isolation or in combination with other spinal, visceral, or soft tissue malformations.

The descriptions of block vertebrae, butterfly vertebrae, hemivertebrae, and Schmorl's nodes as presented in Chapter 5 regarding thoracic spine anomalies hold true for their appearances in the lumbar spine. Refer to Table 5–3 for summaries of these anomalies.

Common anomalies appearing with greatest frequency at the lumbosacral junction include *facet tropism, transitional vertebrae,* and *spina bifida.*

Facet Tropism

Facet tropism ("turning in") refers to the asymmetry of the planes of the facet joint articulations at one spinal level. The facet joints at L5–S1, for example, will each be oriented to a different plane.[66]

Clinical considerations focus on the altered joint biomechanics. Asymmetrical movements will occur at that segment, and adjacent segments will likely accommodate with excessive compensatory motion. Degenerative joint disease of the involved segment and the adjacent segments may be accelerated.

Radiographically, one facet joint space will appear normally radiolucent while the involved facet joint space appears absent, as it is not in the normal plane of evaluation (Fig. 6–44).

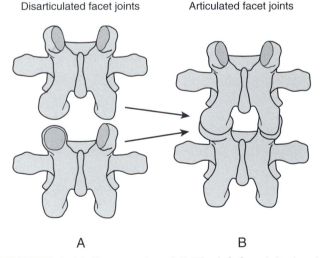

Disarticulated facet joints   Articulated facet joints

A   B

FIGURE 6–44. Facet tropism. (*A*) The left facet joint is oriented in a frontal plane, (*B*) while the right facet joint at the same level is oriented in a sagittal plane.

Transitional Vertebrae[67–69]

Transitional vertebrae are vertebrae that have adopted characteristics of vertebrae from an adjacent spinal region. Transitional vertebrae appear most frequently at the junctions of the spinal curvatures, where the normally marked morphologic changes appearing in the vertebrae of one region compared with the next are most pronounced. The cervicothoracic and thoracolumbar areas may exhibit transitional vertebrae, but the lumbosacral area is the most common region of occurrence.

In the lumbosacral region transitional vertebrae have sometimes been described by the terms "lumbarization of S1" or "sacralization of L5." "Transitional vertebra" encompasses all variations, and, like elsewhere in radiology, the variations are most clearly defined by exact anatomic description of the morphological characteristics.

Most commonly seen is the adoption of sacral characteristics by the L5 vertebra (Figs. 6–45, 6–46). The transverse processes of L5 expand in width and height, appearing more in size like the sacral ala than normal lumbar processes. These enlarged transverse processes may form accessory joints, either unilaterally or bilaterally, with the ilia. The body of L5 usually remains normal in size although the L5–S1 intervertebral disc is generally vestigial.

Clinically, a lumbar transitional vertebra is thought to be insignificant, with no evidence of predisposition to low back pain or role in prolonging low back pain. It is reasonable to assume, however, that the decreased

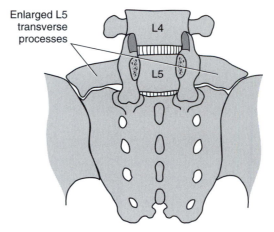

FIGURE 6–45. Transitional L5 vertebra. Note the enlarged transverse processes forming articulations with the sacrum and iliac crests.

mobility caused by accessory articulations and the vestigial disc would cause the adjacent freely moving segments to compensate and predispose those segments to degenerative changes. Furthermore, if the accessory articulations at the transitional segment are unilateral, resultant altered biomechanics of both the transitional segment and adjacent segments may predispose the joints to accelerated degenerative changes.

Radiographically, the AP view will show the en-

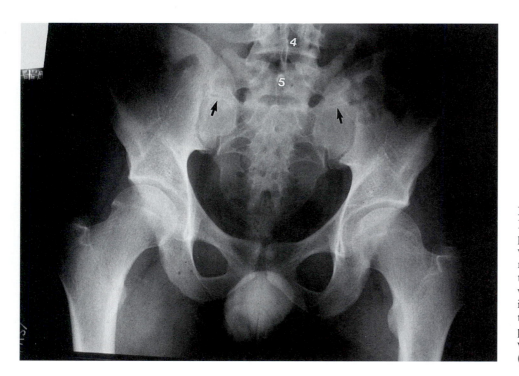

FIGURE 6–46. Sacralization of L5. Note the enlarged transverse processes of L5, expanded in width and height, appearing more in size like the sacral ala than like normal lumbar transverse processes. Additionally, the inferior aspect of the enlarged transverse processus of L5 appears to have formed articulations with the ala of the sacrum (arrows).

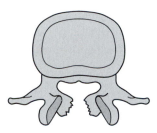

FIGURE 6–47. Spina bifida is a failure of the posterior vertebral arches to unite.

larged transverse processes, the presence of accessory articulations of the transverse processes to the ilia, and the narrowed disc space at L5–S1.

Spina Bifida[70–74]

Spina bifida is a failure of the posterior vertebral arches to fuse (Fig. 6–47). Spina bifida is the most common congenital anomaly of the spine and varies in degrees of severity of neural compromise from no clinical significance to complete paralysis.

Spina bifida occulta (*occulta* meaning "hidden") is the most benign manifestation and is often discovered on radiograph as a purely incidental finding (Figs. 6–48, 6–49). Spina bifida occulta is the failure of the laminae to fuse at midline and form a spinous process. There is no associated neurologic involvement, and the architecture of the vertebra is not weakened. Although uninformed patients may be alarmed at this radiographic finding, it usually holds no clinical significance. Radiographically, the AP view will show a radiolucent cleft between the laminae, and an absent or diminutive spinous process.

Spina bifida vera or *spina bifida manifesta* is the more serious expression of this anomaly, exhibiting a defect in posterior arch fusion large enough to allow protrusion of the spinal cord and its coverings outside of the spinal canal. The sac that forms outside of the body is called a *meningocele* if it contains only cerebrospinal fluid, spinal cord coverings, and nerve roots but the spinal cord remains within the canal. The neurologic deficits are variable in this case and may not be evident at birth but develop in later childhood. A *meningomyelocele* is a sac that contains the meningocele structures plus the spinal cord itself (Fig. 6–50). Complications include serious neurologic deficits, deformities, and hydrocephalus. The most devastating version of spinal cord herniation is the *myelocele* (*rachischisis*). In this case the herniation of the cord and related structures is completely outside and without protective covering of the dura or skin. Infection often leads to infant death.

Radiographically, the AP view will show a wide interpedicular distance, representing the failure of arches to develop. On the lateral film a water density mass may be evident posterior to the bony defect, representing the cerebrospinal fluid within the sac.

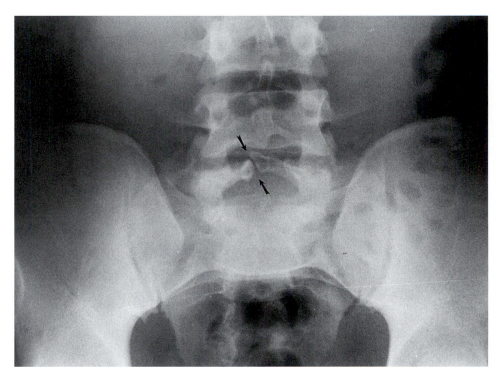

FIGURE 6–48. Spina bifida occulta. An incidental finding during evaluation of the sacroiliac joints in this young man was a developmental failure of the posterior lamina to unite. The arrows mark the radiolucent cleft representing the unfused arch.

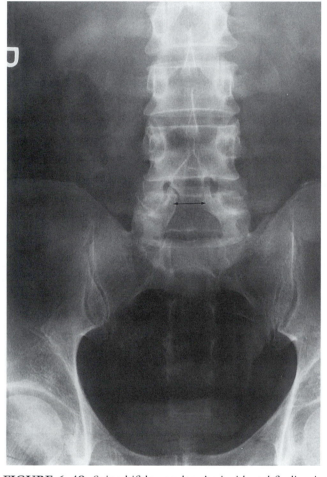

FIGURE 6–49. Spina bifida occulta. An incidental finding in a routine lumbar series in this 41-year-old man was a large radiolucent cleft at L5, representing a failure of the laminae to unite and form a spinous process. The lined arrow extends over the width of the cleft. No clinical symptoms were related to this finding.

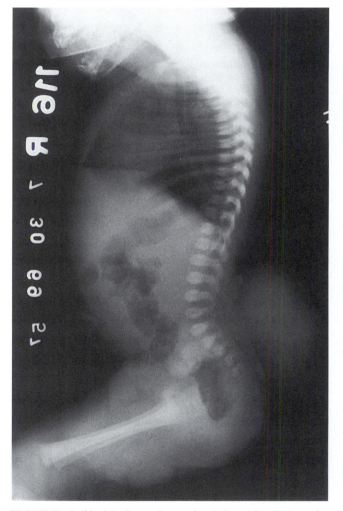

FIGURE 6–50. Myelomeningocele. A large lumbar myelomeningocele is demonstrated on this lateral view of a 2-day-old infant boy.

SUMMARY OF KEY POINTS

1. The routine radiographic evaluation of the lumbar spine includes five projections:
   - **Anteroposterior:** Demonstrates all five lumbar vertebral bodies.
   - **Lateral:** Demonstrates alignment of the lumbar vertebrae and the intervertebral disc spaces.
   - **Right and left obliques:** Demonstrates the facet joint articulations. The "scottie dog" image is seen on this projection.
   - **Lateral L5–S1 spot film:** Demonstrates in greater detail the lumbosacral junction.
2. The routine radiographic evaluation of the sacroiliac joint includes an anteroposterior axial projection, which views both joints simultaneously, and right and left oblique projections, which view each sacroiliac joint individually.
3. Compression fractures of the vertebral bodies are common injuries at the thoracolumbar (T11–L2) region.
4. Spondylolysis refers to a defect at the pars interarticularis. The defect may be secondary to an acute fracture or, more commonly, to a stress fracture due to chronic strain. Radiographically spondylolysis is diagnosed on the oblique projection as a radiolucent streak across the pars interarticularis, often referred to as the image of a collar on a scottie dog.
5. Spondylolisthesis is the anterior displacement of one vertebra upon the stationary vertebra beneath it. Spondylolisthesis may be secondary to spondylolysis or to degenerative joint changes that result in subluxation. The latter is described as degenerative spondylolisthesis or pseudospondylolisthesis.
6. Spinal stenosis is a narrowing of the spinal canal caused by degenerative joint and disc changes. The location of spinal stenosis is divided into three anatomic regions: (1) stenosis of the central canal, (2) stenosis of the intervertebral foramen, and (3) stenosis of the lateral or subarticular recesses. More than one region may be involved at the same intervertebral level. Radiographically, stenosis is suggested by the location of the degenerative changes. Additional studies such as myelography, CT, and MRI can define the amount of encroachment and thecal sac constriction.
7. Intervertebral disc herniation is a protrusion of the nuclear disc material through the confines of the annulus fibrosus. Herniations may occur anteriorly, intravertebrally, or intraspinally. Anterior disc herniations may elevate the anterior longitudinal ligament, instigating osteophyte formation at the anterior and lateral joint margins known as spondylosis deformans. Intravertebral disc herniations may protrude through the vertebral endplates and form osseous cavities known as Schmorl's nodes. Intraspinal herniations generally protrude posterolaterally and have the potential to compress neural elements.
8. Radiography is helpful in the evaluation of sacroiliac joint pathologies such as degenerative joint disease and sacroiliitis. The radiographic assessment is directed to the lower halves of the joints, which are synovial articulations.
9. Ankylosing spondylitis is a progressive inflammatory arthritis characterized by joint sclerosis and ligamentous ossification. The disease usually manifests first in the sacroiliac joints and later ascends through the lumbar and thoracic spines. Early radiographic indicators include abnormal narrowing of the upper halves of the sacroiliac joints and squaring off of the anterior borders of the vertebral bodies,. In later stages syndesmophytes form, bridging vertebral bodies and presenting the characteristic "bamboo spine" image on radiographs.
10. Anomalies appear with some frequency at the lumbosacral spine and are often incidental findings, without significant clinical implications. Examples of anomalies include spina bifida occulta, facet tropism, and transitional vertebrae.

REFERENCES

1. Netter, FH: The Ciba Collection of Medical Illustrations, Vol 8, Part I, Musculoskeletal System. Ciba-Geigy Corporation, Summit, NJ, 1978, pp 15–19.
2. Richardson, JK and Iglarsh, ZA: Clinical Orthopaedic Physical Therapy. WB Saunders, Philadelphia, 1994, pp 120–122.
3. Netter, pp 15–19.
4. Richardson, pp 120–122.
5. Nordin, M and Frankel, VH: Basic Biomechanics of the Musculoskeletal System, ed 2. Lea & Febiger, Malvern, PA, 1989, pp 187–194.

6. Magee, DJ: Orthopedic Physical Assessment, ed 2. WB Saunders, Philadelphia, 1992, pp 170–177.
7. Richardson, pp 126–127.
8. Magee, pp 170, 177.
9. Richardson, pp 125–127.
10. Nordin, pp 192–194, 201–203.
11. Gehweiler, JA, Osborne, RL, and Becker, RF: The Radiology of Vertebral Trauma. WB Saunders, Philadelphia, 1980, pp 24, 38, 51–60.
12. Meschan, I: An Atlas of Normal Radiographic Anatomy. WB Saunders, Philadelphia, 1960, p 420.
13. Magee, pp 199–208.
14. Meschan, pp 416–429.
15. Bontrager, KL: Textbook of Radiographic Positioning and Related Anatomy, ed 3. Mosby Yearbook, St Louis, 1993, pp 218–265.
16. Gehweiler, pp 26–38, 389–390.
17. Wicke, L: Atlas of Radiological Anatomy, ed 5. Lea & Febiger, Malvern, PA, 1994, p 34.
18. Rockwood, CA and Green, DP (eds): Fractures in Adults, Vol 2. JB Lippincott, Philadelphia, 1984, pp 1122–1124, 1156–1158.
19. Weissman, BW and Sledge, CB: Orthopedic Radiology. WB Saunders, Philadelphia, 1986, pp 285–288, 346–397.
20. Greenspan, A: Orthopedic Radiology: A Practical Approach, ed 2. Raven Press, New York, 1992, pp 10.27–10.53.
21. Ibid, p 10.31.
22. Yochum, TR and Rowe, LJ: Essentials of Skeletal Radiology. Williams & Wilkins, Baltimore, 1987, pp 448–450.
23. Schultz, pp 140–143.
24. Salter, RB: Textbook of Disorders of Injuries of the Musculoskeletal System, ed 2. Williams & Wilkins, Baltimore, 1984, p 514.
25. Rockwood, pp 1036–1085.
26. Gehweiler, pp 263–295, 327–375.
27. Weissman, pp 325–326.
28. Greenspan, pp 10.36–10.42.
29. Salter, pp 316–317.
30. Magee, p 207.
31. Richardson, pp 142–144.
32. Yochum, pp 243–272.
33. Meschan, pp 416–420.
34. Brashear, HR and Raney, RB: Shand's Textbook of Orthopaedic Surgery. Mosby, St Louis, 1971, pp 349–352.
35. Gehweiler, pp 401–426, 449.
36. Rockwood, pp 1067–1068.
37. Greenspan, pp 10.43–10.45.
38. Weissman, pp 311–316.
39. Richardson, p 144.
40. Brashear, pp 352–353.
41. Weissman, pp 317–321.
42. Greenspan, p 12.16.
43. Salter, pp 229, 232.
44. Magee, p 172.
45. Richardson, p 148.
46. Nordin, pp 183–186.
47. Brashear, p 338.
48. Salter, p 227.
49. Weissman, pp 297–311.
50. Greenspan, pp 10.46–10.53.
51. Ibid, p 12.14.
52. Gehweiler, pp 296–300.
53. Salter, p 227.
54. Weissman, p 285.
55. Richardson, p 145.
56. Weissman, pp 373–377.
57. Ibid, pp 323–325.
58. Brashear, pp 143–148.
59. Salter, p 201.
60. Richardson, p 146.
61. Magee, pp 170, 205.
62. Brashear, p 348.
63. Salter, pp 132–135.
64. Gehweiler, pp 286–289, 353, 373–375.
65. Greenspan, p 26.1.
66. Magee, p 170.
67. Ibid, p 205.
68. Yochum, pp 121–122.
69. Brashear, p 348.
70. Yochum, pp 118–119, 244–245, 253.
71. Gehweiler, pp 353, 373–375.
72. Brashear, p 348.
73. Salter, pp 132–135.
74. Magee, p 205.

SELF-TEST

Chapter 6

REGARDING FILM A:

1. Identify this projection.
2. Which intervertebral disc spaces are narrowed?
3. The three curving parallel lines that indicate normal vertebral alignment are disrupted. Identify which vertebra is not in normal alignment.
4. Describe the altered position of this vertebra.
5. What altered bony characteristics are present along the anterior margins of several vertebrae? What are some possible clinical or pathological significances of these alterations?

REGARDING FILM B:

6. Identify this projection.
7. Describe the anomaly present. What are some possible clinical or pathological significances of this anomaly?

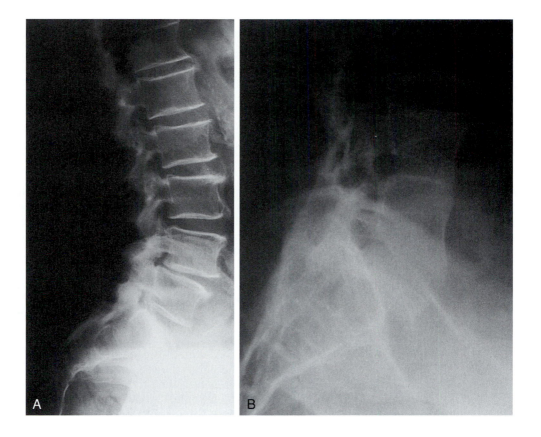

Pelvis and Proximal Femur

The *pelvis* can be considered the keystone of the skeleton, a link between the weight-bearing forces of the trunk and upper body and the ground forces transmitted by the lower body. The structural strength of the pelvis is provided by its substantial osseous components and its relatively rigid ringlike architecture. Trauma to the pelvis requires great force, and fractures here are often associated with serious vascular and visceral complications.

The *femur* is the largest bone in the body. The proximal ends of the femurs articulate with the pelvic acetabuluma to form the hip joints. The hip joints have great structural and ligamentous stability yet permit a wide range of motion. The primary function of the hip joints is to transmit ground forces in the erect skeleton, allowing for maintenance of upright posture and ambulation. The hip joints are common sites for degenerative changes to occur. The proximal femurs are common sites for fracture in the elderly.

The goals of this chapter are first to review osseous radiographic anatomy. Next, to briefly review ligamentous anatomy and joint mobility in order to assist the reader in understanding the functional movement of the hip joints. The routine radiographic evaluation of the pelvis and hip joints follows. Here the reader has an opportunity to interact and learn radiographic anatomy by tracing a radiograph with a marker on a transparency sheet, and then comparing results with the radiographic tracing. An additional goal is to present the radiographic characteristics of some common

fractures and pathologic conditions at the hip joints. A summary is organized into a list of practical points, highlighting the clinical aspects of the chapter. A self-test at the end of the chapter challenges the reader's visual interpretation skills.

RADIOGRAPHIC ANATOMY

Pelvis[1]

The pelvis consists of four bones: two *coxal* (innominate) bones, the *sacrum*, and the *coccyx*. The *ilium*, *ischium*, and *pubis* make up each coxal bone. The fusion of these three components forms the cup-shaped *acetabulum* that accepts the head of the femur to form the *hip joint* (Figs. 7–1, 7–2).

ILIUM

The superior portion of each coxal bone is the ilium. The flared, thin upper portion of the ilium is the *ala*. The upper margin of the ala is the *iliac crest*, extending from the *anterior superior iliac spine (ASIS)* to the *posterior superior iliac spine (PSIS)*. Less prominent landmarks include the *anterior inferior iliac spine (AIIS)*, inferior to the ASIS, and the *posterior inferior iliac spine (PIIS)*, inferior to the PSIS. The inferior portion of the

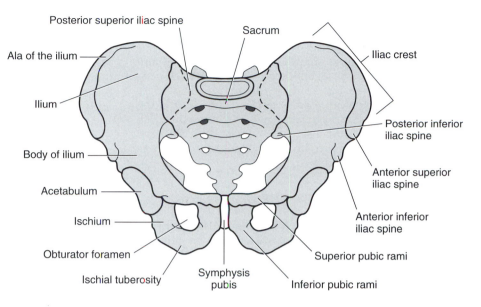

FIGURE 7–1. The bony pelvis.

ilium is the *body*, which includes the upper two-fifths of the acetabulum.

ISCHIUM

The *ischium* is the inferior and posterior portion of each coxal bone. The upper portion of the ischium is the *body*, and it forms the posterior two-fifths of the acetabulum. The lower portion is the *ramus*, ending caudally at the *ischial tuberosity*.

PUBIS

The *pubis* is the inferior and anterior portion of each coxal bone. The *body* of the pubis makes up the antero-

inferior one-fifth of the acetabulum. The *superior rami* extend anteriorly and medially from each body to form the midline *symphysis pubis joint*. The inferior rami extend posteriorly and join with each ischium.

Proximal Femur and Hip Joint[2]

The *proximal femur* is composed of four parts: the *head*, *neck*, *greater trochanter*, and *lesser trochanter* (Fig. 7–3).

HEAD

The head is spherical in shape, covered with cartilage, and has a central depression or *fovea* for attachment of the *capitis femoris ligament*. The head articulates with the acetabulum to form the *hip joint*.

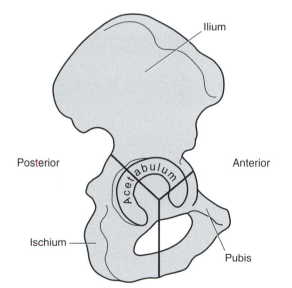

FIGURE 7–2. Each *innominate* bone is formed by the fusion of the ilium, ischium, and pubis bones. The cup-shaped *acetabulum* is formed at the junction of these three components.

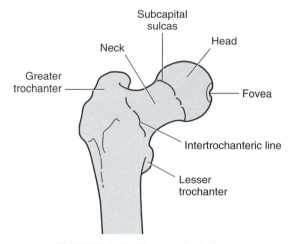

FIGURE 7–3. The proximal femur.

NECK

The head joins the neck at the *subcapital sulcus*. The neck is pyramidal in shape and contains prominent pits for the entrance of blood vessels. The neck connects the head to the *shaft* of the femur. The angle formed at the junction of the neck to the shaft is the *angle of inclination*, and measures in the range of 125 to 135 degrees in adults. The neck is also angled anteriorly on the shaft, approximately 15 degrees in adults. This is called *anteversion*.

GREATER AND LESSER TROCHANTERS

The greater trochanter is a large quadrilateral projection marking the upper lateral end of the femoral shaft. The lesser trochanter is a smaller conical projection marking the junction of the inferior medial neck to the femoral shaft. The *intertrochanteric crest* joins the trochanters posteriorly. The *intertrochanteric line* on the anterior aspect of the femur represents the junction of the neck to the shaft and the site of attachment of the hip joint *capsule*.

HIP JOINTS AND LIGAMENTS

The hip joint is a synovial ball-and-socket joint. The spherical femoral head articulates with the acetabulum which is deepened by a fibrocartilaginous *labrum*. The strong fibrous joint capsule extends from the bony rims and labrum of the acetabulum to the intertrochanteric line just superior to the intertrochanteric crest.

Three ligaments or thickenings of the joint capsule provide stability to the hip joint (Fig. 7–4): (1) the *iliofemoral ligament* lies anteriorly and extends from the AIIS to the intertrochanteric line. It is taut in full extension and promotes stabilization of the pelvis on the femur in erect posture. (2) The *pubofemoral ligament* lies medially and inferiorly and extends from the inferior acetabular rim to the inferior femoral neck. It assists in limiting abduction and extension. (3) The *ischiofemoral*

ligament forms the posterior margins of the capsule and extends from the ischial portion of the acetabulum to the superior femoral neck. Additionally, the *capitis femoris ligament* acts in providing joint stabilization. Extending from the fovea on the femoral head to the acetabular notch, the capitis femoris ligament limits adduction.

JOINT MOBILITY[3]

Mobility at the pelvis occurs at the articulations of the sacroiliac joints and by associated deformation of the fibrocartilaginous *interpubic disc* at the symphysis pubis (see Chapter 6) for sarcoiliac joint mobility.

Mobility at the hip takes places in all three planes. In the sagittal plane approximately 0 to 140 degrees of flexion and 0 to 15 degrees of extension are possible. Abduction ranges from 0 to 30 degrees and adduction ranges from 0 to 25 degrees. When the hip is flexed, 0 to 90 degrees of external rotation and 0 to 70 degrees of internal rotation is possible. Circumduction, or a combination of movement through the elemental planes, is also freely available at the hip joints. Gliding of the articular surfaces upon each other occurs as component movements during all of these motions.

GROWTH AND DEVELOPMENT[4]

Pelvis

At birth a large portion of the pelvis is ossified, but the upper ilium, majority of the acetabulum, lower end of the ischium, and medial end of the pubis are cartilaginous (Fig. 7–5). The junction of the cartilaginous portions of the ilium, ischium, and pubis forms the *triradiate cartilage* that makes up the *acetabular fossa*. By age 10, most of the cartilage has ossified in the coxal

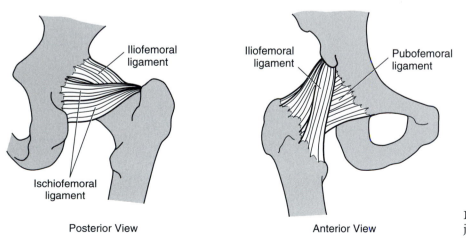

Posterior View   Anterior View

FIGURE 7–4. Ligaments of the hip joint.

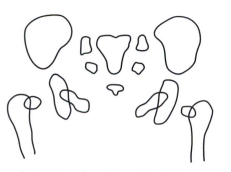

FIGURE 7–5. Tracing of a radiograph of the ossified portions of the pelvis at birth.

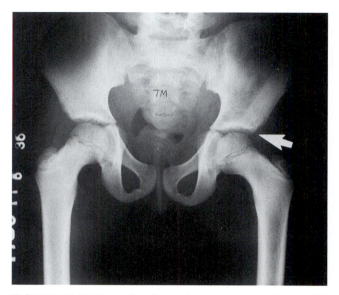

FIGURE 7–7. Normal radiographic appearance of the pelvis of a healthy 7-year-old boy. The innominate bones are ossified with the exception of the triradiate cartilage (arrow) of the acetabular fossa. At the sacrum, the bodies, neural arches, and costal processes have fused over the past 2 years and the sacrum now appears in its gross adult form. The sacroiliac joints remain wide in appearance. At the femurs, the epiphyses for the greater trochanters, which had appeared approximately 2 years earlier, are now well developed and ossified. The epiphyses for the lesser trochanters will appear in another 2 or 3 years. Note the decrease in the angles of inclination of the femoral necks to the femoral shafts compared to the radiograph at age 2.

bones, although the triradiate cartilage remains (Figs. 7–6, 7–7). Secondary centers of ossification appear at puberty. The triradiate cartilage fuses at about age 17, whereas the remaining coxal epiphyses may not fuse until the early 20s.

The shape of the pelvis is similar in males and females until puberty. At that time distinct differences begin and development is modified according to sex Fig. 7–8). The adult male pelvis is usually narrower and less flared, exhibiting an oval or heart-shaped pelvic inlet, and a less-than-90-degree angle of the pubic arch. The adult female pelvis, adapted for childbirth,

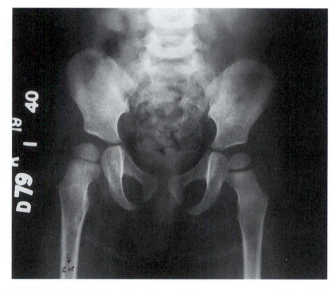

FIGURE 7–6. Normal radiographic appearance of the pelvis of a healthy 2-year-old girl. The majority of the pelvis is ossified, except the acetabulum is primarily cartilaginous. Note the normal appearance of very wide sacroiliac joints and the unfused sacral bodies. At the femur, the epiphysis for the femoral head is well ossified; the epiphyses for the greater and lesser trochanters will not appear for several more years. Note also the large angle of inclination of the femoral neck to the femoral shaft. This angle will progressively decrease with growth and development of the femur.

is usually broader, exhibits a round pelvic inlet, and has an angle of pubic arch greater than 90 degrees. (Fig. 7–9).

Proximal Femur

The shaft of the femur is ossified at birth. Ossification extends to the neck soon after birth. The epiphysis for the head of the femur initiates ossification between 3 and 6 months of age. The epiphysis for the greater trochanter appears between 4 and 5 years of age, and the epiphysis for the lesser trochanter between 9 and 11 years of age. All of these secondary ossification centers fuse in the late teens (see Figs. 7–5, 7–6, 7–7).

The angles of inclination of the femoral neck to the shaft are quite large at birth and decrease with development. At birth the neck-to-shaft angle is approximately 175 degrees. Subsequent growth of the femur decreases the angle to approximately 125 degrees in the adult. Additionally, approximately 40 degrees of anteversion is present at birth, decreasing to approximately 15 degrees in adulthood. Consequently, the acetabulum adapts its obliquity to accommodate the growing femur, exhibiting a 10-degree difference in horizontal orientation from birth to maturity.

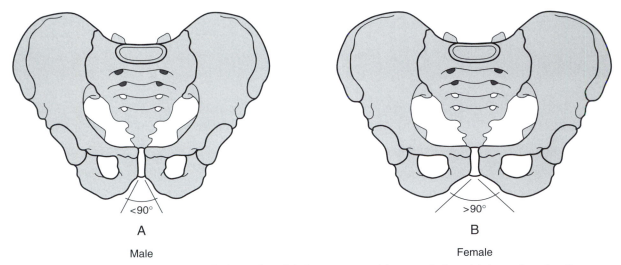

A
Male

B
Female

FIGURE 7–8. (*A*) In general, the male pelvis is narrower, with an oval-shaped inlet and angle of pubic arch less than 90 degrees; in contrast to (*B*) the female pelvis, which is broader, with a rounder inlet and greater angle of pubic arch.

ROUTINE RADIOGRAPHIC EVALUATION[5–9]

Pelvis

Basic: Anteroposterior

The basic radiographic evaluation of the pelvis includes by proximity a basic evaluation of the bilateral hip joints. Thus the *anteroposterior radiograph of the pelvis* provides an *anteroposterior view of both hip joints*. This is advantageous for bilateral comparison purposes. For teaching purposes here, the pelvis and hip will be presented as individual evaluations. Any redundancy hopefully reinforces the learning process.

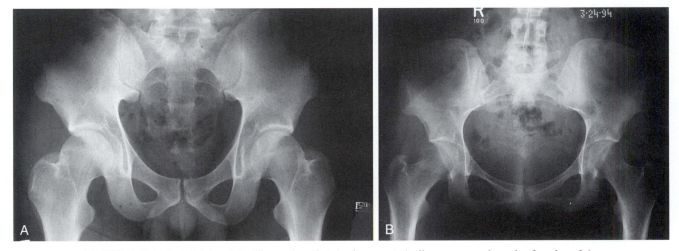

FIGURE 7–9. (*A*) *Male pelvis.* The male pelvis is characteristically narrower than the female pelvis, with an oval or heart-shaped pelvic inlet. (*B*) *Female pelvis.* The female pelvis is characteristically broader than the male pelvis, with a round-shaped pelvic inlet.

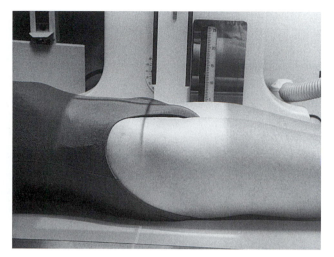

FIGURE 7–10. Patient position for an AP projection of the pelvis.

ANTEROPOSTERIOR (FIGS. 7–10, 7–11, 7–12)

This view demonstrates the entire pelvis, sacrum and coccyx, the lumbosacral articulation, and both proximal femurs and hip joints for comparison purposes. The important observations are:

1. The general architecture of the pelvic girdle appears symmetric on each side of midline.
2. The interpubic cartilaginous disc of the symphysis pubis is represented by a radiolucent potential space.
3. The sacroiliac joints and their potential joint spaces are visible (see Sacroiliac joint, AP Axial, in Chapter 6 for further detail).
4. The hip joints are normally articulated and the femurs exhibit symmetric angles of inclination (see Hip AP for further details).
5. The iliac ala or wings normally become more radio-

lucent at their anterolateral borders owing to thinning of the bony mass.
6. The landmarks of the acetabulum and related structures are referenced by several radiographic lines (Fig. 7–13). Disruptions in these line images may indicate fracture or other abnormality.[10,11]

Radiographic teardrop: An image seen on the medial aspect of the acetabulum, formed by the cortical surfaces of the pubic bone and ischium comprising the anteroinferior aspect of the acetabulum.

Iliopubic (or iliopectineal or arcuate) line: A line from the sciatic notch to the pubic tubercle.

Ilioischial line: A line representing the posteromedial margin of the quadrilateral surface of the iliac bone. Normally this line is tangential to or intersects the radiographic teardrop.

Anterior acetabular rim: Represents the anterior margins of the acetabular cup.

Posterior acetabular rim: Represents the posterior cortical rim of the acetabular cup.

Acetabular roof: Represents the superior cortical aspect of the acetabular cup, which corresponds to the major weight-bearing portion of the acetabulum.

CLINICAL OBJECTIVES

1. Trace each coxal bone.
2. Trace L5, sacrum, and coccyx.
3. Trace the proximal femurs.
4. Trace the acetabulum.
5. Trace the iliopubic, ilioischial, and teardrop lines.
6. Trace the acetabular roof, anterior, and posterior rims.

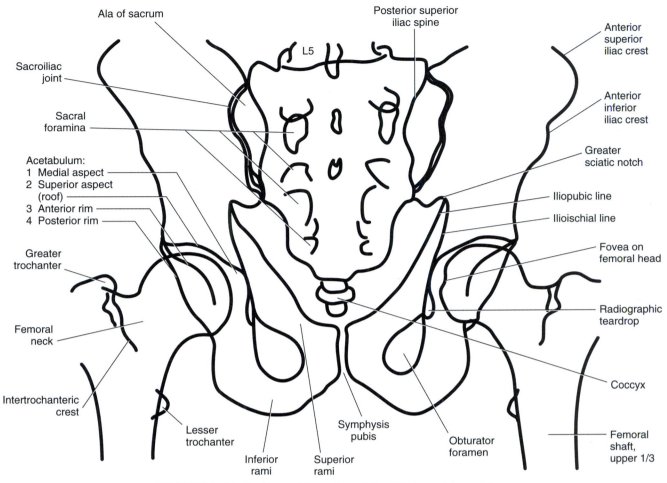

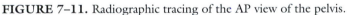

FIGURE 7–11. Radiographic tracing of the AP view of the pelvis.

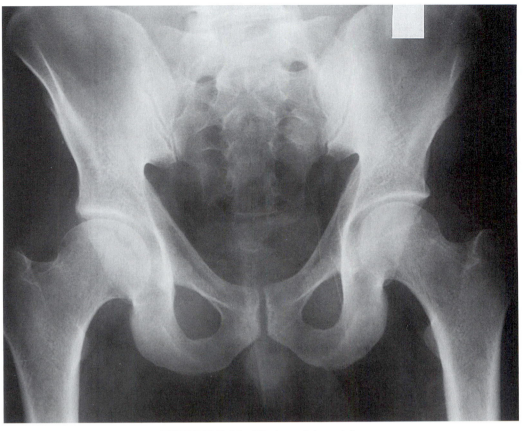

FIGURE 7–12. AP view of the pelvis.

Unilateral Hip and Proximal Femur

Basic: Anteroposterior, unilateral
        Lateral "frog-leg," unilateral

Unilateral hip radiographs are done to obtain greater radiographic detail of the proximal femur, acetabulum, and joint space, or when the interest is confined to one

side, as in the case of fracture and follow-up evaluation. An AP and lateral frog-leg view complete a routine hip evaluation.

Clarification is indicated for the almost standard use of the term "frog-leg," a reference to the position the patient's leg is placed in to provide a lateral view of the proximal femur. "Frog-leg," admittedly nonanatomic, is nonetheless a clear reminder of leg position. The "frog-leg" position defines a supine patient with

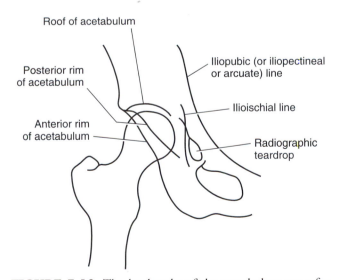

Roof of acetabulum

Posterior rim of acetabulum

Anterior rim of acetabulum

Iliopubic (or iliopectineal or arcuate) line

Ilioischial line

Radiographic teardrop

FIGURE 7–13. The landmarks of the acetabulum are referenced by distinct radiographic line images.

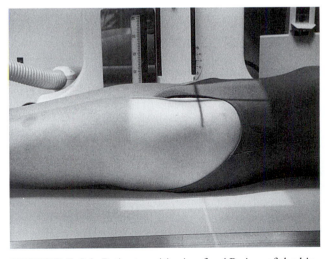

FIGURE 7–14. Patient positioning for AP view of the hip.

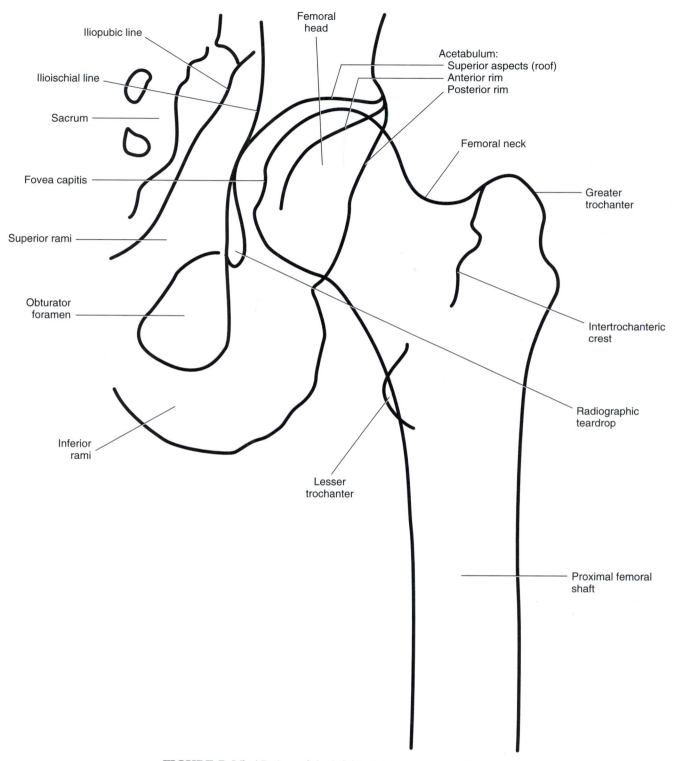

Iliopubic line

Ilioischial line

Sacrum

Fovea capitis

Superior rami

Obturator
foramen

Inferior
rami

Femoral
head

Acetabulum:
Superior aspects (roof)
Anterior rim
Posterior rim

Femoral neck

Greater
trochanter

Intertrochanteric
crest

Radiographic
teardrop

Lesser
trochanter

Proximal femoral
shaft

FIGURE 7–15. AP view of the left hip joint and proximal femur.

a flexed, externally rotated, and laterally abducted hip joint, combined with knee flexion. The radiograph is taken from an AP direction, but the beam actually travels through the medial to lateral aspect of the proximal femur. Thus, a lateral view of the hip, rotated 90 degrees from its position in the AP radiograph, is obtained. The descriptive "frog-leg" is a reminder of this.

In the instance of suspected fracture or trauma to the proximal femur or hip joint, the frog-leg positioning is not done because of the extreme movement it requires. In trauma cases an *axiolateral* or *groin-lateral* is substituted: The involved leg remains in neutral, while the opposite leg is elevated out of the way and the lateral projection is done in a medial-to-lateral direction through the involved proximal femur.

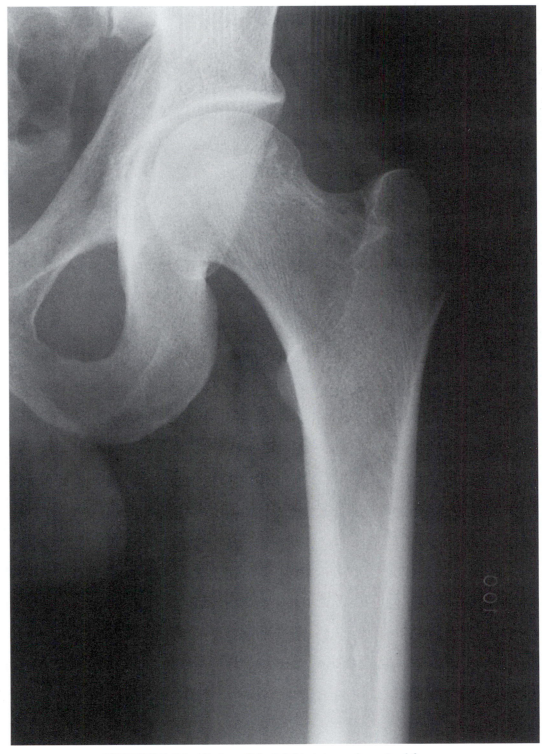

FIGURE 7–16. AP view of the left hip joint and proximal femur.

ANTEROPOSTERIOR (FIGS. 7–14, 7–15, 7–16)

This view demonstrates the acetabulum, femoral head, neck, and proximal one-third of the shaft, the greater trochanter, and the angle of inclination of the femoral neck to the shaft. The important observations are:

1. The patient is positioned supine with the legs straight and the involved lower extremity internally rotated 15 to 20 degrees. This amount of rotation compensates for the normal anteversion of the femoral neck and allows the neck to be visualized *en face*. In correct positioning the lesser trochanter is obscured, or only its tip is showing.

2. The hip joint radiographic joint space should be well preserved. Narrowing of the space indicates degeneration of the articular cartilage.
3. The osseous margins of the femoral head and acetabular cup should be smooth and clearly defined. Sclerotic subchondral areas, narrowed joint space, and osteophytes at the joint margins indicate degenerative joint disease.
4. The ball-and-socket configuration of the hip joint should be obvious. Destruction of normal joint congruity may be caused by various pathologies including avascular necrosis, rheumatoid arthritis, degenerative joint disease, and destructive tumors.
5. The increased density of the cortex of the femoral shaft is normally quite pronounced. Thinning or evaporation of this radiodense image indicates that an abnormal metabolic process is in effect, such as osteoporosis.
6. Trabecular markings of the head and neck normally appear clear and sharp. A washed-out or demineralized appearance may indicate that an abnormal metabolic process is present.
7. The normal angle of inclination of the femoral neck to the shaft is in the range of 125 to 135 degrees. the evaluation of femoral neck fracture, angles less

than this are varus deformities; angles greater than this are valgus deformities.[12]

CLINICAL OBJECTIVES

1. Trace the cetabulum. Identify the roof, anterior, and posterior rims.
2. Trace the proximal femur. Identify head, neck, and shaft.
3. Trace the greater and lesser trochanter and intertrochanteric crest.
4. Trace shade in the increased cortical densities of the neck and shaft.

LATERAL (FROG-LEG) (FIGS. 7–17, 7–18, 7–19)

This view demonstrates the femoral head, neck, and proximal one-third of the shaft, and the greater and lesser trochanters from the *medial* aspect. The important observations are:

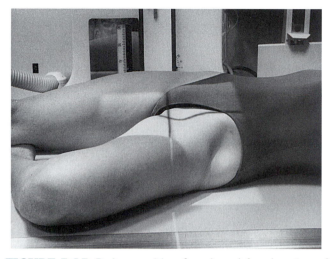

FIGURE 7-17. Patient position for a lateral frog-leg view of the left hip.

1. The hip of the supine patient has been positioned in flexion, external rotation, and lateral abduction. This alters the view of the femur 90 degrees from the AP hip.
2. The femur is now viewed from a medial to lateral aspect. The lesser trochanter is now anterior and the greater trochanter is posterior on this projection. The greater trochanter is thus superimposed behind the neck, and the lesser trochanter is superimposed in front of the neck and extends slightly below the medial border of the femur.
3. The expanse of the femoral head is well exposed.
4. The radiographic image of the acetabulum is unchanged from the AP view.
5. The angle of inclination of the femoral neck to shaft is not visible and the angle of anteversion is distorted; therefore, neither is evaluated on this view.

CLINICAL OBJECTIVES

1. Trace the acetabulum.
2. Trace the proximal femur. Identify head, neck, and shaft.
3. Trace the greater trochanter as it lies superimposed behind the neck.
4. Trace the lesser trochanter as it projects slightly beyond the lower margin of the femur.

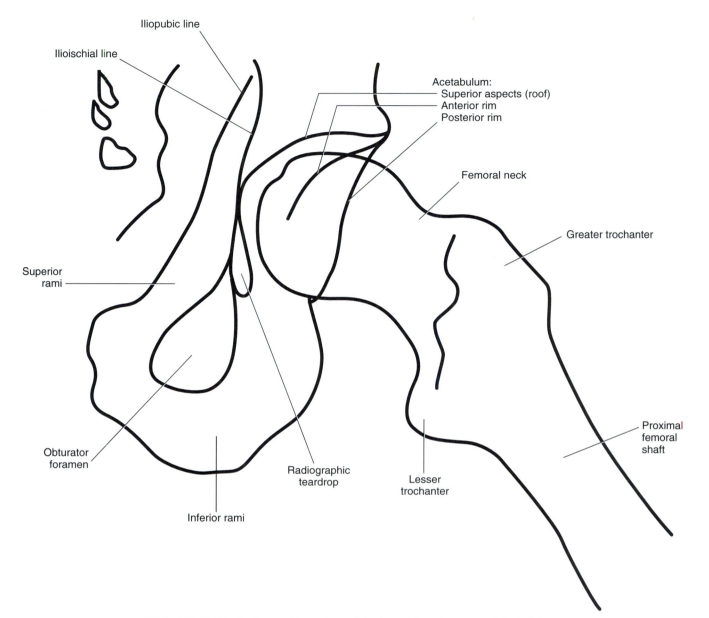

FIGURE 7–18. Radiographic tracing of the lateral frog-leg view of the left hip.

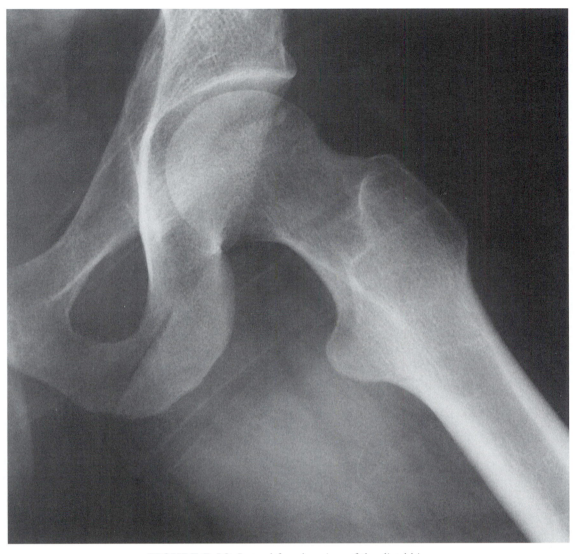

FIGURE 7–19. Lateral frog-leg view of the distal hip.

TRAUMA

Fractures of the Pelvis[13–15]

Fractures of the pelvis are associated with extreme forces and are thus often accompanied by medical complications involving major blood vessels, nerves, and the urinary tract. Most pelvic fractures are readily visible on the AP view of the pelvis, although conventional and computed tomography often assist diagnosis. Numerous ancillary techniques are used to evaluate soft tissue and visceral injuries.

Various classifications of pelvic fractures exist, based on configuration, force mechanisms, or inherent stability. The broadest categorization identifies stable versus unstable fractures. The determination of the stability of the *pelvic ring* is the significant factor in the orthopedic treatment, prognosis, and rehabilitation of the patient. The pelvic ring is defined as the continuous osseous cage formed by the paired coxal bones and the sacrum, including the relatively rigid articulations at the sacroiliac joints and the symphysis pubis.

Stable pelvic fractures do not disrupt any of the joint articulations (Fig. 7–20). Stable fractures include (1) avulsion fractures of the ASIS, AIIS, or ischial tuberosity, commonly seen in athletes owing to forceful or repetitive muscle contraction of the sartorius, rectus femoris, or hamstring attachments, respectively; (2) iliac wing fractures; (3) sacral fractures; and (4) ischiopubic fractures. The last three fractures are usually the result of lateral compression forces or vertical shear forces and falls. Ischiopubic rami fractures are quite common and constitute almost half of all pelvic fractures (Fig. 7–21, 7–22).

Unstable fractures result from disruption at two or more sites on the pelvic ring and are frequently associated with internal hemorrhage. Unstable fractures include (Fig. 7–23) (1) vertical shear or Malgaigne fractures, involving unilateral fractures of the superior and

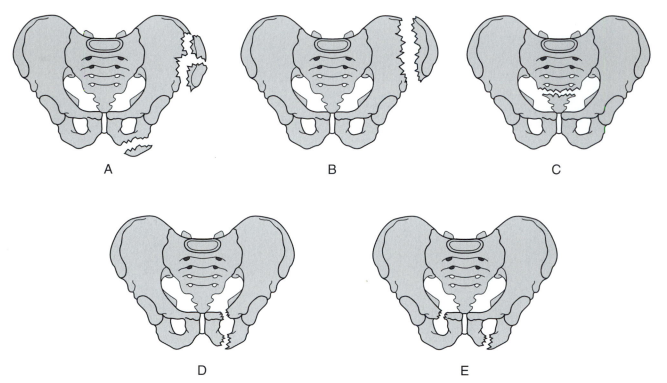

FIGURE 7–20. Examples of *stable* pelvic fractures include (*A*) avulsions of the ASIS, AIIS, or ischial tuberosity; (*B*) iliac wing fractures; (*C*) sacral fractures; and (*D*) ipsilateral and (*E*) contralateral pubic rami fractures.

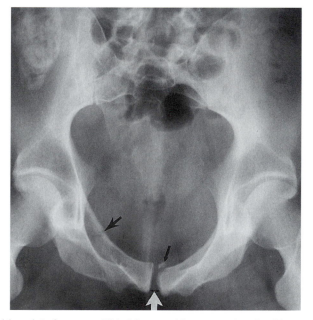

FIGURE 7–21. Stable pelvic fractures. This 29-year-old man was involved in a motor vehicle accident and sustained a fracture to his right superior pubic ramus (large black arrow), and a diastasis, or separation, of the symphysis pubis (white arrow). A small fragment of bone avulsed off the left superior margin of the symphysis pubis (small black arrow).

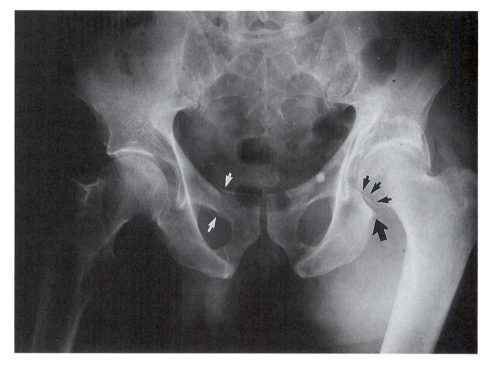

FIGURE 7–22. Stable pelvic fractures. This 55-year-old woman was injured in a motor vehicle accident. She sustained a complete transverse fracture of the right superior pubic rami (white arrows), and on the left side sustained an impaction fracture of the femoral head (3 arrows) and a fracture of the inferior acetabular rim (large black arrow). Note the great amount of swelling at the left hip. These types of fractures at the hip are commonly referred to as "dashboard fractures" because a common mechanism of injury is when the knee strikes the dashboard in a collision and the force is transmitted up the femur and into the acetabulum.

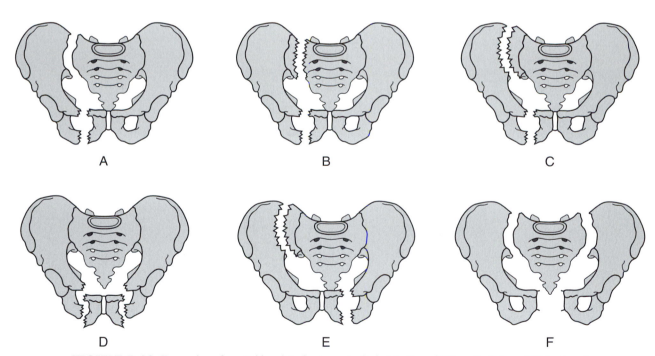

FIGURE 7–23. Examples of *unstable* pelvic fractures include (*A, B,* and *C*) vertical shear (Malgaigne) fractures, involving ischiopubic rami and disruption of an ipsilateral sacroiliac joint, be it (*A*) through the joint itself, (*B*) through a fracture of the sacral wing, or (*C*) a fracture on the iliac bone; (*D*) straddle fractures, involving all four ischiopubic rami; (*E*) bucket-handle fractures, involving an ischiopubic ramus and contralateral sacroiliac joint; and (*F*) dislocations involving one or both sacroiliac joints and the symphysis pubis.

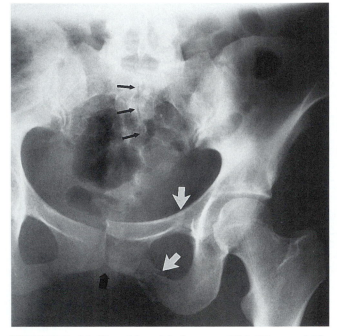

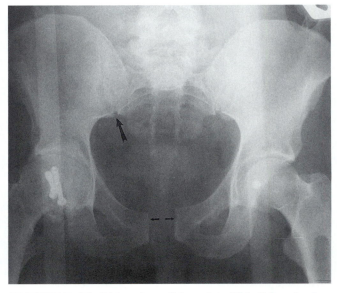

FIGURE 7–24. Unstable pelvic fractures. This 30-year-old female was injured in a motor vehicle accident. She sustained a vertical fracture through the body of the sacrum (3 black arrows), a left-side transverse superior pubic ramus fracture with superior displacement, a left-side comminuted inferior pubic ramus fracture (white arrows), and a diastasis of the symphysis pubis (large black arrow). These injuries constitute an unstable pelvic fracture pattern because more than two sites of the pelvic ring are disrupted.

FIGURE 7–25. Dislocation of the pelvis. This dislocation has occurred unilaterally, involving the right sacroiliac joint (large arrow), and a diastasis or separation of the symphysis pubis (small arrows). Note also the metallic screws in the right hip from a fixation of an old femoral neck fracture, advanced degenerative joint changes of the hip, and multiple loose bodies in the hip joint capsule.

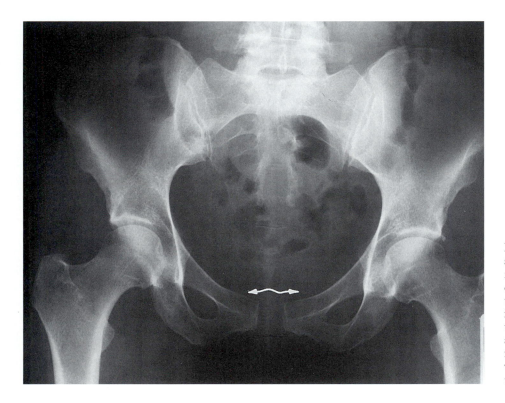

FIGURE 7–26. Diastasis of the symphysis pubis in a 35-year-old female following childbirth. The susceptibility of the ligamentous structures of the symphysis pubis to the increase in ligamentous-relaxing estrogen hormones during pregnancy and during labor may have been a factor in this condition. The wavy white arrow marks the separation of the joint.

inferior pubic rami and disruption of the ipsilateral sacroiliac joint (the damage at the sacroiliac joint may be through the joint itself, or via fracture of the nearby sacral wing or iliac bone); (2) straddle fractures, involving all four ischiopubic rami; and (3) "bucket-handle" fractures, involving an ischiopubic ramus and the contralateral sacroiliac joint. The mechanism of these fractures is often vertical shear, sometimes combined with AP or lateral compression forces (Figs. 7–24, 7–25).

Dislocations are also considered unstable injuries. Dislocations at the pelvis may occur unilaterally, involving one sacroiliac joint and the symphysis pubis, or bilaterally, involving both sacroiliac joints and the symphysis pubis. The bilateral pelvic dislocation is commonly referred to as a "sprung" pelvis. The precipitating force is usually an AP compression that in effect springs open the pelvis like opening a book. Dislocation of the symphysis pubis, also referred to as a *diastasis* or separation, can occur in isolation, as seen in cases of acute trauma, or related to pregnancy or delivery (Fig. 7–26).

Fractures of the Acetabulum[16–18]

Fractures of the acetabulum are sometimes difficult to evaluate on the routine AP pelvis and hip views, because of the superimposition of the femoral head and the configuration of the acetabular cup itself. For this reason, anterior and posterior *oblique* projections are sometimes done to complete the trauma evaluation. Conventional or computed tomography may supplement the plain radiographs, as in evaluation of the pelvis in trauma. Note, however, that the first indication of fracture on the AP pelvis projection may be a disruption in one or more of the six radiographic line images normally visible on that view (see Fig. 7–13).

Classification of acetabular fractures is related to anatomic position. The pelvis is divided into anterior and posterior columns (Fig. 7–27). The anterior column is composed of the iliopubic area, and the posterior column is composed of the ilioischial area. These divisions meet at the midline of the acetabulum. Fractures occurring at the acetabulum are thus defined as[19] (Fig.

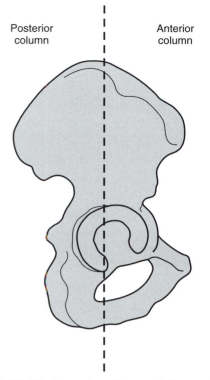

Posterior column   Anterior column

FIGURE 7–27. The innominate bone and the acetabulum are divided into *anterior* and *posterior columns* to reference the location of trauma.

7–28): (1) anterior column fractures, (2) posterior column fractures, (3) transverse fractures, involving both columns, or (4) complex fractures, involving a T-shaped configuration. The terms "anterior lip" or "posterior lip" fractures refer to fracture at the acetabular rims, without extension into the pubic or ischial bones. Posterior lip fractures and posterior column fractures are the most common acetabular fractures and are frequently associated with femoral head impaction or femoral head posterior dislocation (Fig. 7–29). These fractures are often referred to as "dashboard" fractures, as they result from the knee contacting the dashboard in a motor vehicle accident (see Fig. 7–22).

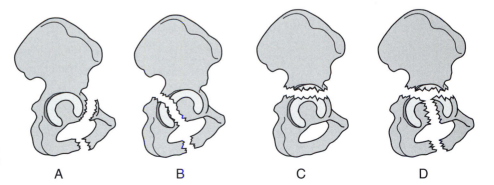

FIGURE 7–28. Classification of acetabular fractures. (*A*) Anterior column. (*B*) Posterior column. (*C*) Transverse, involving both columns. (*D*) Complex or T-shaped, involving both columns.

A   B   C   D

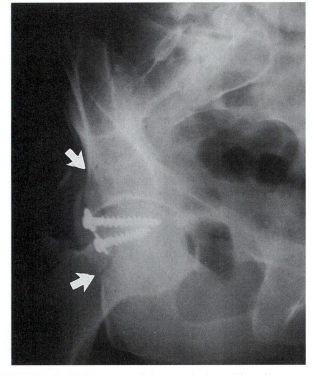

FIGURE 7–29. Fracture of the acetabulum. The white arrows mark the extent of the fracture line through the posterior lip of the acetabulum. Two metallic screws have been used to fixate the fragment in place.

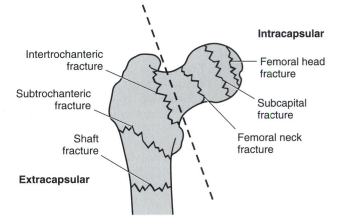

FIGURE 7–30. Fractures of the proximal femur are broadly divided into *intracapsular* and *extracapsular* sites. Intracapsular fractures are especially vulnerable to posttraumatic vascular complications because of the injury potential of blood vessels in close proximity.

Fractures of the Proximal Femur[20–22]

The incidence of proximal femur fractures is highest in elderly women with osteoporotic structural weakness. Falls are the most frequent cause of fracture, although the bone may fracture first from a normal weight-bearing force, precipitating the fall. Acute fractures from trauma are uncommon in children and young adults, due to the inherent strength of this bone. Great force is required to fracture the proximal femur in these age groups, and the healing process is often complicated. Stress fractures in the proximal femur may be seen in young adults, and these are usually associated with athletic overuse (e.g., distance running).

The radiographic evaluation of proximal femur fractures is usually complete on the AP and lateral frog-leg projections. If the involved extremity cannot withstand extreme movement, the *axiolateral* or *groin-lateral* is substituted for the lateral frog-leg projection. Conventional tomography or radionuclide bone scan may supplement the plain radiographs, especially in evaluation of subtle or impacted fractures.

Proximal femur fractures are commonly referred to as "hip" fractures. Although the term is not exactly untrue, it is too general to be useful for clinical management decisions. Proximal femur fractures can be most broadly divided into *intracapsular* and *extracap-*

sular fractures (Fig. 7–30). The distinction in these two groups is not only anatomic location but also designates which fractures are prone to vascular disruption and healing complications, thus affecting surgical treatment choices and prognosis.

INTRACAPSULAR FRACTURES

Intracapsular fractures of the proximal femur are located within the hip joint capsule. This includes the femoral head, the subcapital area, and the femoral neck regions (Fig. 7–31). Intracapsular fractures are fraught with complications owing to the frequently associated tearing of the *circumflex femoral arteries*. These vessels form a ring at the base of the neck, and ascending branches supply the neck and head. Only a minor blood supply is available through the arteries in the capitis femoris ligament at the femoral head. Thus the primary blood supply to the neck and head is dependent on the integrity of these vessels. The proximity of the vascular configuration is readily susceptible to injury when this region is fractured. Posttraumatic complications include avascular necrosis, delayed union, and nonunion.

Surgical treatment varies depending on the amount of displacement and stability of the fracture site, and additional factors including age, health and prior functional status of the patient. Pins, nails, compression screws, and sideplate and screw combinations are some devices used for internal fixation. Stable, impacted fractures may not require surgical intervention. Severe fractures with probable vascular interruption may require resection and replacement arthroplasty.

EXTRACAPSULAR FRACTURES

Extracapsular fractures of the proximal femur occur below the distal attachment of the joint capsule and

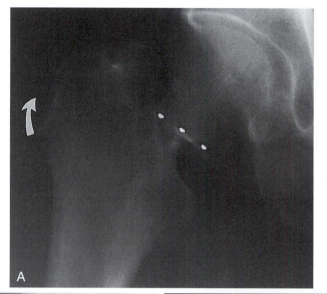

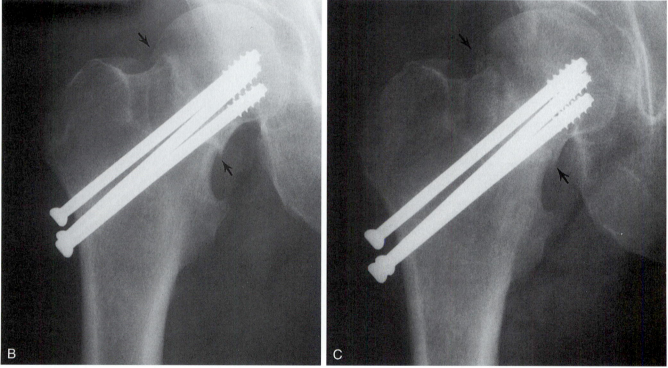

FIGURE 7–31. Femoral neck fracture. This 52-year-old male injured his hip in a fall off a truck bed as he was unloading furniture. (*A*) Anteroposterior view of the right hip shows a complete fracture of the femoral neck with superior displacement. The open arrows mark the borders of the femoral neck just proximal to the fracture site. (*B*) Restoration of alignment and good compression is obtained via fixation with three compression screws. The black arrows mark the extent of the fracture line. (*C*) Follow-up films 9 weeks later show no evidence of healing. The fracture line remains radiolucent and no new bone growth is noted. The delayed union of this fracture is most likely caused by the damage sustained by the major blood vessels in this region. All intracapsular fractures are susceptible to complications in healing because of the frequently associated tearing of the circumflex femoral arteries. It can be assumed that the major displacement of the fracture fragments at the time of injury contributed to the severity of the damage to the vessels.

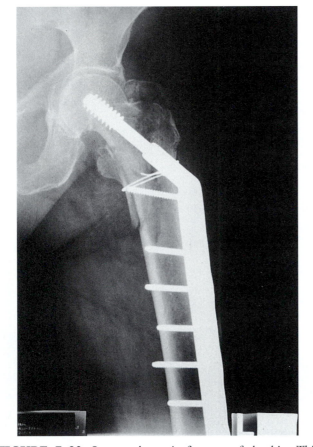

FIGURE 7–32. Intertrochanteric fracture of the hip. This postoperative film demonstrates fracture fixation via a side plate and screw combination device. The fracture line is evident, extending diagonally through the intertrochanteric region to the proximal femoral shaft. Some comminution is evident, and a large fragment on the medial shaft is noted. The soft tissue outlines of adipose tissue and swelling are clearly seen.

include the trochanteric region. Unlike the intracapsular fractures, this region's blood supply is not precarious or prone to injury. The trochanteric region is supplied by branches from the circumflex artery and also from nearby muscle attachments. Posttraumatic complications such as avascular necrosis or nonunion are rare.

Extracapsular fractures are divided into two subgroups: *intertrochanteric* and *subtrochanteric* fractures (see Fig. 7–30). Like fractures in general, these groups are further subdivided and described according to the obliquity of the fracture line and the number of fracture fragments present. Intertrochanteric fractures are located in the region between the greater and lesser trochanters, often extending diagonally from one to the other (Fig. 7–32). Subtrochanteric fractures occur below the intertrochanteric line, at the level of the lesser trochanter or immediately distal to it.

Surgical internal fixation includes sideplate and screw combinations or intermedullary rods.

ABNORMAL CONDITIONS

Degenerative Joint Disease of the Hip[23,24]

Osteoarthritis, or degenerative joint disease, is the most common disease affecting the hip joints. Characteristic of osteoarthritis in general, the etiology may be *primary*, developing without a clear precursor or *secondary*, directly related to some predisposing trauma or pathologic condition. Secondary osteoarthritis in the hip may be due to a variety of pre-existing conditions such as fracture, Paget's disease, epiphyseal disorders, congenital dislocation, avascular necrosis, or other inflammatory arthritides.

The radiographic features of hip joint osteoarthritis include the three general radiographic hallmarks of joint space narrowing, sclerotic subchondral bone, and osteophyte formation at the joint margins (Fig. 7–33). Additionally, osteoarthritis in the hip joint will exhibit

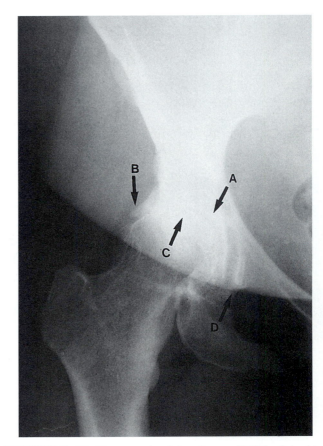

FIGURE 7–33. Degenerative joint disease (DJD) of the hip. The radiographic hallmarks of DJD are: A, decreased joint space; B, osteophyte formation at joint margins; and C, sclerosis of a subchondral bone; D, the large arc of increased density is the adipose tissue of the abdomen of this obese patient. (From Richardson and Iglarsh,[24] with permission.)

a fourth hallmark. Degeneration of the articular carti-lage causes microfractures in the subchondral bone, al-lowing intrusion of synovial fluid into bone. As a re-sult, cysts are formed, which show up radiographically as distinctive subarticular radiolucent lesions. In the acetabulum, these cysts are called *Egger's cysts*[25] (see Fig. 2–49).

Another feature of osteoarthritis in the hip joint is the migration of the femoral head. Destruction of the articular cartilage alters normal joint congruity be-tween the femoral head and acetabulum. The most common pattern of altered surface relationship is for the femoral head to migrate to or articulate in a supero-medial position, relative to its normal position (see Fig. 2–39).

Similar to other joints affected by osteoarthritis, the severity of degenerative changes evident on radio-graph does not always correlate with the severity of the clinical symptoms. Pain, stiffness, and function loss may be of a greater degree than radiographic evidence would seem to justify, and conversely, symptoms may be moderate in the presence of severe radiographic changes.

Conservative treatment of hip joint osteoarthritis is designed with the goals of decreasing pain, restoring flexibility and strength, and preserving functional ac-tivities and ambulation. Surgical treatment is neces-sary in severe cases of osteoarthritis and may include wedge osteotomy to alter joint biomechanics and pro-mote weight-bearing on an uninvolved surface of the femoral head, femoral head and neck resection and hemiarthroplasty to replace a degenerative femoral head, or total hip arthroplasty to replace the degener-ative femoral head and degenerative acetabulum (Figs. 7–34, 7–35).

Rheumatoid Arthritis of the Hip[26,27]

Rheumatoid arthritis is a progressive, systemic, au-toimmune inflammatory disease primarily affecting synovial joints. Incidence is three times greater in women, and onset is most common in young adult-hood. Characteristically, the small joints of the hands and feet, primarily the proximal interphalangeal joints, exhibit symptoms first, but the large joints of the ex-tremities may also be involved.

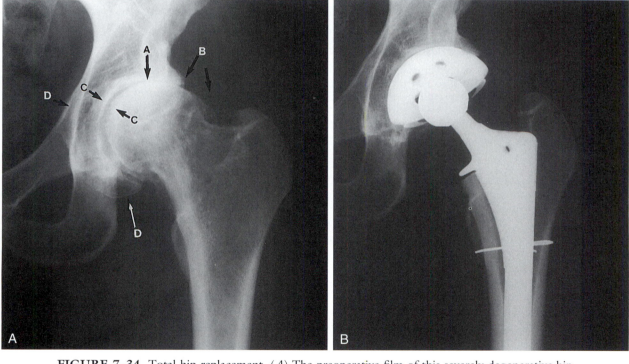

FIGURE 7–34. Total hip replacement. (*A*) The preoperative film of this severely degenerative hip joint of a 44-year-old man demonstrates the classic signs of degenerative joint disease: A, Narrowed joint space with superior migration of the femoral head; B, osteophyte formation at the joint margins of both the acetabulum and femoral head; C, sclerosis of subchondral bone on both sides of the joint surface; D, acetabular protrusio, a bony outpouching of the acetabular cup in response to the pro-gressive superior and medial migration of the femoral head. (*B*) Postoperative film shows a total hip arthroplasty. Both the acetabular and femoral portions of the joint have been resected and replaced with prosthetic components.

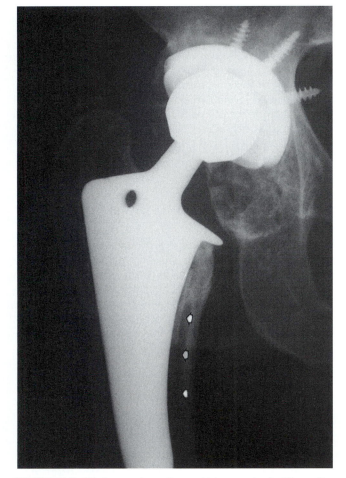

FIGURE 7–35. Loosening of a total hip prosthesis. The radiolucent streak paralleling the medial aspect of the stem of the femoral component (open arrows) represents space within the shaft of the femur caused by unwanted movement of the femoral prosthesis.

Regardless of the joints involved, rheumatoid arthritis is identified on radiograph by these distinctive abnormal features[28] (see Fig. 2–25):

1. Osteoporosis of periarticular areas, becoming more generalized with advancement of the disease
2. Symmetric and concentric joint space narrowing
3. Articular erosions, located either centrally or peripherally in the joint
4. Synovial cysts located within nearby bone
5. Periarticular swelling and joint effusions.

In the hip joint, osteoporosis is often first seen at the femoral head. Concentric joint space narrowing will promote an axial migration of the femoral head into the acetabulum, sometimes causing *acetabular protrusio*, a pouching of the acetabulum into the pelvis (Fig. 7–36). Articular erosions become evident when the joint surfaces lose their optimal congruity. The spherical shape of the femoral head becomes distorted, and the acetabulum loses its cuplike appearance. Synovial cysts may be located in proximity to the joint, at the acetabulum or femoral head. Joint effusions may be difficult to identify on plain radiographs and are best demonstrated on MRI.

Distinctive from osteoarthritis, rheumatoid arthritis has minimal reparative processes. Thus, radiographic features such as sclerotic subchondral bone and osteophyte formation, hallmarks of osteoarthritis, are not features of rheumatoid arthritis. The same radiograph may show characteristics of both processes, however, as both processes may occur at a joint as separate entities. Remissions and exacerbations are typical in rheumatoid arthritis. Destructive changes from a prior exacerbation can cause mechanical stresses that predispose the joint to secondary osteoarthritic processes while the joint is in remission from the rheumatoid arthritis.

Avascular Necrosis of the Proximal Femur[29-34]

Avascular necrosis of the proximal femur is a complicated disease process initiated by an interruption of blood supply to the femoral head causing bone tissue death. The etiology of femoral head avascular necrosis it may be related to trauma including overuse, various conditions such as prolonged steroid use, alcoholism, or renal disorders that predispose its deveopment, or it may simply appear idiopathically (Fig. 7–37).

Posttraumatically, avascular necrosis is commonly associated with femoral neck fractures (Fig. 7–38). The greater the severity and displacement of the fracture, the greater the chance of avascular necrosis's developing. Other direct trauma to the joint, such as contusions or dislocations, are less frequently associated with avascular necrosis but have the potential to develop avascular necrosis if the blood vessels become torn or sustain prolonged compression in the injury.

Idiopathic avascular necrosis of the femoral head

FIGURE 7–36. Acetabular protrusio. (*A*) The hip joints of this 79-year-old female with rheumatoid arthritis also show characteristics of osteoarthritis, since both processes may occur at a joint as separate entities; additionally, destructive changes from a prior rheumatoid exacerbation can cause mechanical stresses that predispose the joint to secondary osteoarthritic processes while the joint is in a remission from the rheumatoid arthritis. The striking feature of this film, however, is the large acetabular protrusio of the right hip joint (outlined with small black triangles). This bony, pouching of the acetabulum into the pelvis is a result of concentric joint space narrowing and axial migration of the femoral head. (*B*) After total hip arthroplasty, the deformity of acetabular protrusio is still evident.

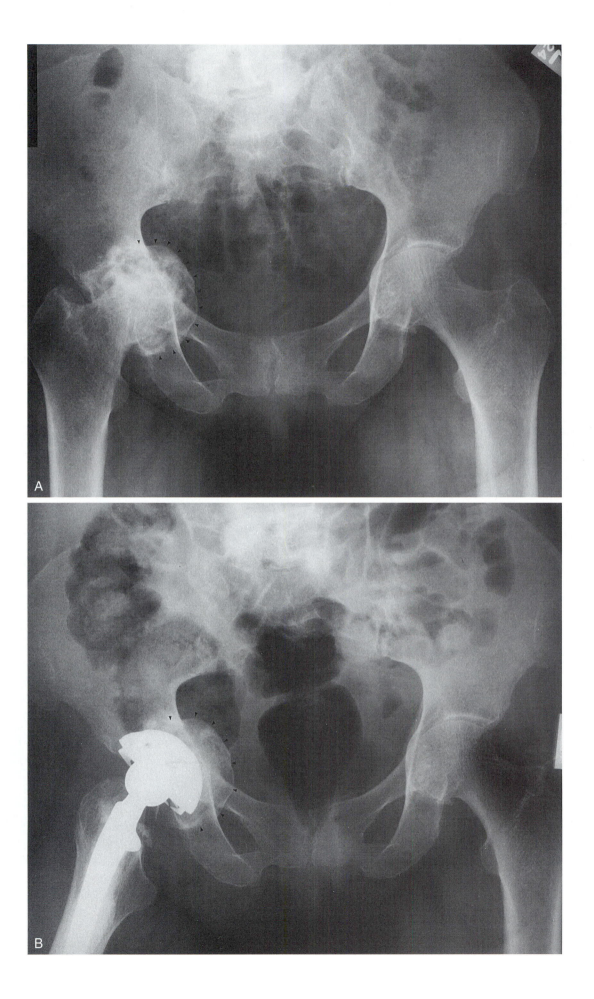

233

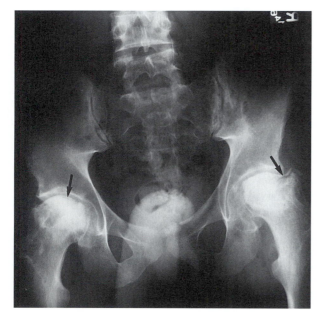

FIGURE 7–37. Avascular necrosis of bilateral femoral heads with crescent sign. This 38-year-old male had been on steroid therapy for the management of chronic obstructive lung disease for several years prior to the development of avascular necrosis bilaterally in the femoral heads. This radiograph shows the late stages of avascular necrosis with advanced deformities. Note the loss of the ball-and-socket configuration of the hips secondary to progressive collapse of the bone. The left hip shows greater deformity than the right. The arrows point to the crescent sign, a radiolucent line paralleling the articular surface that represents collapse of necrotic subchondral bone.

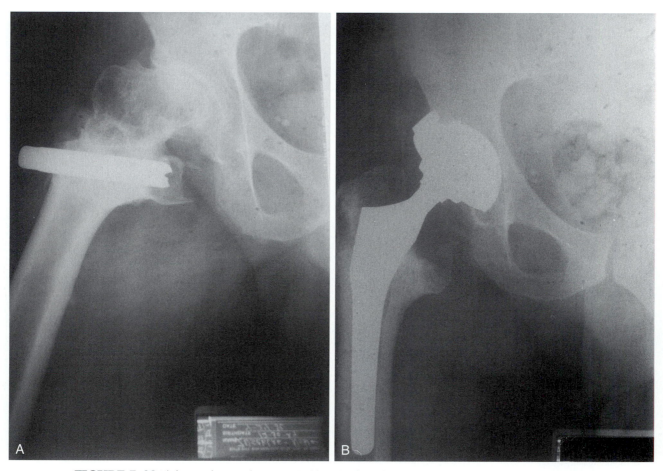

FIGURE 7–38. Advanced avascular necrosis (AVN) of the femoral head, resected. (*A*) This 72-year-old male underwent a hip pinning several years earlier to fixate a femoral neck fracture. Healing was complicated by vascular interruption. The femoral head became necrotic and over the years progressively collapsed until the hip joint was no longer functional and ambulation was severely impaired. (*B*) The femoral head was resected, and a total hip arthroplasty performed. The postoperative film shows the femoral component articulated in the acetabular cup. (From Richardson and Iglarsh,[24] pp. 653 and 673, with permission.)

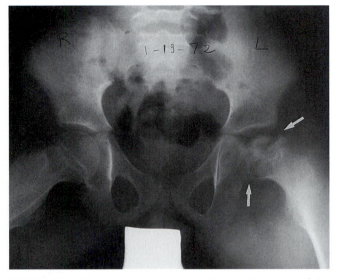

FIGURE 7–39. Legg-Calvé-Perthes disease. Necrosis of the secondary epiphysis of the femoral head developed idiopathically in this 11-year-old boy. Note the flattening and irregularity of the femoral head. The irregular densities and sclerotic patches of the femoral head represent the late-healing fibrous replacement and reossification stage of the disease (arrows).

may occur in children or adults, and then often appears bilaterally. The prognosis in children is much more favorable, and successful results are often achieved with conservative treatment, which may include prolonged non-weight-bearing, traction, bracing, casting, and exercise. The prognosis in adults is more variable and may or may not require surgical intervention. Legg-Calvé-Perthes disease is necrosis of the secondary epiphysis of the femoral head seen predominantly in young boys, the average age about 6 years old (Fig. 7–39). The literature refers to this condition as either an idiopathic avascular necrosis, or also associates it with subtle trauma, synovitis, infection, or metabolic bone disease.

The course and prognosis of this avascular necrosis at the femoral head is highly variable. The events from initial avascularity through revascularization, reossification, and remodeling may take several years, if not arrested at any stage. Generally, the prognosis is better in younger patients who possess a healthier, more adaptable blood supply. Successful healing under conservative treatment is common in the younger patients. Surgical intervention is often necessary in older patients and may include drilling into the femoral head to hasten revascularization, grafting healthy bone into

FIGURE 7–40. Early and late stages of avascular necrosis, crescent sign. The unfortunate young man in Fig. 7–37 who had developed avascular necrosis of both femoral heads secondary to prolonged steroid use also developed necrotic changes in the proximal humerus. It is interesting to note that the crescent sign demonstrated in Fig. 7–37 in the advanced stages of AVN at the hips is usually the first radiographic sign of impending necrotic changes at any joint. These films that were available of the patient's shoulder exhibit this finding clearly. (*A*) The arrow points to the radiolucent line paralleling the superior rim of the humeral head, subjacent to the articular surface. This represents the collapse of the necrotic subchondral bone. (*B*) Follow-up films 1 year later show flattening and irregularity of the humeral head, and irregular densities and sclerotic patches in the humeral head, representing the late stages of avascular necrosis.

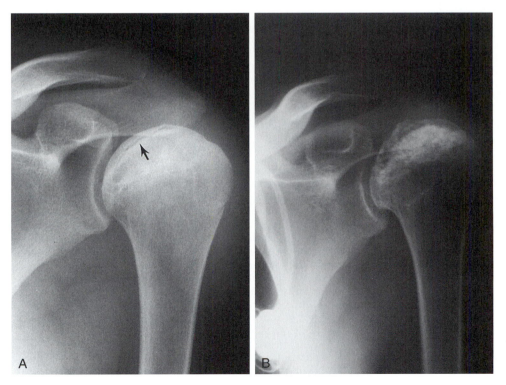

the drill holes to assist the repair process, varus dero-
tation osteotomy to provide a viable weight-bearing
surface on the femoral head or, as a last resort, osteotomy and replacement arthroplasty.

Radiographic evaluation in the initial stages of avascular necrosis may appear normal for several weeks.
One of the first radiographic signs, appearing as early
as 4 weeks postinjury, is a radiolucent crescent image,
representing the collapse of the necrotic subchondral
bone of the femoral head (Fig. 7–40). This crescent sign
appears parallel to the superior rim of the femoral
head, subjacent to the articular surface. Sclerosis and
cyst formation at the femoral head are other characteristic signs of the initial necrotic processes and healing

TABLE 7–1 Radiologic Staging of Avascular Necrosis of the Femoral Head

Stage	Criteria
0	Normal x-ray film, normal bone scan, and MRI
I	Normal x-ray film, abnormal bone scan, or MRI
	A. Mild (<15%)
	B. Moderate (15–30%)
	C. Severe (>30%)
II	Sclerosis and/or cyst formation in femoral head
	A. Mild (<15%)
	B. Moderate (15–30%)
	C. Severe (>30%)
III	Subchrondral collapse (crescent sign) without flattening
	A. Mild (<15%)
	B. Moderate (15–30%)
	C. Severe (>30%)
IV	Flattening of head *without* joint narrowing or acetabular involvement
	A. Mild (<15% of surface and <2 mm depression)
	B. Moderate (15–30% of surface *or* 2–4 mm depression)
	C. Severe (>30% of surface or >4 mm depression)
V	Flattening of head *with* joint narrowing and/or acetabular involvement
	A. Mile
	B. Moderate } (determined as above plus estimate of acetabular involvement)
	C. Severe
VI	Advanced degenerative changes.

From Richardson, JK and Iglarsh, ZA: Clinical Orthopaedic Therapy. WB Saunders, Philadelphia, 1994, p. 359.

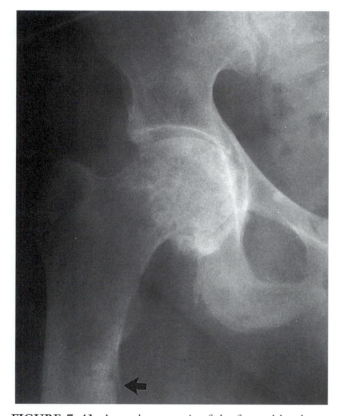

FIGURE 7–41. Avascular necrosis of the femoral head, pre-
deformity. Two disease processes are markedly evident in this
AP view of the hip. First, the overall density of the pelvis and
femur (below the head) appears severely demineralized. The
cortices of the femoral shaft are diminished, and the width of
the femoral neck and shaft appear abnormally wide. These findings are characteristic of osteomalacia, a hypocalcification disorder of bone. The fluffy sclerosis throughout the femoral head
is characteristic of the reossification attempts of the bone secondary to AVN. Note that although the joint spaces have narrowed and the femoral head has migrated superomedially, the
configuration of the femoral head is, at this point, still rounded
and has not undergone any collapse or deformity, although this
will undoubtedly occur in the future. The arrow points to an
incomplete transverse fracture on the medial side of the femoral
shaft. The configuration of this incomplete fracture (similar to
a greenstick fracture in a child) is likely to be related to the
altered density of the bone secondary to the osteomalacia.

attempts taking place (Fig. 7–41). These radiographic
signs can be distinguished from the similar characteristic signs of osteoarthritis by the normal preservation
of the radiographic joint space, which is not involved
in the necrotic process. In advanced stages of avascular
necrosis, the femoral head will collapse, or appear flattened, because of structural weakness and impaired
ability to withstand weight-bearing forces. The entire
femoral head and neck will become more radiodense
because of new bone attempting to heal the microfractures of the trabeculae and calcification of necrotic
marrow. Eventually the progressive collapse of the
femoral head will alter joint surface congruity and involve the acetabulum. At this advanced stage the joint
space will be markedly compromised.

Radiologists identify the stages of progression of the
disease by the presence of the foregoing signs. Table
7–1 provides a summary of the radiologic staging of
avascular necrosis of the femoral head. The drawback
of plain-film radiologic evaluation of avascular necrosis is the absence of findings until several weeks into
the disease process. In contrast, radionuclide bone
scans identify increased uptake at the site of the lesion
soon after injury. Currently, however, MRI is considered the study of choice for early sensitivity and specificity in diagnosing avascular necrosis.

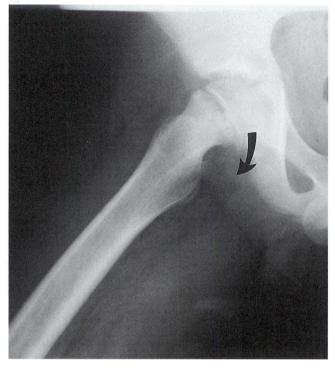

FIGURE 7–42. Slipped femoral capital epiphysis. This lateral frog-leg view of the right hip of a 10-year-old boy demonstrates the posterior, medial, and inferior displacement of the epiphysis of the femoral head as is characteristic for this condition. The weakness of the epiphyseal plate that permits this displacement is theorized to be related to an imbalance between the growth and sex hormones.

Slipped Femoral Capital Epiphysis[35,36]

Slipped femoral capital epiphysis is the most common disorder of the hip in adolescence. A weakening of the epiphyseal plate at the junction of the femoral neck and head allows the head to displace posteriorly, medially, and inferiorly from the neck. The etiology is unknown but is theorized to be related to an imbalance between the growth and sex hormones, which weaken all epiphyseal plates. The extreme shear and weight-bearing forces inherent to the functioning of this specific joint render it vulnerable to displacement. The onset is insidious and often coincides with growth spurts at puberty. The disorder appears twice as often in boys, and obesity and delayed maturation are common characteristics in affected individuals of either sex.

Clinical symptoms include vague patterns of pain in the hip or knee area, limited hip range of motion, antalgic gait, and limb length shortening. Conservative treatment is not generally successful, and surgical fixation is usually necessary to prevent further slippage and stabilize the physis.

Radiographic abnormalities will coincide with the amount of slippage present. Radiographic signs on the AP projection include a blurring and widening of the physis, and a decreased height of the epiphysis relative to the contralateral hip. The lateral frog-leg projection best demonstrates the amount of epiphyseal displacement (Figs. 7–42, 7–43).

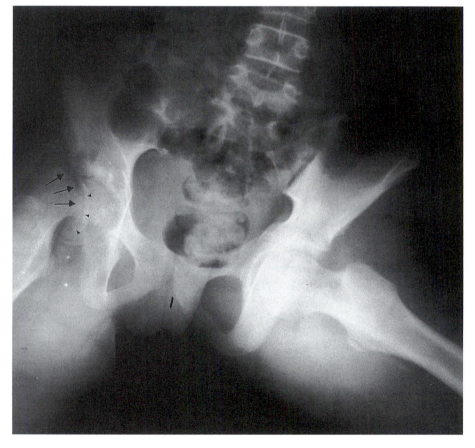

FIGURE 7–43. Slipped femoral capital epiphysis (SFCE). This AP view of the hips in a young teenager shows the severe posterior, medial, and inferior displacement of the femoral head characteristic for SFCE. In normal positioning of the femoral head, the small triangles would line up with the points of the arrows on the femoral neck.

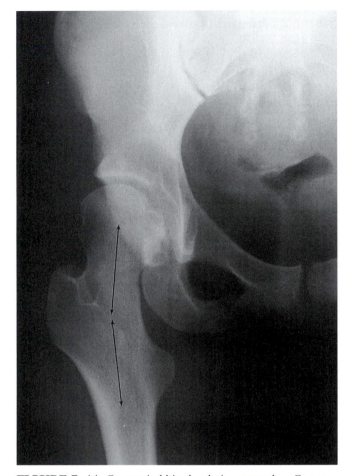

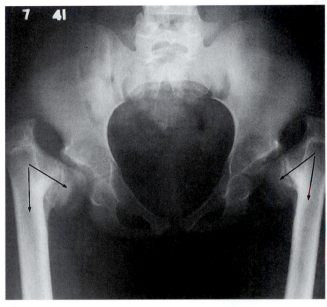

FIGURE 7–45. Congenital hip dysplasia, coxa vara. Congenital abnormalities in the configuration of the acetabulum and proximal femur are present bilaterally in this teenager. The extremely small angles of inclination (line arrows) of the femoral heads to the femoral shafts are described as coxa vara deformities.

FIGURE 7–44. Congenital hip dysplasia, coxa valga. Congenital abnormalities in the configuration of the acetabulum in the proximal femur are seen in this 20-year-old female. Note the abnormally wide angle of inclination of the femoral neck to the femoral shaft (line arrows), described as coxa valga.

Congenital Dislocation of the Hip[37–39]

The hip joint is the most common site of congenital dislocation and presents challenging diagnostic and treatment issues. Early diagnosis and treatment is necessary in infancy, prior to ambulation, to promote normal joint development and prevent the debilitating consequences of later degenerative changes (Figs. 7–44, 7–45).

The etiology of congenital hip dislocation may be genetic, hormonal, or mechanical, as related to the fetus position in utero. The presentation of the disorder is variable. *Congenital hip dysplasia* defines an altered joint relationship caused by an abnormal acetabulum and a deformed proximal femur. This term is used broadly to describe the predisposing condition of the hip joint leading to subluxation and dislocation, or to encompass all variations of the disorder. *Congenital*

subluxation of the hip defines an abnormal joint relationship with a partial preservation of joint contact. A congenital subluxation also permits the hip joint to be dislocatable with minimal force. *Congenital dislocation* of the hip defines complete displacement of the femoral head from the acetabulum, although it remains within the confines of the joint capsule.

Treatment in the newborn consists primarily of splinting to maintain reduction of the joint and allow normal articulation to develop. Over 6 months of age, treatment options include continuous skin traction for several weeks, or surgical intervention, including acetabular or intertrochanteric osteotomy, inverted labrum removal, or adductor tenotomy (Fig. 7–46). Rehabilitation needs are extensive and include strengthening, stretching, positioning, and functional skill development.

The head of the femur is not ossified in the infant, and the ossification center for the femoral head epiphysis does not appear until 3 to 6 months of age. Therefore, the radiographic evaluation of this disorder is not assessed by direct visualization but by evaluating a series of drawn lines and intersecting angles relating the ossified portions of the pelvis to the ossified femoral shaft. From these measurements the depth of the acetabulum and the orientation of the cartilaginous femoral head are determined (Figure 7–47).

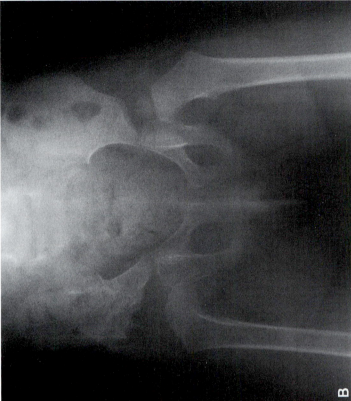

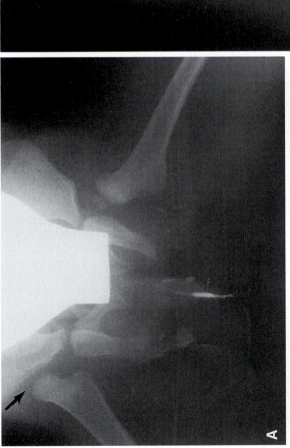

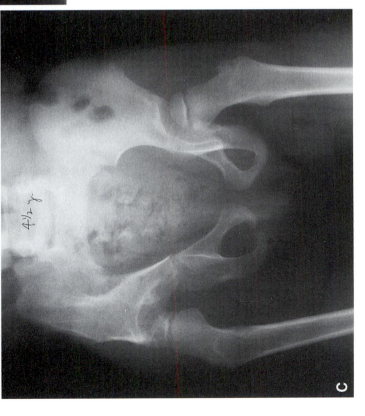

FIGURE 7–46. Surgical correction of congenital hip dysplasia in a toddler. (*A*) Arrow points to the congenital deformity of the hip joint in this 16-month-old boy. For comparison, note the configuration of the normal hip joint on the left. This film was made preoperatively. (*B*) This follow-up film was made at 22 months of age. The child had undergone a posterior iliac osteotomy to create an acetabular fossa. Note the delay in the ossification of the femoral capital epiphysis on the right. (*C*) Follow-up film made when the child was 4½ years of age shows relatively satisfactory results. The proximal femur is adequately articulated in the surgically sculpted acetabulum, and the hip is functional for all ambulatory activities.

239

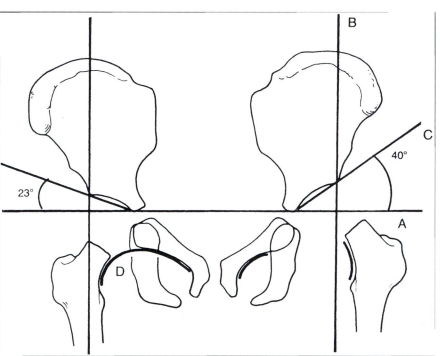

FIGURE 7–47. Radiologic signs of congenital hip dislocation. A horizontal line (*A*) is drawn through the junctions of the iliac, ischial, and pubic bones at the center of the acetabulum (Hilgenreiner's line). A perpendicular line (*B*) is drawn through the outer border of the acetabulum (Perkins' line). The secondary ossification center of the femoral head (or, in its absence, the medial metaphyseal beak of the proximal femur) should lie within the inner lower quadrant formed by the intersection of these lines. The acetabular index, a measure of acetabular depth, can be estimated by inscribing a line (*C*) joining the inner and outer edges of the acetabulum. The angle formed by this line and line A is normally less than 30 degrees. Increased angles indicate acetabular hypoplasia. Shenton's line (*D*) is inscribed along the inferior border of the femoral neck and inferior border of the superior pubic ramus. It is ordinarily smooth and unbroken. Proximal displacement of the femoral head in congenital hip dislocation results in interruption of line D. (From Richardson, JK and Iglarsh, ZA: Clinical Orthopaedic Physical Therapy. WB Saunders, Philadelphia, 1994, p. 366.)

SUMMARY OF KEY POINTS

1. The routine radiographic evaluation of the pelvis includes two projections that also serve to evaluate both hip joints simultaneously:
   - **Anteroposterior:** Demonstrates the entire pelvis and bilateral femurs in the anatomic position.
   - **Anteroposterior bilateral frog-leg:** Demonstrates the lateral aspects of the proximal femurs by positioning the hips in flexion, abduction, and external rotation.
2. Six line images are viewed on the AP projection to reference the normal position of the acetabulum and related osseous structures. The lines are: the radiographic teardrop, the iliopubic line, the ilioischial line, the anterior acetabular rim, the posterior acetabular rim, and the acetabular roof. Disruptions in these line images may indicate fracture, dislocation, or pathology.
3. The normal ball and socket configuration of the hip joints should be obvious on the anteroposterior projection. Destruction of normal joint congruity may be caused by various pathologies including avascular necrosis, rheumatoid arthritis, degenerative joint disease, or destructive tumors.
4. Fractures of the pelvis are broadly classified as stable fractures, in which no joint articulations are disrupted, or unstable fractures, in which two or more articulation sites on the pelvic ring are disrupted.
5. Ischiopubic rami fractures, which in themselves are stable fractures, comprise approximately half of all pelvic fractures.
6. Acetabular fractures are classified by anatomic position into fractures: (1) of the anterior column or (2) the posterior column or that (3) are transverse through both columns or (4) complex, involving a "T" shaped configuration. Posterior column fractures, including the posterior rim of the cup, are most common and are frequently associated with femoral head impaction or posterior dislocation. Radiographic assessment is sometimes difficult on the routine projections due to superimposition of the femoral head and the configuration of the acetabular cup. Oblique projections or ancillary techniques such as CT or conventional tomography may supplement the routine films.

7. Proximal femoral fractures can be classified by their anatomic location relative to the hip joint capsule. Intracapsular fractures, including femoral head, subcapital, and femoral neck fractures, are located within the hip joint capsule and are often complicated by vascular disruption potentially progressing to avascular necrosis. Extracapsular fractures, including subtrochanteric and intertrochanteric fractures, are located outside the capsule, and vascular complication is rare. The incidence of proximal femoral fractures is highest in elderly women owing to osteoporotic-induced structural weakness at the fracture site.

8. Degenerative joint disease is a common affliction at the hip joints. Radiographic hallmarks of DJD at the hip joints are like those of other synovial joints, including (1) joint space narrowing, (2) sclerotic subchondral bone, and (3) osteophyte formation at joint margins. Additional signs of DJD at the hip joints include radiolucent cysts known as Egger's cysts, formed by intrusion of synovial fluid into microfractures in the subchondral bone, and superior migration of the femoral head due to articular cartilage loss and altered joint surface relationships. Note that the amount of radiographic evidence of degenerative joint disease may not always correlate with the severity of clinical symptomatology.

9. Rheumatoid arthritis at the hip joints is evidenced radiographically by the bilateral presence of (1) demineralization of the femoral head, (2) concentric joint space narrowing, (3) axial migration of the femoral head into the acetabulum, sometimes causing acetabular protrusio and (4) articular erosion loss of the ball-and-socket joint configuration. Reparative processes signified by subchondral sclerosis and osteophyte formation (hallmarks of DJD) are not present.

10. Avascular necrosis of the proximal femur is the terminal stage of a series of events initiated by interrupted circulation to the femoral head. The entire course of the disease from initial avascularity to revascularization, new bone growth, and remodeling may span from several weeks to years, if not arrested at any given stage. It is associated posttraumatically with intracapsular hip fractures, but can also be seen idiopathically in both children and adults. Earliest detection is by radionuclide bone scans or MRI. Radiographic diagnosis is not conclusive until several weeks into the disease process. The earliest radiographic indicator is the crescent sign, a radiolucent image representing collapse of the necrotic subchondral bone of the femoral head. Late stage AVN is hallmarked by increased radiodensity of the femoral head and neck, and progressive collapse of the femoral head.

11. Slipped femoral capital epiphysis is the most common disorder of the hip in adolescence, appearing twice as frequently in males. Weakening of the epiphyseal plate at the junction of the femoral head and neck allows the femoral head to displace posteriorly, medially, and inferiorly. The frog-leg projection best demonstrates the amount of displacement.

12. The hip joint is the most common site of congenital dislocation. Early diagnosis and treatment are necessary in infancy, prior to ambulation, to promote normal joint development. Radiographic evaluation cannot be assessed by direct visualization due to lack of ossification in infant hip joint. Evaluation is done by measuring the lines and intersecting angles relative to the ossified portions of the pelvis and femoral shaft.

REFERENCES

1. Netter, FH: The Cibia Collection of Medical Illustrations, Vol 8, Part I, Musculoskeletal System. Ciba-Geigy Corporation, Summit, NJ, 1978, pp 16–19.
2. Ibid, pp 99–93.
3. Nordin, M and Frankel, VH: Basic Biomechanics of the Musculoskeletal System, ed 2. Lea & Febiger, Malvern, PA, 1989, p 137.
4. Meschan, I: An Atlas of Radiographic Anatomy. WB Saunders, Philadelphia, 1960, pp 216–218.
5. Weissman, B and Sledge, C: Orthopedic Radiology. WB Saunders, Philadelphia, 1986, pp 335–346.
6. Greenspan, A: Orthopedic Radiology: A Practical Approach, ed 2. Raven Press, New York, 1992, pp 7.1–7.8.
7. Bontrager, KL: Textbook of Radiographic Positioning and Relted Anatomy, ed 3. Mosby, St. Louis, 1993, pp 217–270.
8. Fischer, HW: Radiographic Anatomy: A Working Atlas. McGraw-Hill, New York, 1988, pp 81–85.
9. Wicke, L: Atlas of Radiographic Anatomy, ed 5. Lea & Febiger, Malvern, PA, 1994, pp 46–50.
10. Weissman, pp 341–343.
11. Greenspan, p 7.12.
12. Ibid, p 7.3.
13. Ibid, pp 7.8–7.16.

14. Weissman, pp 346–368.
15. Rockwood, CA and Green, DP (eds): Fractures in Adults, Vol 2, ed 2. JB Lippincott, Philadelphia, 1984, pp 1093–1210.
16. Greenspan, pp 7.13–7.16.
17. Weissman, pp 360–368.
18. Rockwood, pp 1161–1165.
19. Greenspan, p 7.14.
20. Ibid, pp 7.17–7.24.
21. Weissman, pp 369–373.
22. Rockwood, pp 1211–1356.
23. Greenspan, pp 12.1–12.5.
24. Richardson, JK and Iglarsh, ZA: Clinical Orthopedic Physical Therapy. WB Saunders, Philadelphia, 1994, pp 386–390.
25. Greenspan, p 12.2.
26. Ibid, pp 13.4–13.20.
27. Weissman, p 404.
28. Greenspan, pp 13.4–13.5.
29. Rockwood, pp 1215–1216, 1255–1256, 1275.
30. Weissman, pp 418–422.
31. Greenspan, p 7.17.
32. Richardson, pp 383–385.
33. Weissman, pp 418–439.
34. Yochum, TR and Rowe, LJ: Essentials of Skeletal Radiology, Vol 2. Williams & Wilkins, Baltimore, 1987, pp 978–986.
35. Richardson, pp 381–383.
36. Greenspan, p 27.14.
37. Richardson, pp 369–374.
38. Greenspan, pp 27.3, 27.9.
39. Yochum, pp 127–132.

SELF-TEST

Chapter 7

REGARDING FILM A:

1. Identify this projection.
2. Based on the bony configuration of the pelvis and the pelvic inlet, would you guess this patient is male or female?

REGARDING FILM B:

3. What is the most striking feature of the bilateral hip joint spaces?
4. Describe the position of the femoral heads in relationship to the acetabulum.
5. What is the term used to describe the altered configuration of the acetabulum?
6. Does a degenerative process or an inflammatory process appear to be responsible for the changes visible at the hip joints?

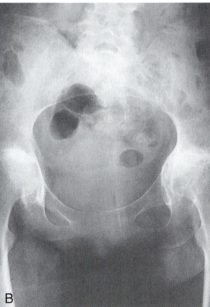

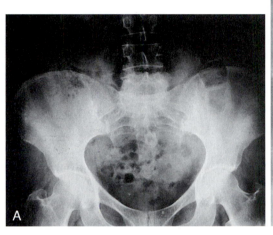

CHAPTER **8**

Knee

The knee has been subjected to more clinical investigation and scientific research than any other joint in the body.[1] A reason for this may be the enormous number of patients with knee disorders.

The complex arthrokinematics of the knee are dictated by its osseous architecture, ligamentous structures, interposed menisci, and interrelated muscular actions. The functioning of the knee allows for great stability while at the same time permitting great mobility. This mechanical compromise enables the knee to withstand tremendous weight-bearing and load transmission forces while promoting ambulatory freedom. The knee's unique anatomy, combined with its exposed location between the two longest bones of the body, does, however, predispose the knee to various injuries, trauma, and other pathologies.

The knee is well demonstrated on the routine radiographic evaluation. Most fractures and degenerative processes are adequately defined via plain films. Injuries to the soft tissues of the knee, which occur with great frequency, are generally diagnosed with ancillary techniques. At present, magnetic resonance imaging is usually the study of choice with respect to evaluation of the soft tissues.

The goals of this chapter are first to provide a review of osseous and radiographic anatomy. Next, a brief review of ligamentous anatomy and joint mobility is presented. The routine radiographic evaluation of the knee follows. Here the reader has an opportunity to interact and learn radiographic anatomy by tracing a radiograph with a marker on a transparency sheet and then comparing results with the radiographic tracing. Examples of common traumas follow, as does a discussion on degenerative joint disease. The chapter concludes with examples of congenital deformities seen with frequency at the knee joint. The summary is organized into a list of practical points that highlight the clinical aspects of the chapter. A self-test challenges the reader's visual interpretation skills.

RADIOGRAPHIC ANATOMY

Osseous Anatomy[2]

The knee joint, or *tibiofemoral joint*, is formed by the articulation of the distal end of the femur to the proximal end of the tibia (Figs. 8–1, 8–2). Adaptive congruency of the articular surfaces is made possible by the interposed *menisci*. Associated with the knee joint are the *patellofemoral joint*, an articulation between the

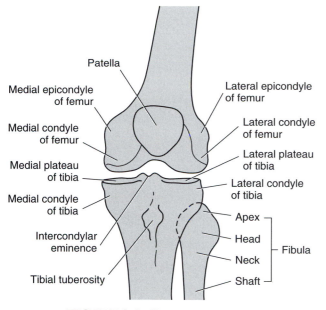

FIGURE 8–1. Knee, anterior aspect.

anterior aspect of the femur and the patella, and the *tibiofibular joint*, an articulation between the lateral aspect of the tibia and the fibular head.

Distal Femur: Anteriorly, the distal femur exhibits *medial and lateral condyles* separated by the *patellar surface*, also known as the *trochlear groove* or *intercondylar sulcus*. Posteriorly, the femoral condyles are divided by the deep *intercondylar fossa*. *Medial and lateral epicondyles* are prominences serving as sites of muscle attachments.

The *patella* is a large sesamoid bone embedded in the *quadriceps tendon*. The smooth articular surface

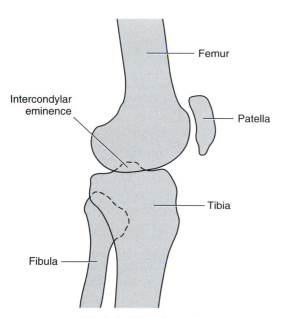

FIGURE 8–2. Knee, lateral aspect.

has multiple facets for efficient load distribution mechanisms during its tracking actions on the trochlear groove. The outer anterior surface is convex and roughened. The broad superior surface is the *base*, and the pointed inferior surface is the *apex* of the patella.

Proximal Tibia: The proximal tibia exhibits *medial and lateral condyles*, which superiorly form the flared articular surface, the *tibial plateau*. Located between the condyles on the tibial plateau is the *intercondylar eminence* or *tibial spine*, composed of two small pointed prominences, the *intercondylar tubercles*. The lateral condyle has a facet on its posteroinferior surface for articulation with the head of the fibula. At the midline of the anterior proximal tibia, just distal to the condyles, is the *tibial tuberosity*, a prominence serving as the distal attachment of the patellar ligament. Beginning distally from this point is the *anterior crest* of the tibia. This sharp ridge represents the anterior surface of the tibial shaft and extends to the medial malleoli.

Fibula: The fibula is the non-weight-bearing bone of the lower extremity. The proximal end of the fibula is the *head*, which articulates with the tibia. The superior tip of the head is the *apex* or *styloid process*. The tapered region inferior to the head is the fibular *neck*. The long slender shaft of the fibula ends distally as the lateral malleoli at the ankle.

Ligamentous Anatomy[3]

There are four major stabilizing ligaments of the knee joint (Fig. 8–3): the *medial collateral*, the *lateral collateral*, the *anterior cruciate*, and the *posterior cruciate*. Other various minor ligaments and the muscular complexes provide additional stability.

The *medial collateral ligament*, also known as the *tibial collateral ligament*, arises from the medial epicondyle of the femur and extends to the medial condyle and medial surface of the tibia. Fibers of the medial collateral ligament blend with the joint capsule and medial meniscus. The medial collateral ligament is the prime stabilizer against valgus stresses, in either flexion or extension.

The *lateral collateral ligament*, also known as the *fibular collateral ligament*, arises from the lateral epicondyle of the femur and extends to the fibular head. The lateral collateral ligament is extra-articular in that it does not blend with the joint capsule or lateral meniscus. The lateral collateral ligament plays a role in defending the knee against varus stresses.

The *anterior cruciate ligament* arises from the nonarticular area of the tibial plateau just anterior to the intercondylar eminence and extends to the posterior medial aspect of the lateral femoral condyle. The anterior cruciate lies entirely within the joint capsule. This ligament functions as the primary restraint against anterior tibial displacement.

The *posterior cruciate ligament* is also contained

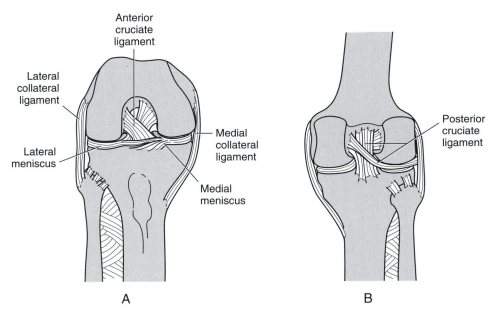

FIGURE 8–3. Major ligaments of the knee joint. (*A*) Anterior view. (*B*) Posterior view.

within the joint capsule, arising from behind the intercondylar eminence and extending to the lateral aspect of the medial femoral condyle. The posterior cruciate is the primary stabilizer against posterior tibial displacement.

The *patellar ligament*, also referred to as the *patellar tendon*, extends from the apex of the patella to the tibial tuberosity (Fig. 8–4). The patella ligament can be considered a continuation of the common tendon of the quadriceps muscle group.

JOINT MOBILITY[4]

The knee functions as a specialized hinge joint, permitting a wide range of flexion and extension movement in the sagittal plane. Accessory rotational mobil-

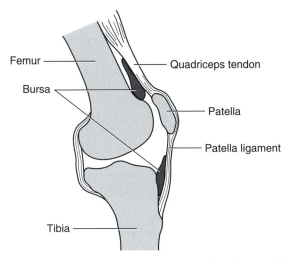

FIGURE 8–4. The patella is embedded within the quadriceps tendon. The distal extension of the quadriceps tendon is the *patella ligament.*

ity is present in the transverse plane. Normal values for active motion range from 0 degrees of extension, or 10 degrees of hyperextension, to 145 degrees of flexion. Tibial rotation is possible to 45 degrees both medially and laterally when the knee is positioned in flexion. Abduction and adduction in the frontal plane are similarly affected by the amount of joint flexion, reaching a maximum of a few degrees each when the knee is flexed in the 0 to 30 degrees range.

The tibiofemoral joint arthrokinematics follow the orthopedic rules for convex-concave surfaces. That is, the motions of knee extension and flexion occur via a combined movement of rolling and gliding of the femoral convex surfaces to the tibial concave surfaces. The specific actions of the articular surfaces depend on whether the joint is functioning in closed or open chain kinetic state, and whether flexion or extension is occurring.

The patellofemoral joint functions as a saddle type of joint. The primary motion is a gliding or tracking action along the trochlear groove. In knee extension the patella is positioned at the superior end of the trochlear groove, and during flexion the patella will track or glide caudally in the trochlear groove. The patella glides distally a distance of approximately 7 centimeters from full knee extension to flexion. Both medial and lateral patellar facets contact the femur at extension and through 90 degrees of flexion. Beyond 90 degrees the patella rotates, or tilts, and remains in contact with only the medial femoral condyle. At full knee flexion, the patella sits deep in the trochlear groove.

The patellofemoral joint mechanics are mediated directly or indirectly by the pull of the quadriceps muscle on the patella. Proximally, the angulation of the hip joint, or distally, the mechanics of the foot, may alter the angle of pull of the quadriceps on the patella, known as the ''Q'' *angle* (Fig. 8–5). The Q angle is determined by the intersection of the line of pull of the quadriceps with the line connecting the center of the

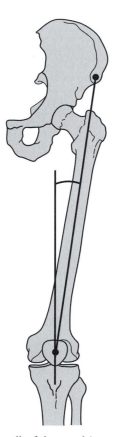

FIGURE 8–5. The pull of the quadriceps on the patella is described as the *Q angle*. It is measured by the angle formed by the intersection of a line drawn from the center of the patella to the tibial tuberosity and a line drawn from the center of the patella to the anterior superior iliac spine.

patella to the center of the tibial tuberosity. The normal Q angle is approximately 10 degrees, and values greater than this may indicate a predisposition to inadequate patellar tracking and resultant instability. The patella itself serves to lengthen the lever force arm of the quadriceps and allows for a wider distribution of femoral compressive forces. Maladaptive mechanics

at the patellofemoral joint can lead to painful conditions and functional disability of the knee joint.

The proximal tibiofibular joint is a gliding type of synovial joint. Limited movement is available between the lateral tibial condyle and the head of the fibula. Note that the distal tibiofibular joint is not synovial but is a syndesmotic joint that is slightly movable.

GROWTH AND DEVELOPMENT[5]

At birth the secondary epiphyseal centers for the distal femur and the proximal tibia are present and can be identified as ossified structures on radiograph (Fig. 8–6). The secondary epiphyseal center for the head of the fibula does not appear until approximately 3 years of age. The patella is not visible on radiographs until it begins ossification at approximately 4 years of age. The physis of each long bone continues to grow progressively and the epiphyseal plates finally fuse post-puberty at approximately 16 to 18 years of age. Women generally show earlier skeletal maturity than men (Fig. 8–7).

ROUTINE RADIOGRAPHIC EVALUATION[6–10]

Knee

Basic: Anteroposterior (AP)
Lateral
Axial or tunnel view of the intercondylar fossa
Axial view of the patellofemoral joint

The routine radiographic evaluation of the knee includes the above four projections and encompasses examination of the tibiofemoral, patellofemoral, and tibiofibular joints. The proximal third of the tibial and fibular shafts are also usually apparent. Radiographic evaluation of the entire length of the tibia and fibula is

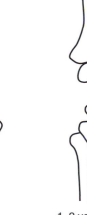
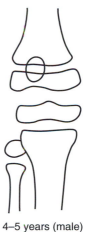

FIGURE 8–6. Radiographic tracings of ossification of the knee at varying ages from birth through 18 years. (Adapted from Meschan,[5] p. 218.)

Birth   1–2 years (male)   4–5 years (male)   18 years (male)

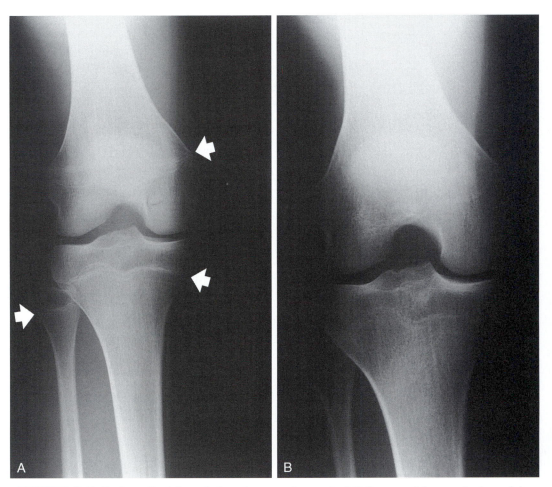

FIGURE 8–7. Fusion of epiphyseal plates in normal growth. (*A*) Intercondylar notch view of the knee in a 17-year-old male shows the presence of partially fused epiphyseal plates at the distal femur, proximal tibia, and proximal fibula (arrows). (*B*) Intercondylar notch view of the same teenager 1 year later shows normal growth and maturation changes. The epiphyseal plates have completely fused but the growth lines are still evident, especially across the proximal tibia.

done on a separate lower leg examination, with both proximal and distal articulations visible on one radiograph.

The *AP projection* of the knee provides information regarding the distal femur, proximal tibia, joint articulation, and fibular head. The patella is not well demonstrated in this view, as it is superimposed over the distal femur.

The *lateral* projection of the knee allows for assessment of the patellar-femoral relationship in profile, and examination of the suprapatellar bursa and quadriceps tendon.

The *axial* or *tunnel view of the intercondylar fossa* is useful in examining the intercondylar notch, posterior aspect of the femoral condyles, and the intercondylar eminence of the tibial plateau.

The *axial view of the patellofemoral joint* visualizes the patella and the patellofemoral joint tangentially, across the plane of the patellofemoral joint. This provides information regarding the joint surfaces, and how the patella is positioned in the intercondylar fossa.

Anteroposterior (Figs. 8–8, 8–9, 8–10)

This view demonstrates the distal femur, proximal tibia, the tibiofemoral articulation, and the head of the fibula. The important observations are:

1. The patella is superimposed over the distal femur. The inferior pole of the patella normally lies at the level of the joint line.
2. The tibiofemoral radiographic joint space is normally well defined in both the medial and lateral compartments.
3. The articular surface of the tibial plateau is seen end-on, with only minimal surface area visualized.

4. The medial half of the fibular head is superimposed behind the tibia.
5. Normal radiographic contrast between the bones and soft tissues should be evident. Trabecular markings and cortical margins should appear distinct.

CLINICAL OBJECTIVES

1. Trace the distal femur, identifying medial and lateral condyles.
2. Trace the proximal tibia, identifying the medial and lateral condyles and intercondylar eminence.
3. Trace the patella.
4. Trace the proximal fibula.

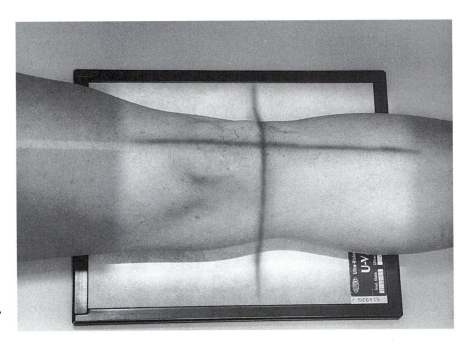

FIGURE 8–8. Patient position for AP view of the knee.

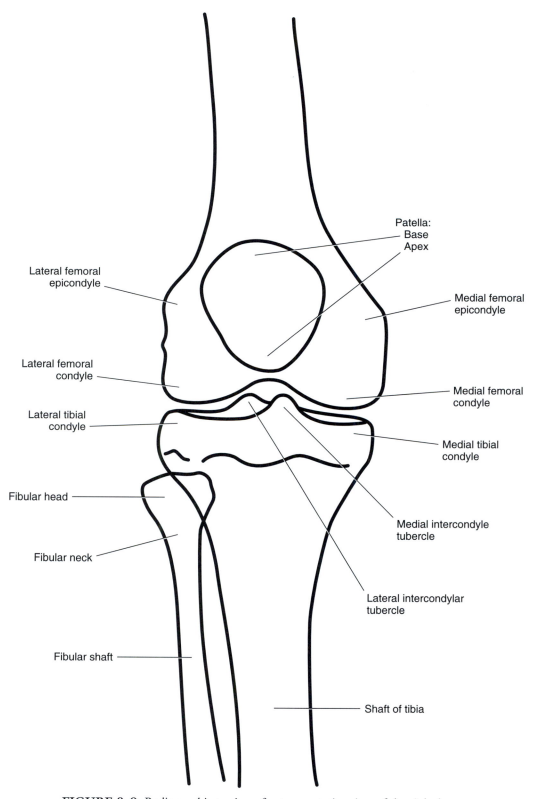

Lateral femoral
epicondyle

Lateral femoral
condyle

Lateral tibial
condyle

Fibular head

Fibular neck

Fibular shaft

Patella:
Base
Apex

Medial femoral
epicondyle

Medial femoral
condyle

Medial tibial
condyle

Medial intercondyle
tubercle

Lateral intercondylar
tubercle

Shaft of tibia

FIGURE 8–9. Radiographic tracing of anteroposterior view of the right knee.

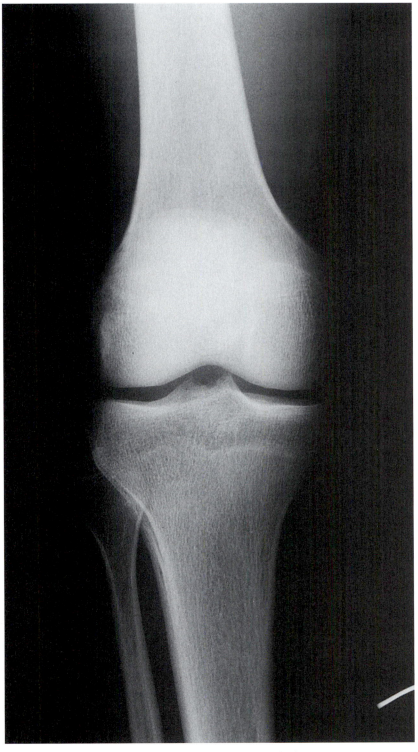

FIGURE 8–10. AP view of the right knee.

Lateral (Figs. 8–11, 8–12, 8–13)

This view demonstrates the patellofemoral joint in profile, the suprapatellar bursa, the quadriceps tendon, and the patellar tendon. The important observations are:

1. The knee is flexed approximately 20 degrees on a standard lateral.
2. The x-ray beam is directed through the knee in a medial to lateral direction, thus a portion of the fibular head is superimposed behind the tibia.
3. In true lateral positioning the femoral condyles will be directly superimposed over one another. If positioning is not exact, each femoral condyle will cast an outline.
4. The tibial medial and lateral condyles are also superimposed on one another. The intercondylar eminence projects above the tibial plateau and is partly superimposed by the femoral condyles.

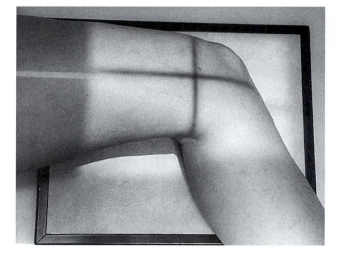

FIGURE 8–11. Patient position for lateral view of the knee.

5. The relationship of the patella to the femur is examined. Abnormally superior positioning of the patella is termed *patella alta.* Abnormally inferior positioning of the patella is termed *patella baja.*
6. The relationship of the length of the patella to the length of the patella ligament is examined. The length of the patella is measured from its base to its apex. The length of the patellar ligament is measured from its attachment at the patellar apex to the tibial tuberosity. These distances are normally approximately equal, and normal variance does not exceed 20 percent. More than 20 percent variation indicates an abnormal patellar position.[11]
7. Normal radiographic contrast between the bones and soft tissues should be evident. The cortical margins of the long bones and the patella should be distinct.
8. The suprapatellar bursa normally images as a thin, radiolucent strip just posterior to the quadriceps tendon. The bursa becomes distended with joint effusion and images as an oval-shaped density in the presence of joint injury.
9. The fabella, a small sesamoid bone located in the posterior joint capsule at the insertion of the lateral head of the gastrocnemius muscle, is noted in up to 18 percent of the population. When present, it will be seen as a small, oval-shaped density in the posterior soft tissues. Abnormal conditions, such as joint effusion or arthritis, may displace the fabella.[12]

CLINICAL OBJECTIVES:

1. Trace the distal femur.
2. Trace the proximal tibia and the proximal fibula, partially superimposed.
3. Trace the patella. Measure and compare the length of the patella to the length of the patellar tendon.

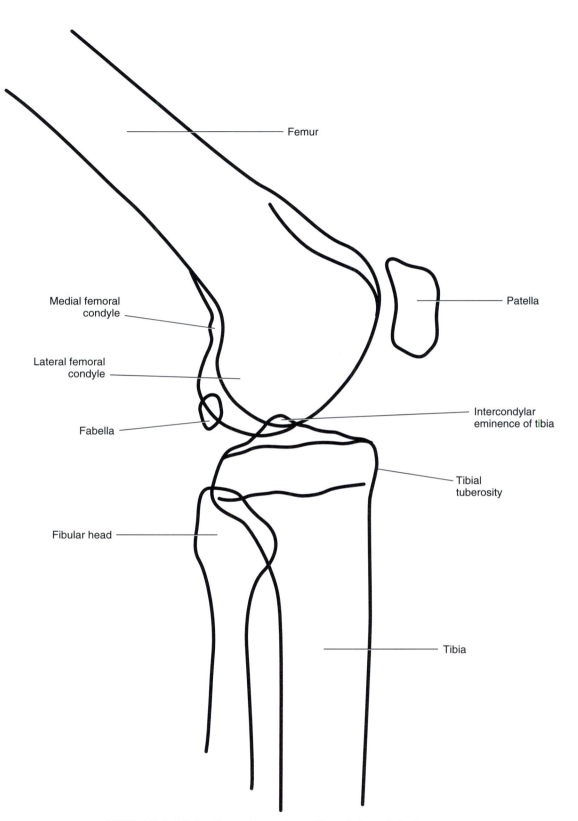

FIGURE 8–12. Radiographic tracing of lateral view of the knee.

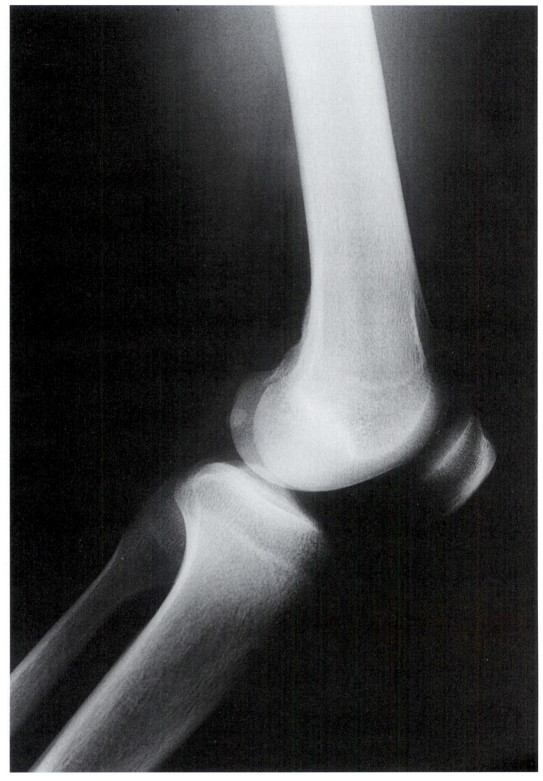

FIGURE 8–13. Lateral view of the knee.

Axial or Tunnel View of the Intercondylar Fossa (Figs. 8–14, 8–15, 8–16)

This view demonstrates the intercondylar fossa, the posterior aspects of the femoral and tibial condyles, the intercondylar eminence of the tibia, and the tibial plateaus. The important observations are:

1. The patient is prone and the knee is flexed approximately 40 degrees in this projection. The x-ray beam enters from a posterior to anterior direction.

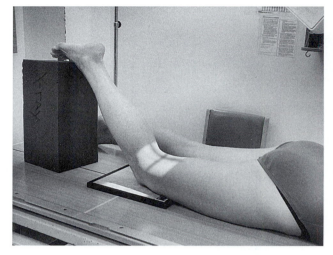

FIGURE 8–14. Patient position for axial view of the intercondylar fossa of the knee.

2. The patella is superimposed behind the distal femur.
3. The intercondylar fossa should appear open and its surface visualized.
4. The tibial articular surface should be partially visible. Both tibial spines of the intercondylar eminence should be visible.
5. The fibular head is partially superimposed over the proximal tibia.

CLINICAL OBJECTIVES

1. Trace the distal femur. Identify the medial and lateral condyles and the intercondylar fossa.
2. Trace the proximal tibia. Identify the medial and lateral condyles and the intercondylar eminence.
3. Trace the fibula.
4. Trace the patella superimposed behind the femur.

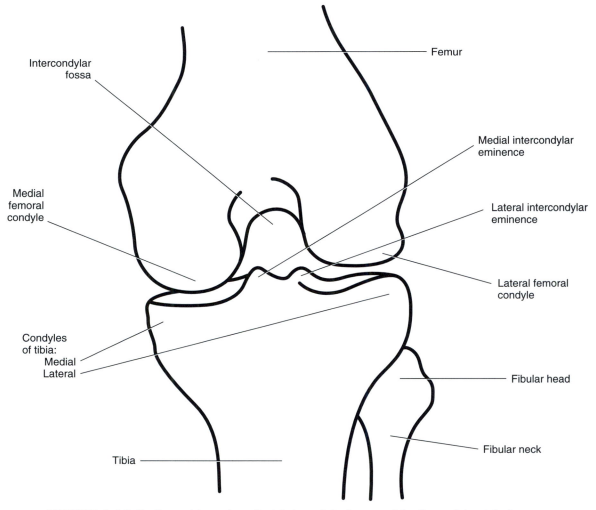

Femur

Medial intercondylar eminence

Lateral intercondylar eminence

Lateral femoral condyle

Fibular head

Fibular neck

Intercondylar fossa

Medial femoral condyle

Condyles of tibia:
Medial
Lateral

Tibia

FIGURE 8–15. Radiographic tracing of axial view of the intercondylar fossa of the right knee.

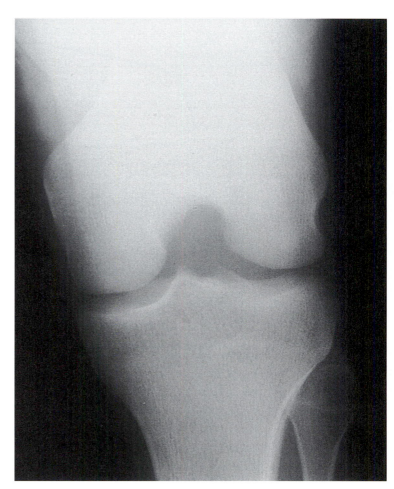

FIGURE 8–16. Axial view of the intercondylar fossa of the right knee.

Axial View of the Patellofemoral Joint (Figs. 8–17, 8–18, 8–19A)

This view demonstrates an axial view of the patellofemoral joint space and the articular surfaces of the patella and the femur. The important observations are:

1. The patient is positioned supine and the knee is flexed 45 degrees. The x-ray beam enters parallel to the patellofemoral joint space, or *tangentially* across the joint surface.
2. The articular surface of the patella should be smooth and distinct. Two superimposed borders may be imaged due to the irregular topography of the articular surface.
3. On this view, the medial and lateral facets of the patella are visible. Usually the medial facet is smaller than the lateral, and may show a more steeply sloped contour.
4. The intercondylar sulcus is identified as the groove between the distal femoral condyles.
5. This view can be used to detect subtle subluxations of the patella. Merchant described two measurements that can be used to determine normal positioning of the patella:[13,14]

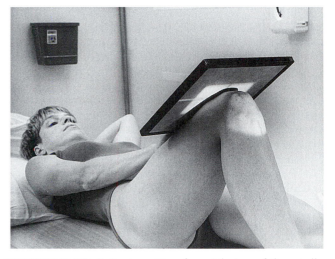

FIGURE 8–17. Patient position for axial view of the patellofemoral joint.

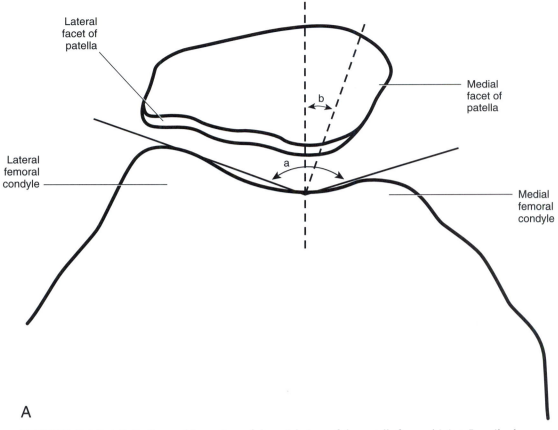

Lateral
facet of
patella

Medial
facet of
patella

Lateral
femoral
condyle

Medial
femoral
condyle

A

FIGURE 8–18. (*A*) Radiographic tracing of the axial view of the patellofemoral joint. Inscribed are the sulcus angle (a), and the congruence angle (b). (*B*) Axial view of patellofemoral joint.

The sulcus angle: Lines are drawn from the highest points of the femoral condyles to the deepest point of the trochlear groove. This angle has a normal value of 138 degrees, plus or minus 6 degrees. Shallow sulcus angles (those with greater measurements) may be related to recurrent patellar dislocations.

The congruence angle: This angle helps to define the position of the patella within the intercondylar sulcus. First, a reference line is drawn bisecting the sulcus angle. A second line is drawn from the apex of the sulcus angle to the most posterior or lowest point on the patellar articular ridge. If the second line is *medial* to the reference line, the resultant congruence angle formed is assigned a *negative* value. If the second line is *lateral* to the reference line, the resultant congruence angle is assigned a *positive* value. Merchant's study found an average congruence angle of −6 degrees in normal subjects. A congruence angle of +16 degrees or more was associated with lateral patellar subluxation or other patellofemoral disorders.

In evaluating the patellofemoral relationship, remember that this projection can only provide information specific to the position of knee flexion. A radiograph cannot provide information regarding the dynamic joint relationship but only information re-

garding one point in the range of motion. Additional tangential views are suggested at 30, 60, and 90 degrees of knee flexion to assist in diagnosing subtle subluxations.

CLINICAL OBJECTIVES

1. Trace the patella. Identify the medial and lateral surfaces.
2. Trace the femoral condyles. Identify the medial and lateral surfaces.
3. Trace and measure the sulcus angle.
4. Trace and measure the congruence angle.

Additional Views Related to the Knee

AP & LATERAL OF LOWER LEG

The radiographic evaluation of the *lower leg* is a separate examination from the knee. Both the knee and

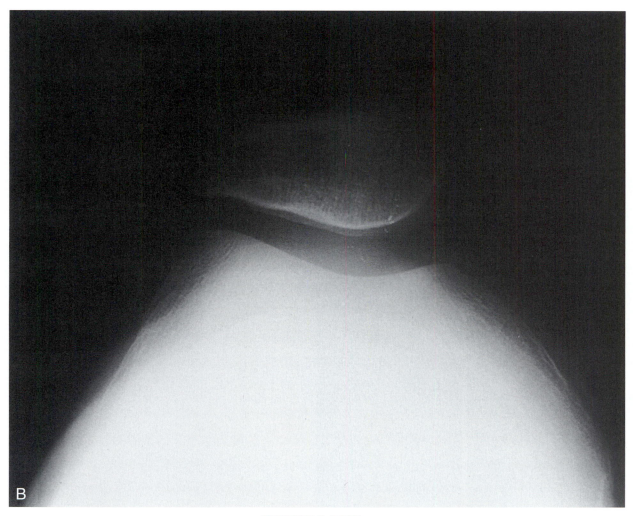

FIGURE 8–18(B).

ankle joints will, however, be included in routine AP and lateral radiographs (see Figs. 8–19B, C).

TRAUMA

The location of the knee joint at the junction of two long weight-bearing bones predisposes it to various types of injuries. The most common injuries to the knee joint involve the soft tissues, including the ligaments, menisci, and cartilage. Less common than soft tissue injuries but still seen frequently are fractures of the distal femur and proximal tibia. Dislocations are less common than fractures. The etiology of most knee injuries is related to direct trauma sustained during athletic activities or in motor vehicle accidents. Acute injuries occur most frequently in the teenage and adult age groups.[15]

Radiographs adequately diagnose most fractures. Many ancillary imaging studies are used in conjunction with plain films in diagnosing trauma at the knee. Bone scans assist in identifying subtle fractures. Conventional tomography assists in evaluating tibial pla-

teau and osteochondral fractures. Magnetic resonance imaging has almost completely replaced the use of arthrography in the diagnosis of ligamentous and meniscal tears.[16]

A discussion of common fractures, ligamentous injuries, and meniscal tears follows.

Fractures of the Distal Femur[17,18]

Fractures of the distal femur are classified by location as either *supracondylar*, *intercondylar*, or *condylar* fractures (Fig. 8–20).

Supracondylar fractures are fractures occurring at a site superior to the femoral condyles (Fig. 8–21). Fracture patterns associated with supracondylar fractures are comminution, impaction, or linear, with or without displacement.

Intercondylar fractures are located in the region between the medial and lateral femoral condyles. The fracture pattern appearing in this instance is commonly referred to as a "Y" fracture, as the condyles are split apart from each other and from the shaft. Con-

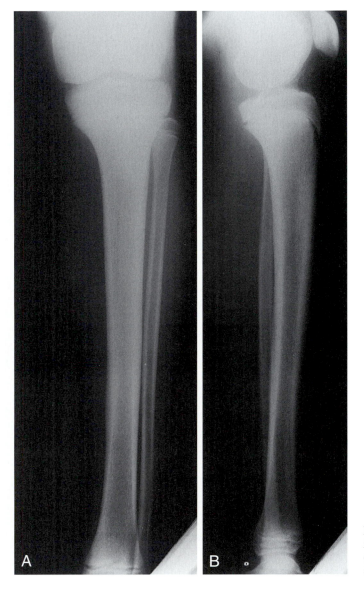

FIGURE 8–19. Routine radiographic examination of the leg includes AP (*A*) and lateral (*B*) views covering the entire length of the tibia and fibula, and the proximal and distal joint articulations.

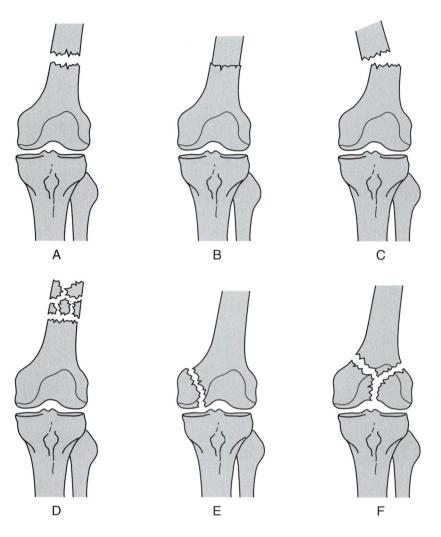

FIGURE 8–20. Fractures of the distal femur can be classified as supracondylar (*A*) nondisplaced, (*B*) impacted, (*C*) displaced, (*D*) comminuted; (*E*) condylar; or (*F*) intercondylar. (Adapted from Greenspan,[7] p. 8.14.)

dylar fractures are usually linear and involve only one femoral condyle.

Treatment of distal femur fractures may involve continuous skeletal traction via pinning through the tibial shaft, or open reduction and internal fixation. Complications include the formation of joint and soft tissue adhesions, and posttraumatic degenerative joint disease.

The radiographic assessment of distal femur fractures is usually complete on the routine AP and lateral projections of the knee. Conventional tomography may assist in evaluating the depth and extent of the fracture lines.

Fractures of the Proximal Tibia[19–21]

Fractures of the proximal tibia in adults occur most frequently at the medial and lateral tibial plateaus, with the lateral plateau more often involved (Fig. 3–15). Varus or valgus forces combined with axial compression will cause the hard femoral condyle to be

driven into the softer tibial plateau. This action will compress and depress the tibial articular surface and subchondral bone into the underlying cancellous bone. Thus, fractures of the tibial plateaus are actually *impaction fractures*.

Joint instability is a commonly associated complication of tibial plateau fractures. The varus and valgus forces acting on the knee also frequently rupture the collateral ligament contralateral to the fracture site, producing instability in the joint. Significant depression of one plateau will also cause joint instability due to the loss of the buttressing effect of the tibial plateau to the femoral condyle. This instability may occur despite intact ligaments.

Treatment of tibial plateau fractures varies dependent on the amount of tibial depression and comminution. Closed reduction with continuous pin traction is used in treatment of the elderly. Younger patients may require open reduction and internal fixation, and this can involve elevating and internally fixating the depressed plateau and filling the underlying defect with bone grafts. Complications of treatment include the formation of joint and soft tissue adhesions due to

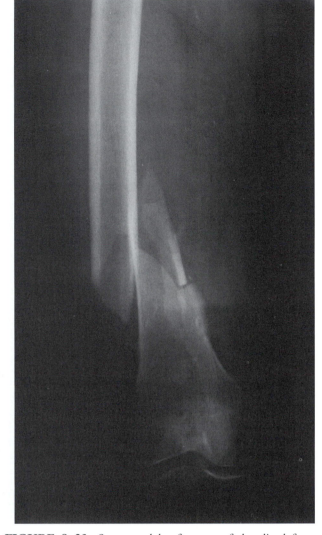

Type I: A nondisplaced vertical split fracture of the lateral tibial plateau, caused by a pure valgus force

Type II: A local depression of the lateral tibial plateau, caused by a combination of axial and valgus forces

Type III: A displaced vertical split fracture with depression at the lateral plateau, caused by a combination of valgus and axial forces, often associated with proximal fibula fracture

Type IV: A displaced depressed fracture of the medial plateau, caused by varus and axial forces

Type V: A vertical split fracture of the anterior or posterior aspect of the tibial plateau, caused by axial forces

Type VI: Displaced, comminuted fractures of both condyles, caused by axial forces, often associated with proximal fibula fractures

Note that proximal tibial fractures in children occur in entirely different patterns due to the uniqueness of growing bone. Areas predisposed to fracture are the epiphyseal growth plate and the metaphyseal region, which is composed of extensively remodeled new endosteal trabecular bone and more fenestrated laminar cortical bone, both of which predispose to compression injury (Fig. 8–23).

Fractures of the Patella[23–25]

The patella is vulnerable to two different types of injury. The superficial and anterior location of the patella predisposes it to *direct trauma* from falls or blows. Additionally, the position of the patella within the quadriceps tendon subjects it to *indirect trauma* from tension forces (Fig. 8–24).

In direct trauma, the patella fractures as it is compressed against the femur (Fig. 8–25). The most frequently seen fracture pattern is a transverse linear fracture line through the mid-region of the bone. Vertically oriented fracture lines and comminution are also seen. Fractures of the patella may be displaced or nondisplaced.

Avulsion fractures of the patella happen as a result of indirect trauma. A sudden and forceful contraction of the quadriceps while the knee is in flexion is the precipitating mechanism of injury. An example of this occurring is seen in the attempt of a person to keep himself or herself from falling after tripping.

Treatment of patella fractures often requires open reduction and internal fixation with wires followed by straight leg casting. Severe comminution with little hope of restoring a functional articular surface requires excision of the fracture fragments and reconstruction of the quadriceps expansion. Complications include posttraumatic degenerative joint disease of the patellofemoral joint, if the patella is present. If the patella has been excised, chronic loss of a percentage of knee extension strength is a significant functional problem.

FIGURE 8–21. Supracondylar fracture of the distal femur. This 83-year-old woman was injured while involved in a motor vehicle accident. The fracture is severely comminuted. The major fracture line extends obliquely through the lower third of the femoral shaft.

prolonged immobilization, pressure on the popliteal nerve due to the injury itself or from casting, and post-traumatic degenerative joint disease.

The radiographic assessment of tibial plateau fractures often requires conventional tomography in addition to the routine radiographic assessment. The expanse of the tibial plateau necessitates the imaging of various depths possible on tomography to accurately determine the extent of the fracture line or the amount of depression present across the plateaus.

The Hohl classification system of tibial plateau fractures identifies six common fracture patterns and their predisposing force mechanisms (Fig. 8–22)[22]:

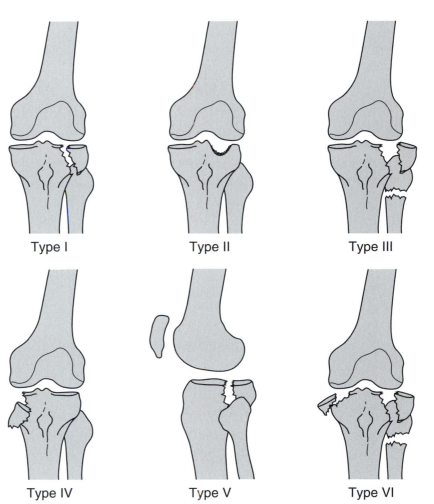

Type I   Type II   Type III

Type IV   Type V   Type VI

FIGURE 8–22. (*Type I–Type VI*) The Hohl classification of tibial plateau fractures. (Adapted from Greenspan,[7] p. 8.15.)

Radiographic assessment of patellar fractures includes tangential, lateral, and oblique views. Conventional tomography is a commonly used ancillary technique.

Subluxations and Dislocations of the Patella[26–28]

Chronic subluxations of the patella are much more common than true dislocations. Extensive literature exists devoted to patellar tracking dysfunctions, extensor mechanism deficiencies, and pathognomonic biomechanical factors present at the patellofemoral joint or acting on the joint, all of which can contribute to the predisposition for the initial subluxation or dislocation and the susceptibility for recurrent subluxation or dislocation. While the diagnosis of a chronically subluxing/dislocating patellofemoral joint may be clinically evident by history or physical examination, radiographs are necessary to determine if osteochondral fragments or fractures are present, to assist in the di-

agnosis of subtle subluxations, or to provide information regarding the joint articular surfaces and joint congruity at different points in the range of motion.

When evaluating the subluxing/dislocating patellofemoral joint via radiographs, multiple views are necessary. No single view can demonstrate all of the articular surfaces. Also, in functional reality, even multiple views cannot define the dynamic relationship of the patella to the femoral intercondylar sulcus during movement. However, multiple views can provide a great deal of information. The recommended projections for evaluating subluxation are not standard and vary among authors. Multiple tangential and lateral views made at varying degrees of flexion are suggested, as are other weight-bearing AP and oblique views. In the clinical management of this condition, a systemic radiologic approach correlated with patient history and physical findings best serves to aid clinical decision making.

Acute traumatic dislocations of the patellofemoral joint are rare (Fig. 8–26). (Although the patients with recurrent subluxations/dislocations had to have an initial episode, they also typically have abnormal bio-

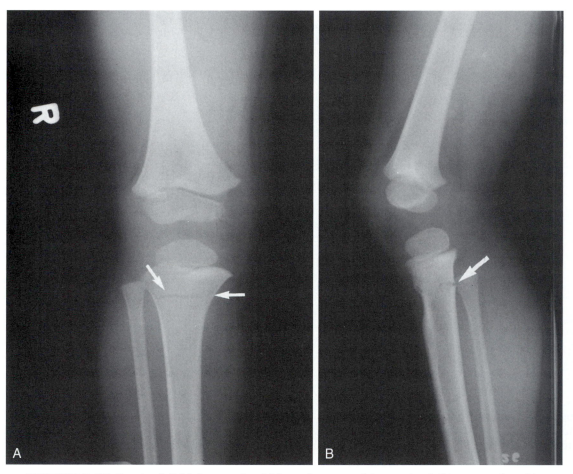

FIGURE 8–23. Proximal tibial fracture. In children, the areas of the proximal tibia most vulnerable to fracture are the epiphyseal growth plate and the metaphyseal region, which is composed of newly remodeled bone and is predisposed to compression injury. This 3½-year-old boy fell off a jungle gym and sustained a transverse, greenstick-type fracture through a metaphysis of the proximal tibia. (*A*) The AP view of the knee demonstrates the transverse linear fracture site (arrows). (*B*) The lateral view of the knee localizes the fracture site to the posterior margin of the proximal metaphysis. The fracture line breaks through the posterior cortex but does not extend to the anterior cortex (arrow). Although this fracture appears simple, any fracture in this region in growing bone can develop undesirable sequelae, namely angulation and deformity secondary to overgrowth at the healed fracture site. (It is interesting to note the absence of the image of the patella, which does not begin ossification until 4 years of age.)

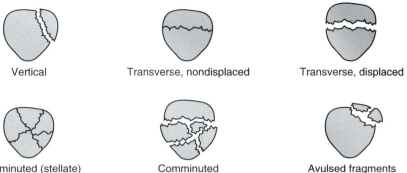

Vertical | Transverse, nondisplaced | Transverse, displaced

Comminuted (stellate) nondisplaced | Comminuted displaced | Avulsed fragments

FIGURE 8–24. Examples of patellar fractures. (Adapted from Greenspan,[7] p. 8.18.)

mechanics that may have increased susceptibility and predisposed the event.[29]) In patients with "normal" patellofemoral configuration, normal strength, and normal alignment of the joint and extensor mechanism, a relatively severe injury is necessary to produce a patellofemoral dislocation. The usual mechanism is a direct blow to a flexed knee, as in a motor vehicle accident, or a powerful quadriceps contraction superimposed on a rotary or valgus force at the knee, as when a runner is cutting to the direction opposite his or her planted foot. Radiographs are necessary prereduction and postreduction to identify avulsed bony or cartilaginous fragments or fractures.

Fractures and Dislocations of the Proximal Fibula[30]

Fractures of the fibula result from three mechanisms of injury: a direct blow, a twisting injury to the ankle, or a varus stress to the knee. Fractures are classified by location at the fibular head, neck, or shaft. Associated injuries are frequently seen, including injury to the peroneal nerve, the anterior tibial artery, and the interosseous membrane. Associated tibial fractures, located at the same level as the fibular fracture or distally at the ankle, are also seen. Fibular fractures usually heal without difficulty; however, if a fibular fracture heals before a tibial fracture at the same level, the fibula may prevent the necessary compression at the tibial site, leading to tibial nonunion.

The proximal fibula may be subluxed or dislocated from acute trauma such as a direct blow or a striking of the lateral aspect of the leg in a fall, or from chronic excessive torsional stresses originating at the ankle causing hypermobility at the superior tibiofibular joint. Diagnosis is made on plain films by a bilateral comparison of the joints. The AP projection demonstrates lateral displacement of the involved proximal fibula with widening of the proximal interosseous space (Fig. 8–27). The lateral view of the involved joint demonstrates greater overlap of the fibula on the tibia in comparison to the uninvolved joint.

Fractures of the Articular Cartilage[31–33]

Impaction forces or combinations of shear, rotation, and impaction forces at the knee joint may injure the articular cartilage or the underlying subchondral bone. Injuries involving the articular cartilage are referred to as *chondral fractures*. Compressions of the subchondral bone are referred to as *subchondral fractures*. The tibial plateau, tibial condyles, femoral condyles, or patella may be involved.

These fractures may be extremely subtle but are suspected in the presence of a clinical history including an acute traumatic episode combined with clinical symptoms of joint effusion, pain, and localized tenderness. The severity of the injury may range from only a minor indentation of the articular cartilage to a portion of the articular cartilage becoming detached, often taking with it a piece of subchondral bone. A partially attached fragment is referred to as an *osteocartilaginous flap*, and a segment that is completely detached and floating freely about the joint is an *osteochondral fragment* (Fig. 8–28).

Osteochondritis dissecans is the presence of avascular necrosis at the site of an osteochondral fracture, osteocartilaginous flap, or the detached osteochondral fragment (Fig. 8–29). Osteochondritis dissecans appears predominantly in older children and young adults, affecting males with greater frequency. The femoral condyles are the most common location. The etiology is debated; acute trauma, chronic trauma, and pre-existing abnormalities in the epiphyses are all suspected as playing a role in the development of this condition.

Treatment of the foregoing conditions may be conservative, consisting of limited weight-bearing and joint movement, or may require surgical intervention to remove a fragment or fixate a large fragment back in place.

The radiologic assessment of chondral fractures is incomplete with plain films and requires arthrography or magnetic resonance imaging (MRI) for full evaluation of the articular cartilage. Osteochondral fractures may be visualized on plain films, especially if the frag-

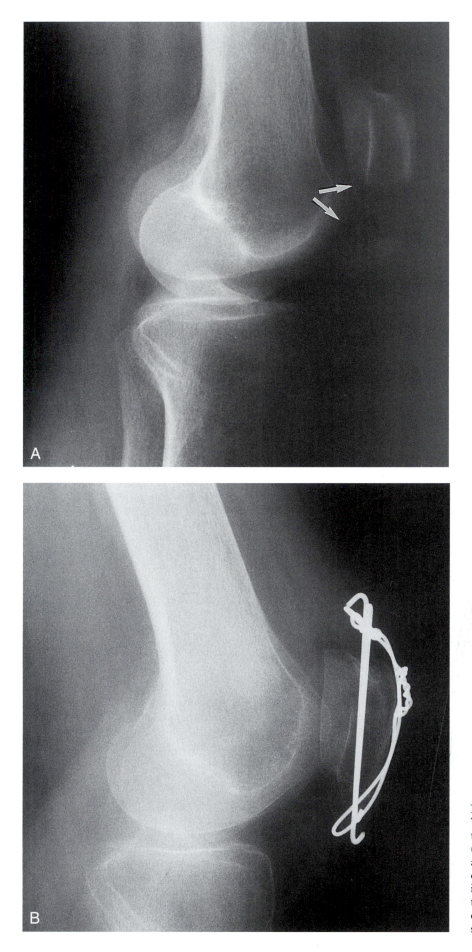

FIGURE 8–25. Fracture of the patella. This very active 68-year-old woman fractured her patella in a fall off her rollerskates. (*A*) Lateral view of the knee demonstrates a transverse linear fracture line through the distal third of the patella. The white arrows indicate the wide displacement of the fracture fragments. (*B*) Follow-up films demonstrate pin-and-wire fixation devices and successful healing of the fracture site.

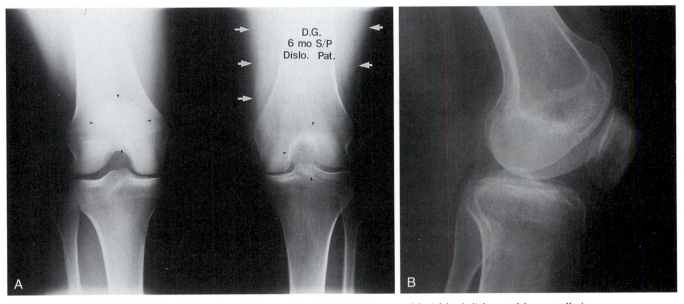

FIGURE 8–26. Dislocation of the patella. (*A*) This 16-year-old girl had dislocated her patella in a skateboarding accident. Follow-up films made 6 months after injury show patella baja, an abnormally inferior position of the patella secondary to extensor mechanism insufficiency. The black triangles denote the abnormal position of the patella on the patient's left and the normal position of the patella on the patient's right. The white arrows indicate the diminished soft tissue shadow representing a decrease in the bulk of the quadriceps muscle group. Compare with the uninvolved right thigh shadow for normal soft tissue image. Besides muscle atrophy, note the disuse atrophy of bone by comparing the increased radiolucency of the proximal tibia and distal femur on the involved extremity with that of the uninvolved extremity. This demineralization of bone is directly related to the prolonged disuse of the extremity. (*B*) Lateral view of the left knee demonstrates the abnormal inferior position of the patella.

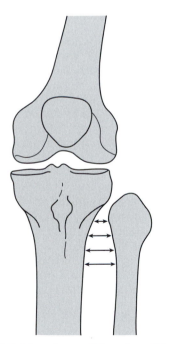

FIGURE 8–27. Subluxation or dislocation of the proximal tibiofibular joint is apparent on the anteroposterior projection by the wide proximal interosseous space.

ment has become detached. Osteochondritis dissecans, as with other examples of avascular necrosis, may show no abnormalities on early stage plain films and is best evaluated with bone scan or MRI.

Tears of the Menisci[34,35]

Meniscal tears occur during shear, rotary, and compression forces that abnormally stress the fibrocartilaginous tissues. The medial meniscus is more frequently injured than the lateral meniscus due to its greater peripheral attachment and decreased mobility, impairing its ability to withstand imposed forces. The lateral meniscus is more prone to injury, however, if the developmental abnormality, often referred to as a *discoid meniscus*, is present. A discoid lateral meniscus is an enlarged, thickened meniscus, theorized to be caused by repetitive movements. An abnormally wide lateral radiographic joint space is evident on the AP knee projection if this condition exists.

The most common meniscal tears are vertically oriented through the tissue; a longitudinal extension of a vertical tear is called a *bucket handle tear* (Fig. 8–30). Degenerative tears in the older age groups are usually horizontally oriented.

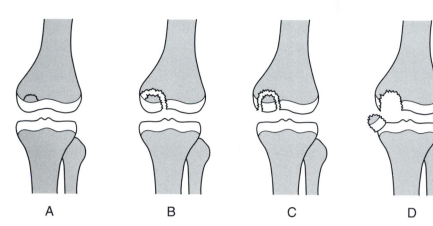

A   B   C   D

FIGURE 8–28. Examples of chondral fractures: (*A*) Osteochondral body with intact articular cartilage; (*B*) osteocartilaginous flap; (*C*) detached osteochondral fragment; (*D*) detached osteochondral fragment in joint. Avascular necrosis if any of these lesions is termed *osteochondritis dissecans*. (Adapted from Greenspan,[7] p. 8.23.)

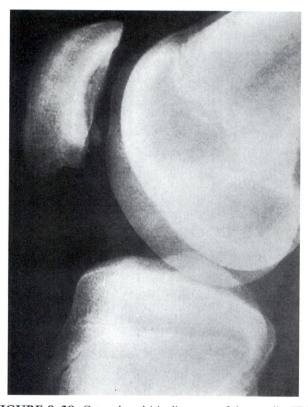

FIGURE 8–29. Osteochondritis dissecans of the patella. This 15-year-old boy presented with complaints of being unable to extend the right knee completely after weight-bearing for the past 2 years. During the past 6 months there had also been slight swelling of the knee. This lateral view of the knee demonstrates a well-defined radiolucency on the articular surface of the patella representing cartilaginous and bony sequestrum. An osteochondral flap, or a partially attached fragment of necrotic bone, is visible at the distal end of the radiolucency. The necrotic bone was surgically debrided. (From Eiken, M: Roentgen Diagnoses of Bones: A Self-Teaching Manual. FADLS Forlag AS, Copenhagen, 1975, p. 28, with permission.)

Treatment generally involves surgical intervention as the torn fragment will disrupt normal knee functioning. Total meniscectomies are uncommon unless the entire meniscus is involved. Partial meniscectomies excise the torn portion of the meniscus and preserve as much of the meniscus as possible. Surgical repair of tears is possible in smaller, peripherally located tears where good vascularity is present.

Because cartilaginous tissue is indistinct on plain radiographs, routine radiographic assessment may only expose joint effusion, secondary to the intra-articular damage. Arthrography with contrast was the definitive diagnostic study in the past but has been almost completely replaced by MRI (Fig. 8–31).

Tears of the Collateral Ligaments[36,37]

The medial collateral ligament is typically injured as a result of a valgus force. The lateral collateral is injured resulting from a varus force. The medial ligament is the more commonly injured collateral and is often associated with tears of the joint capsule and medial meniscus, to which it is firmly attached. Severe injuries will further damage the anterior cruciate ligament, and this combination of injuries is referred to as *O'Donoghue's unhappy triad* (Fig. 8–32). Treatment in the case of isolated tears may be conservative with controlled motion bracing and extensive rehabilitation. Surgical repair is often required in more involved injuries, followed by extensive rehabilitation.

Radiographic assessment includes the evaluation of joint instability via stress films. To evaluate the integrity of the medial collateral ligament a valgus force is applied at the knee and an AP projection is done. Excessive widening of the medial joint space is consistent with a diagnosis of medial collateral ligament tear.

Arthrographic evaluation of a medial collateral ligament tear will show a leak of contrast material at the tear site. Chronic tears may heal and eventually ossify, and then the characteristic *Pellegrini-Stieda* lesion will be evident on the AP projection as a calcification at the site of old injury.

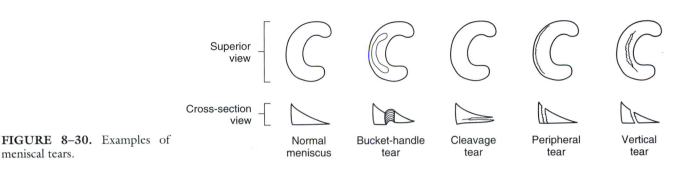

FIGURE 8–30. Examples of meniscal tears.

Superior view | Cross-section view — Normal meniscus / Bucket-handle tear / Cleavage tear / Peripheral tear / Vertical tear

Tears of the Cruciate Ligaments[38,39]

Isolated tears to the cruciate ligaments are uncommon. The collateral ligaments, capsule, and menisci are frequently associated injuries. Common mechanisms of injury to the posterior cruciate ligament involve external forces that strike the anterior aspect of the knee, as in dashboard injuries. Common mechanisms of injury to the anterior cruciate ligament involve noncontact forces that place great valgus and rotary stresses on the knee, as when an athlete suddenly decelerates and turns.

Treatment depends on the amount of joint instability, the amount of associated structural damage, and the patient's desired activity level. Treatment at the conservative end may include controlled motion bracing and extensive rehabilitation; surgical intervention may include direct, primary repairs of the injured tissues, or reconstructive procedures using tendon grafts, followed by extensive rehabilitation.

The plain film radiographic assessment of cruciate ligament injuries may be able to identify an avulsed portion of bone at the attachment site of a collateral (Fig. 8–33). Generally, however, the study of choice is MRI.

Trauma of the Patellar Ligament[40,41]

Two similar conditions related to trauma occur at either end of the patellar ligament (Fig. 8–34). *Sinding-Larsen-Johansson* disease refers to a disorder at the proximal patellar attachment, and *Osgood-Schlatter* disease refers to a disorder at the distal patellar attachment. These disorders are mechanical in etiology, possibly initiated by trauma such as a fall, and are not true disease processes. The repetitive irritation from tension forces generated by quadriceps activity postinjury is theorized to be a factor in the development of these conditions. Adolescents, predominantly males, are most frequently affected.

Sinding-Larsen-Johansson disease is a traction separation with fragmentation of the inferior pole of the patella (Fig. 8–35). Calcification and ossification often appear in the patellar ligament when the condition has become chronic.

Osgood-Schlatter disease is a traction apophysitis at

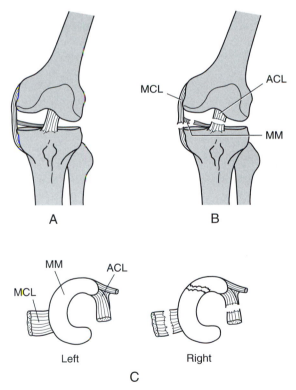

FIGURE 8–32. (*A–C*) The "terrible triad," a combination of injuries to the medial meniscus, medial collateral ligament, and anterior cruciate ligament, viewed in two different perspectives. (*A*) Intact ligaments stretched by valgus force. (*B*) Rupture of MCL, ACL, and MM. (*C*) *Left* normal relationship of MCL, ACL, and MM, superior view, *right*, rupture of MCL, ACL, and MM, superior view.

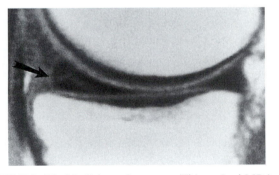

FIGURE 8–31. Medial meniscus tear. This sagittal MR image of the knee shows a tear of the medial meniscus. Note the high-intensity signal of the tear, which extends into the inferior surface of the meniscus (arrow). (From Greenspan,[7] p. 8.29, with permission.)

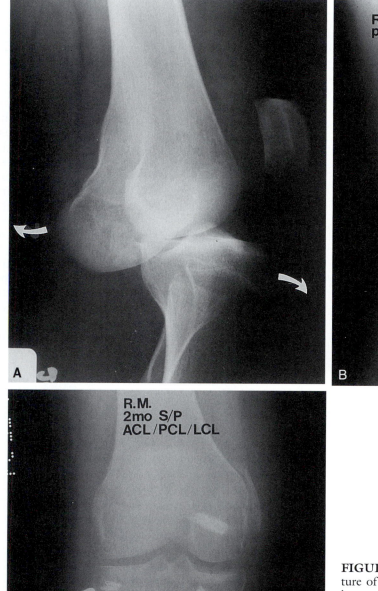

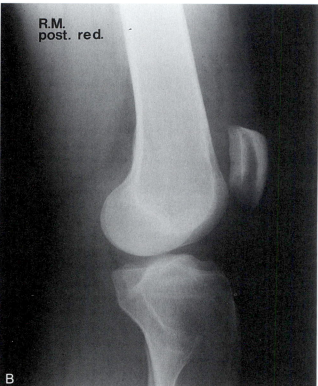

FIGURE 8–33. Anterior dislocation of the knee with rupture of ligaments. This 22-year-old man was injured when he was thrown from a horse he was trying to saddle break and the horse fell on him. (*A*) Lateral view of the knee shows the anterior displacement of the tibia in relation to the distal femur. (*B*) Lateral film made after reduction demonstrates normal articulating relationships and absence of any fractures. Note the great amount of capsular effusion and soft tissue swelling. (*C*) Although the patient did not sustain any fractures, he did rupture several ligaments. This AP film demonstrates the prosthetic devices used to surgically fixate and reconstruct the attachments of the anterior cruciate ligament, posterior cruciate ligament, and lateral collateral ligament. This patient was fortunate that he escaped neurovascular injury during the initial accident. About half of all knee dislocations involve some degree of damage to the popliteal artery or peroneal nerve.

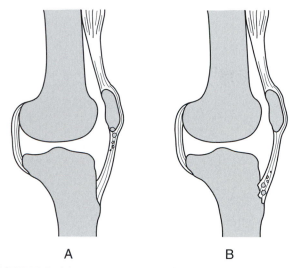

A   B

FIGURE 8–34. Representation of traction apophysitis with fragmentation in the patellar ligament (*A*) at the inferior patella pole, known as *Sinding-Larsen-Johansson* disease, and (*B*) at the tibial tuberosity, known as *Osgood-Schlatter* disease.

the tibial tubercle (Fig. 8–36). Chronic irritation from tension forces generated by the quadriceps (often due to repeated jumping and running on hard surfaces) enlarge and deforms the tubercle.

Treatment consists of limited activity, modalities to control inflammation and pain, and protective padding to prevent further impact to the knee. Surgical excision of large calcified areas may be necessary.

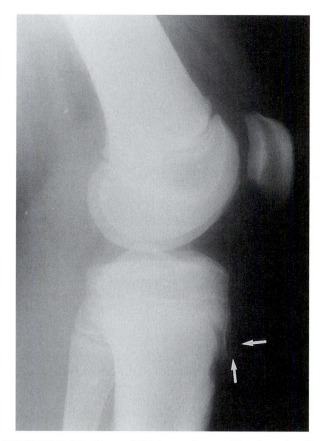

FIGURE 8–36. Osgood-Schlatter disease. This lateral radiograph of the knee demonstrates calcification and ossification with the patellar ligament at its attachment to the tibial tubercle (arrows). The patient is an 11-year-old boy who is an avid basketball player.

Both disorders present clinically with soft tissue swelling, pain, and localized tenderness. The lateral radiograph usually establishes the diagnosis as bone fragmentation, and ossification within the tendon is obvious at either location.

DEGENERATIVE JOINT DISEASE[42–44]

Degenerative joint disease (DJD) or osteoarthritis of the knees is present to some degree in the majority of people over age 55. Repetitive mechanical and compressive stresses from occupational, recreational, athletic, and normal activities of daily living over many decades typically result in osteoarthritic changes. Also, secondary osteoarthritic changes are a long-term sequela of previous fracture, meniscal, or ligamentous injury. The characteristic radiographic signs of osteoarthritis at the knee are similar to other large joints and include (1) decreased radiographic joint space, (2) sclerosis of subchondral bone, (3) osteophyte formation at joint margins, and (4) subchondral cyst formation (Fig. 8–37). The routine radiographic examination sufficiently demonstrates these changes.

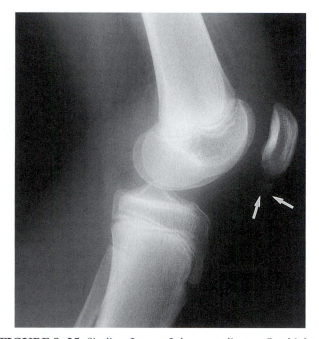

FIGURE 8–35. Sinding-Larsen-Johansson disease. On this lateral view of the knee, calcification and ossification within the patellar ligament is apparent just distal to the patella (arrows). The patient is a 13-year-old girl who is an avid clogging and tap dancer.

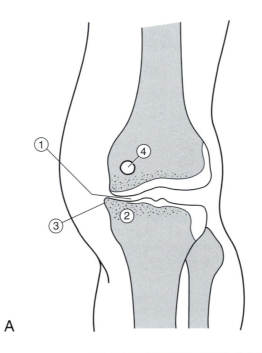

A

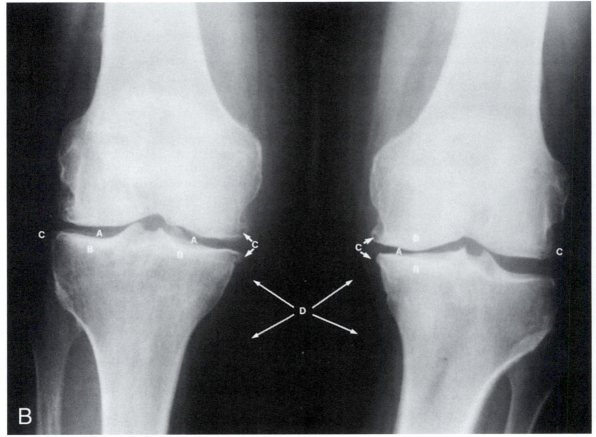

B

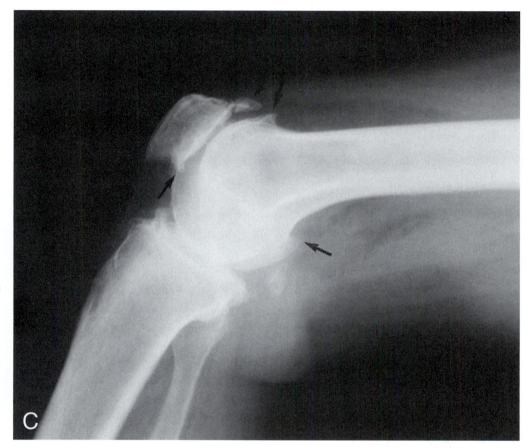

FIGURE 8–37. Degenerative joint disease of the knees. (*A*) Representation of radiographic hallmarks of osteoarthritis: (1) decreased joint space, (2) sclerotic subchondral bone, (3) osteophyte formation at joint margins, and (4) subchondral cyst formation. (*B*) AP weight-bearing view of bilateral knees in an elderly male demonstrates the characteristic hallmarks of advanced DJD: A, Narrowed joint spaces. Note the extreme narrowing of the medial compartment of patient's left knee. B, Sclerosis of subchondral bone; C, osteophyte formation at joint margins; D, joint deformity secondary to loss of articular cartilage thickness and altered joint congruity. Note the soft tissue outline of both extremities, which show a medial bulging at the joint line combined with a bow leg or valgus deformity secondary to the medial angulation and slight rotation of the tibia. This deformity is more pronounced on patient's left lower extremity. (*C*) On this lateral view of the knee, note DJD of the patellofemoral joint with flattening of the patellar articular surface and marked spur formation at the patella margins and the margins of the femoral condyles (arrows). The irregularly shaped density in the soft tissue of the popliteal fossa is the fabella.

The location of osteoarthritis at the knee is often described by the knee's anatomic compartments. The *medial compartment* of the knee refers to the articulation between the medial femoral and tibial condyles. The *lateral compartment* of the knee refers to the articulation between the lateral femoral and tibial condyles. The patellofemoral articulation is also referred to as a compartment, and is susceptible to osteoarthritic changes as well (Figs. 8–37B, C). Advanced osteoarthritis of the lateral or medial compartments alters the congruity of the articular surfaces and may cause a varus or valgus type deformity, respectively, visible both on films and clinically (Fig. 8–38).

Note that, similar to osteoarthritis at any joint, the severity of the radiographic findings of knee joint osteoarthritis do not always correlate with the severity of pain and functional loss experienced by the patient (Chapter 2). Marked radiographic changes may be seen in a patient experiencing minimal pain or func-

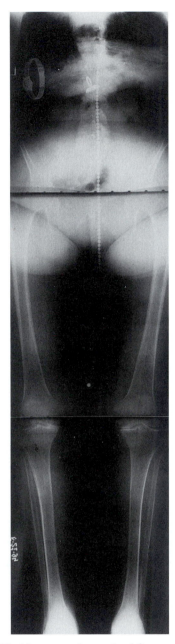

FIGURE 8–38. Alignment determined from standing views of the entire lower extremity. This weight-bearing view assists the surgeon preoperatively in determining the amount of varus or valgus deformity present secondary to the osteoarthritic knee joint, and planning for the amount of surgical correction required. Various types of surgical procedures can correct knee joint deformities including tibial osteotomy, in which a wedge of bone is removed from the proximal tibia in order to realign the leg and reduce and redistribute stresses over the largest possible articular surface; and total joint arthroplasty, which resects the involved articular surfaces and replaces them with artificial fibial, femoral, and patellar prosthesis. Note that whatever procedure is chosen, it is likely that the leg length will be altered postoperatively. It is desirable in the patient's rehabilitation that this is compensated for in order to prevent further mechanical stresses in the other joints of the kinetic chain. This can be achieved simply by utilizing a heel lift in the shoe of the shorter leg.

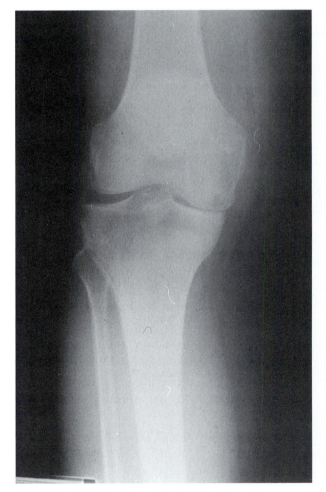

FIGURE 8–39. This AP weight-bearing film of the right knee demonstrates advanced osteoarthritic changes of the medial compartment of the knee with a valgus deformity of the leg. The patient's activity was impaired because of severe pain, so she elected to undergo a total joint replacement. (From Richardson and Iglarsh,[1] p. 650, with permission.)

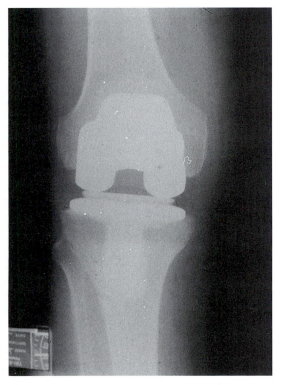

FIGURE 8–40. Postoperative AP view of the knee demonstrating the femoral and tibial components of the artificial joint. (From Richardson and Iglarsh[1] p. 650, with permission.)

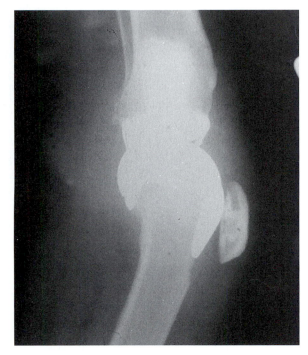

FIGURE 8–41. Postoperative lateral view demonstrates the femoral, tibial, and patellar prosthetic components. Note that the *articular surface* of the patella is replaced; a small stem drilled into the midportion of the patella anchors the surface to the patient's own patella. (From Richardson and Iglarsh,[1] p. 651, with permission.)

tional loss, and minor radiographic changes may exist in a patient with debilitating pain. Osteoarthritis that has progressed to the point where pain and loss of joint function debilitates ambulation may require surgical intervention. Total joint arthroplasty (total knee replacement) is a surgical procedure that replaces the articular surfaces of the femur, tibia, and patella (Figs. 8–39, 8–40, 8–41). Extensive rehabilitation post–joint replacement restores normal strength and functional motion to the knee. Complications of this procedure include bone fracture, instability, infection, and loosening of the prosthesis.[45]

ANOMALIES[46,47]

As discussed previously, congenital or developmental anomalies can generally be grouped into categories related to a structure's failure to develop, arrested development, or the development of accessory bones. At the knee an additional grouping is needed, regarding the deformity that may be present within the bone itself, as in the example of congenital limb bowing. Common examples of knee and lower extremity congenital deformities are genu valgum, genu varum, and genu recurvatum.

Genu Valgum

Genu valgum denotes the angular deformity of the lower extremities commonly referred to as "knock-knees." The distal ends of the tibia are spaced widely apart when the knees are approximated (Figs. 8–42, 8–43). The condition becomes most obvious when the child begins to ambulate. The etiology may be familial,

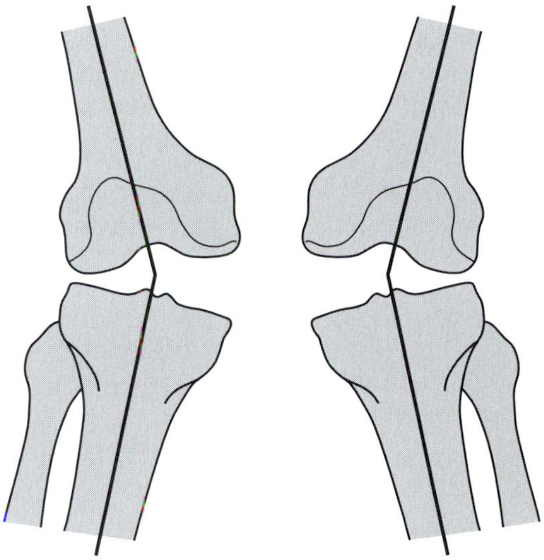

FIGURE 8–42. Genu valgum, or "knock knees," is an angular deformity of the lower extremities, whereby the ankles are spaced widely apart when the knees are approximated.

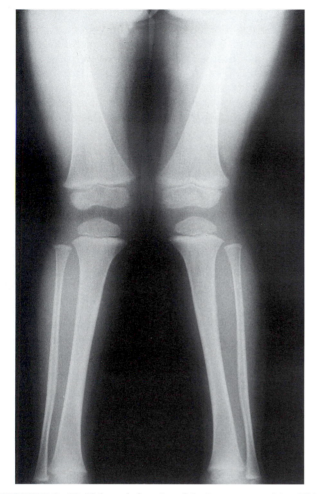

FIGURE 8–43. Valgus deformity of the lower extremities. This AP weight-bearing view of the lower extremities in a 3-year-old boy shows the approximation of the knees and wide spacing of the ankles in extension, as is characteristic with genu valgum.

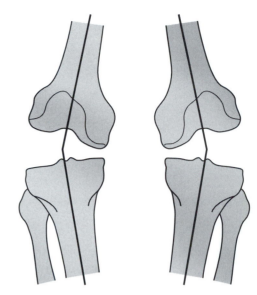

FIGURE 8–44. Genu varum, or "bow legs," is an angular deformity of the lower extremities, whereby the knees are spaced widely apart when the ankle malleoli are in contact.

related to hip or foot positioning, associated with trauma to the epiphyseal plate, fractures, or neurologic deficits, or may be idiopathic.

Treatment and prognosis depend on the etiologic factors and the severity of the angulation. Conservative treatment for mild cases may consist of orthotic correction of foot pronation and exercise to address flexibility and strength deficits. Surgery may be required in more severe cases to restore normal joint articulation. The AP radiograph, enlarged in scope to view the entire lower extremity, adequately demonstrates this deformity.

Genu Varum

Genu varum is the angular deformity of the lower extremities commonly referred to as "bowlegs." The

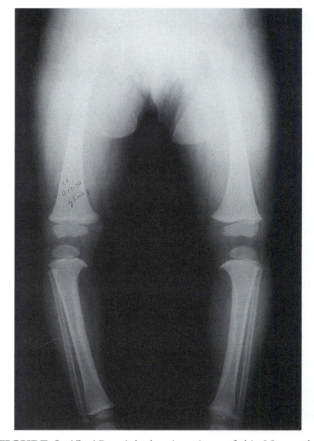

FIGURE 8–45. AP weight-bearing views of this 18-month-old girl demonstrate bilateral genu varum. This symmetric, apparent bowing is common in many toddlers and is usually outgrown in childhood. See Figure 8–46 for follow-up film.

knees are spaced widely apart when the ankle malleoli are in contact (Fig. 8–44). It is common for a certain amount of apparent bowing to be present in infants and toddlers, and this *physiologic bowing* will be symmetric and is usually outgrown during childhood, decreasing progressively as the child ages (Figs. 8–45, 8–46).

The etiology of genu varum may also be highly varied, related to renal or dietary rickets, epiphyseal injury, osteogenesis imperfecta, or osteochondritis, known as Blount's disease.

Blount's disease, in contrast to physiological bowing, is a developmental anomaly in which the medial proximal tibial epiphysis, epiphyseal plate, and metaphysis are deformed by growth arrest (Fig. 8–47). It commonly appears bilaterally at the knee between the ages of 1 and 3, but may also appear, usually unilaterally, in early adolescence. Treatment is often successful with bracing, although osteotomy may be required to achieve normal joint alignment.

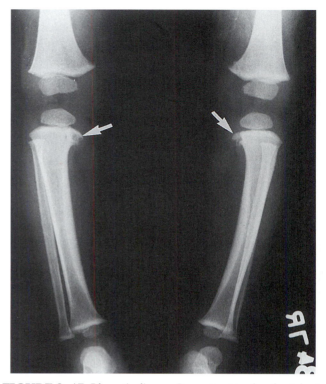

FIGURE 8–47. Blount's disease. In contrast to the physiologic bowing as seen in Fig. 8–45 and 8–46, the lower-extremity bowing seen in this 18-month-old is secondary to a developmental anomaly in which the medial proximal tibial epiphysis, epiphyseal plate, and metaphysis are deformed by growth arrest. Note the bony irregularities of this region seen bilaterally (arrows).

Radiographically, the deformity of the lower extremities will be evident on the AP projection. Developmental physiologic bowing of the extremities is distinguished from other disease processes by the normal appearance of cortical bone, epiphyses, plates, and metaphyses. Both the femoral and tibial medial and lateral cortical shafts will exhibit gentle bowing. In contrast, Blount's disease will show deformity, depression, and possibly early fusion at the medial tibial epiphysis and metaphysis.

Genu Recurvatum

Genu recurvatum is excessive hyperextension of the knee (Figs. 8–48, 8–49, 8–50). Etiologies are varied and numerous, and may be familial, idiopathic, or related to neurologic and muscular deficits.

Treatment and prognosis are dependent on the etiologic factors but is usually conservative, using bracing and exercise to restore alignment and muscular balance. The lateral radiograph demonstrates this deformity.

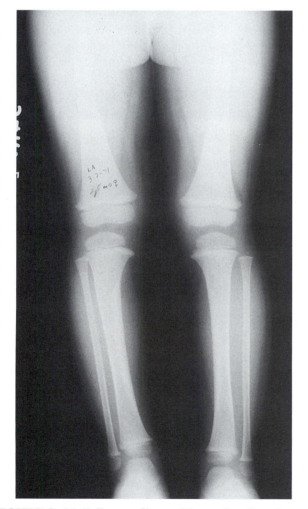

FIGURE 8–46. Follow-up films at 29 months of age demonstrate that a natural correction of the bowing has occurred.

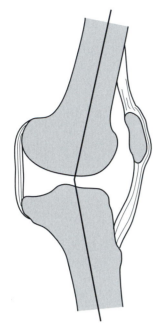

FIGURE 8–48. Genu recurvatum, or extreme hyperextension of the knee, is obvious on the lateral view of the joint.

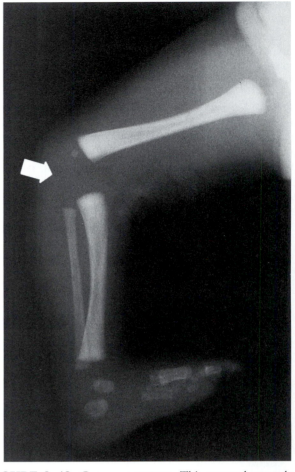

FIGURE 8–49. Genu recurvatum. This unusual example of genu recurvatum is seen in a radiograph of a 2-day-old infant. The arrow points to the *posterior* knee joint, which is in a position of extreme hyperextension.

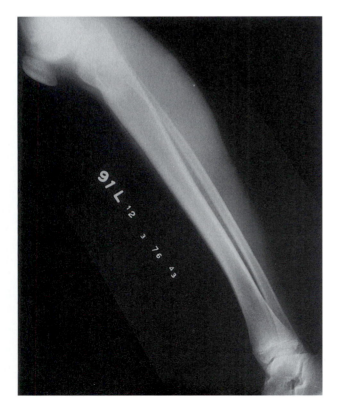

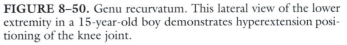

FIGURE 8–50. Genu recurvatum. This lateral view of the lower extremity in a 15-year-old boy demonstrates hyperextension positioning of the knee joint.

SUMMARY OF KEY POINTS

1. The routine radiographic evaluation of the knee includes four projections:
   - **Anteroposterior:** Demonstrates the tibiofemoral joint, distal femur, and proximal tibia. The patella is obscured as it is superimposed over the distal femur
   - **Lateral:** Demonstrates the patellofemoral joint in profile, the expanse of the quadriceps and patellar tendon, and the suprapatellar bursa
   - **Axial of the intercondylar fossa:** Demonstrates the intercondylar fossa, the posterior aspect of the femoral condyles, and the intercondylar eminence of the tibial plateau
   - **Axial of the patellofemoral joint:** Demonstrates the patella and the articular relationship of the patellofemoral joint at one point in the range of motion
2. In regard to trauma at the knee, the most frequently seen injuries involve the soft tissues of the joint including the menisci, collateral ligaments, and cruciate ligaments. Soft tissue trauma is usually diagnosed via arthrography or MRI. Fractures at the knee are diagnosed via radiography, conventional tomography, and radionuclide bone scans.
3. Fractures of the distal femur are classified by anatomic location as supracondylar, intercondylar, or condylar fractures.
4. Fractures of the proximal tibia occur most frequently at the tibial plateaus with the lateral plateau most often involved. The Hohl classification system identifies six common fracture patterns and their predisposing force mechanisms.
5. The patella is vulnerable to two types of injury: fracture sustained from a direct blow or avulsion fracture sustained from forceful contraction of the quadriceps.
6. Osteochondral fractures are fractures at the articular cartilage or the underlying subcondral bone. Osteochondritis dissecans is avascular necrosis at the site of an osteochondral fracture. Radiographic assessment of osteochondral pathology is usually incomplete with plain films, so ancillary studies such as arthrography, computed tomography, and MRI are used to fully evaluate the articular cartilage.
7. Sinding-Larsen-Johansson disease and Osgood-Schlatter disease are mechanical traction disorders of the proximal and distal patellar ligament attachment sites, respectively. In chronic stages, the lateral radiograph will reveal bone fragmentation and calcification within the affected area of the patellar ligament.
8. Degenerative joint disease at the knee is hallmarked radiographically by (1) decreased joint space, (2) sclerotic subchondral bone, (3) osteophyte formation at joint margins, and (4) subchondral cyst formation. The location of DJD in the knee is sometimes described as existing at the medial compartment, involving the medial aspect of the tibiofemoral joint, or at the lateral compartment, involving the lateral aspect of the tibiofemoral joint. The patellofemoral joint is also susceptible to DJD.
9. Common knee and lower extremity congenital deformities include genu valgum or "knock-knees," genu varum or "bowlegs," and genu recurvatum or hyperextended knees. Valgus and varus deformities may also develop in adulthood secondary to altered joint congruity resulting from destructive joint processes, such as osteoarthritis.

REFERENCES

1. Richardson, JK and Iglarsh, ZA: Clinical Orthopaedic Physical Therapy. WB Saunders, Philadelphia, 1994, p 400.
2. Netter, FH: The Ciba Collection of Medical Illustrations, Vol 8, Part I, Musculoskeletal System. Ciba-Geigy Corp, Summit, NJ, 1978, pp 106–108.
3. Ibid, p 100.
4. Nordin, M and Frankel, VH: Basic Biomechanics of the Musculoskeletal System, ed 2. Lea & Febiger, Malvern, PA, 1989, pp 115–134.
5. Meschan, I: An Atlas of Normal Radiographic Anatomy. WB Saunders, Philadelphia, 1960, pp 54, 218.
6. Weissman, B and Sledge, C: Orthopedic Radiology. WB Saunders, Philadelphia, 1986, pp 497–517.
7. Greenspan, A: Orthopedic Radiology: A Practical Approach, ed 2. Raven Press, New York, 1992, pp 8.1–8.13.
8. Bontrager, KL: Textbook of Radiographic Positioning and Related Anatomy, ed 3. CV Mosby, St Louis, 1993, pp 169–216.
9. Fischer, HW: Radiographic Anatomy: A Working Atlas. McGraw-Hill, New York, 1988, pp 26, 27, 33, 46.
10. Wicke, L: Atlas of Radiographic Anatomy, ed 5. Lea & Febiger, Malvern, PA, 1994, pp 54–61.
11. Greenspan, p 8.2.
12. Weissman, p 514.
13. Ibid, p 515.
14. Greenspan, p 8.6.
15. Ibid, p 8.1.
16. Ibid, p 8.13.
17. Ibid, p 8.14.
18. Rockwood, CA and Green, DP: Fractures in Adults, Vol 2, ed 2. JB Lippincott, Philadelphia, 1984, pp 1429–1443.
19. Ibid, pp 1453–1477.
20. Greenspan, p 8.15.
21. Weissman, pp 54–58.
22. Greenspan, p 8.15.
23. Rockwood, pp 1444–1452.
24. Weissman, pp 552–553.
25. Greenspan, p 8.18.
26. Rockwood, pp 1495–1502.
27. Weissman, pp 514–516, 534–535.
28. Rockwood, pp 1495–1502.
29. Ibid, p 1496.
30. Ibid, p 1478.
31. Greenspan, pp 8.20–8.25.
32. Weissman, pp 550–552.
33. Rockwood, pp 1511–1519.
34. Greenspan, pp 8.27–8.31.
35. Richardson, pp 426–428.
36. Rockwood, pp 1520–1548.
37. Greenspan, p 8.30.
38. Ibid, 8.32–8.33.
39. Rockwood, pp 1520–1548.
40. Greenspan, pp 8.18–8.19.
41. Richardson, p 436.
42. Greenspan, p 12.2.
43. Weissman, pp 539–546.
44. Richardson, pp 430, 476.
45. Weissman, pp 563–581.
46. Salter, RB: Textbook of Disorders and Injuries of the Musculoskeletal System, ed 2. Williams & Wilkins, Baltimore, 1983, pp 105–110, 308.
47. Brasher, RH and Raney, RB: Shand's Handbook of Orthopaedic Surgery, ed 9. Mosby, St Louis, 1978, pp 403–405.

SELF-TEST

Chapter 8

FILMS A, B, AND C BELONG TO THE SAME PATIENT.

1. Identify each of the three <u>projections</u>.
2. In film A, an arrow points to a small oval-shaped area of <u>increased density</u>. Would you guess this object lies <u>inside or outside of the joint capsule</u>? What helps you determine this?
3. Name one possibility this object may represent.
4. Which <u>compartments</u> of the knee shows <u>degenerative changes</u>?
5. Describe those <u>degenerative changes</u> present.

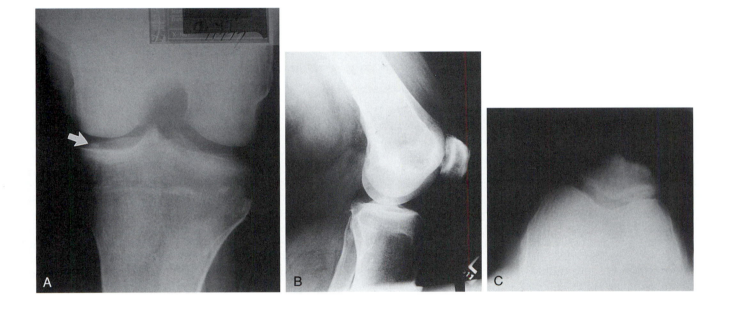

Ankle and Foot

Injuries to the ankle and foot occur with great frequency. The ankle is the most commonly injured major weight-bearing joint in the body, and fractures of the foot make up 10 percent of all fractures.[1]

Ankle injuries may involve the bones or soft tissue structures of the joint, including the ligaments, tendons, and syndesmosis. Often a combination of bone and soft tissue damage is present in an injury. The routine radiographic evaluation generally is sufficient for diagnosing fractures and can at times determine ligamentous injury on the basis of disrupted joint relationships or fracture configuration. If routine films are normal, stress films may be obtained to further evaluate suspected ligamentous injury. Additionally, various ancillary imaging studies are important in accurately defining both the bone and soft tissue damage of many ankle injuries.

Most foot injuries are sufficiently evaluated on the routine radiographs of the foot. Special tangential views are occasionally used in assessment of the subtalar joint and the sesamoid bones at the toes. Ancillary imaging studies such as conventional and computed tomography (CT) may be used in evaluating complex and cartilaginous fractures, tenography and magnetic resonance imaging (MRI) for evaluation of ligamentous injury, and radionuclide bone scan for identification of stress fractures.

The goals of this chapter are first to present an overview of osseous radiographic anatomy. A brief description of ligamentous anatomy and joint mobility is presented to assist the reader in understanding the mechanisms of injury in this region. The routine radio-graphic evaluation of the ankle and foot follows. Here the reader has the opportunity to interact and learn radiographic anatomy by tracing a radiograph with a marker on a transparency sheet and then comparing the results with the radiographic tracing. Brief discussion, illustrations, and films of common trauma follow. The chapter concludes with examples of common foot deformities. The summary is organized into a list of practical points highlighting the clinical aspects of the chapter. A self-test challenges the reader's visual interpretation skills.

RADIOGRAPHIC ANATOMY

Osseous Anatomy[2]

The *ankle joint* is formed by the articulation of the *distal tibia* and *fibula* with the *talus* (Fig. 9–1). The distal end of the tibia is distinguished by a broad articular surface, the *tibial plafond*, an elongated medial process, the *medial malleolus*, an expanded process at the anteromedial aspect, the *anterior tubercle*, and a posterior marginal rim, sometimes called the third or *posterior malleolus*. The distal end of the fibula, the *lateral malleolus*, is slightly posterior to and reaches below the level of the medial malleolus, extending alongside the talus. The inferior contours of the distal tibia and fibula combine to form a deep socket, or *ankle mortise*, into which the upper end of the talus fits. This articulation is the *talocrural joint*, or ankle joint proper.

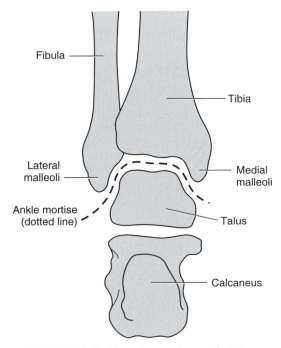

FIGURE 9–1. The talocrural or ankle joint.

The foot consists of 26 bones. There are 7 *tarsals*, 5 *metatarsals*, and 14 *phalanges* (Fig. 9–2).

TARSALS

The tarsals include the talus, *calcaneus, cuboid, navicular*, and three *cuneiforms*. The talus is the second largest tarsal and is key in transmitting weight-bearing forces from the ankle to the foot. The *body* of the talus articulates in the talocrural joint. The superior surface of the body is referred to as the *talar dome*. The talar *neck* lies anterior to the body. The talar *head* articulates with the navicular anteriorly and the calcaneus inferiorly. The *subtalar joint*, or *talocalcaneonavicular joint*, defines the complex articulation between the talus, calcaneus, and navicular bones.

The calcaneus is the largest tarsal bone. The posteroinferior aspect is the *tuberosity* or heel. A medial process and larger lateral process extend from either side of the tuberosity. The prominent *sustentaculum tali* is a process extending from the medial proximal aspect of the calcaneus. The calcaneus articulates with the talus and the cuboid. The superior articulation with the talus forms the *talocalcaneal joint*. The anterior articulation with the cuboid forms the *calcaneocuboid joint*. A depression on the superior surface of the calcaneus, the calcaneal sulcus, corresponds with a groove on the inferior surface of the talus, the sulcus tali, to form the *tarsal sinus*.

The cuboid is located on the lateral aspect of the foot, articulating with the calcaneus posteriorly, the base of

the fourth and fifth metatarsals anteriorly, and the third cuneiform medially. Occasionally the cuboid will also form an articulation with the navicular.

The navicular lies on the medial side of the foot, articulating with the talus posteriorly, forming the *talonavicular joint*, and the three cuneiforms anteriorly.

The cuneiforms are designated by number or by position. All three articulate with the navicular posteriorly and with each other adjacently. Anterior articulations with the metatarsals form the *tarsometatarsal joints*. The first or medial cuneiform articulates with the base of the first and second metatarsal; the second or middle cuneiform articulates with the base of the second metatarsal; the third or lateral cuneiform articulates with the second, third, and fourth metatarsals, and with the cuboid laterally.

METATARSALS

The metatarsals are numbered from one to five beginning on the medial side of the foot. Each metatarsal is composed of a small distal *head*, a long, slender *shaft*, and a broad proximal *base*. The head of the first metatarsal articulates with two *sesamoid bones* on its inferior surface. The base of the fifth metatarsal supports a distally projecting *tuberosity*. Articulations between adjacent metatarsals form *intermetatarsal* joints. Articulations between the metatarsal heads and the proximal phalanges form the *metatarsalphalangeal joints*.

PHALANGES

The phalanges, toes, or digits are numbered from one to five beginning on the medial or great toe side of the foot. The first phalanx is distinctive in that it is is composed of only a *proximal* and *distal phalanx*. The remaining phalanges each additionally possess a middle phalanx. The distal phalanges of the second through fifth digits are usually quite small and sometimes difficult to identify on radiograph.

The foot is often divided into three anatomic segments referred to as the *hindfoot, midfoot*, and *forefoot*. The hindfoot is composed of the talus and calcaneus. The midfoot is composed of the remaining tarsal bones. The forefoot is composed of the metatarsals and phalanges. The hindfoot is separated from the midfoot by the *transverse tarsal joint* (consisting of the talonavicular and calcaneocuboid joints) commonly called *Chopart's joint*. The midfoot is separated from the forefoot by the *tarsometatarsal joint*, commonly called the *Lisfranc joint*.

Ligamentous Anatomy[3,4]

Three principal sets of ligaments stabilize the ankle joint: the *medial collateral ligament, lateral collateral liga-*

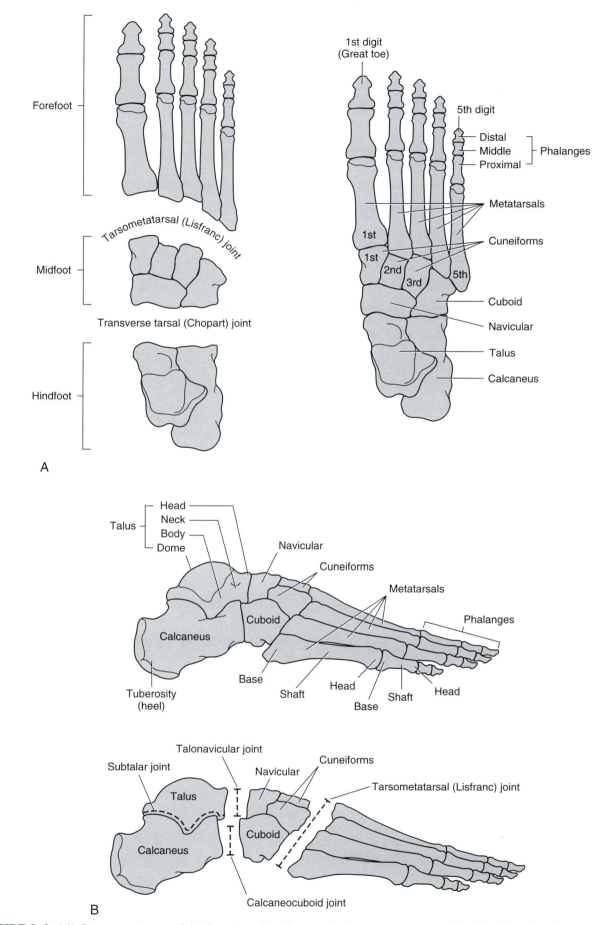

FIGURE 9–2. (*A*) Osseous anatomy of the foot from dorsal aspect. (*B*) Osseous anatomy of the foot from lateral aspect.

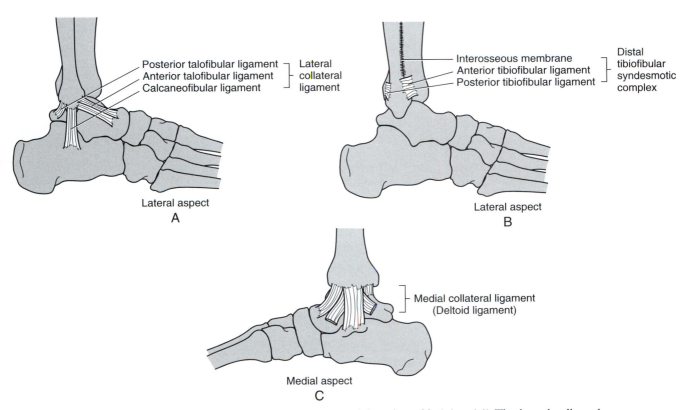

FIGURE 9–3. Three principal sets of ligaments stabilize the ankle joint: (*A*) The lateral collateral ligament, (*B*) the distal tibiofibular syndesmotic complex, and (*C*) the medial collateral (deltoid) ligament.

ment, and the *distal tibiofibular syndesmotic complex* (Fig. 9–3).

The medial collateral ligament, also known as the deltoid ligament, consists of a variable number of superficial and deep bands expanding in a fanlike shape from the medial malleoli to the talus, navicular, and sustentaculum tali of the calcaneus. This ligament possesses great tensile strength and is rarely injured in isolation.

The lateral collateral ligament is the collective name for three distinct ligamentous bands extending from the lateral malleoli to the talus and calcaneus: the anterior talofibular, posterior talofibular, and calcaneofibular ligaments. The lateral collateral ligament is injured with much greater frequency than the medial collateral ligament.

The distal tibiofibular syndesmotic complex is considered to be one of the most important stabilizing structures of the ankle, crucial in maintaining the width and stability of the ankle mortise. This complex is comprised of three structures: the *anterior tibiofibular ligament*, the *posterior tibiofibular ligament*, and the *inter-*

osseous membrane, which binds the fibular and tibial shafts together.

The ligamentous support of the foot is fairly extensive. Muscular action, in concert with the ligaments, maintains the various arches of the foot and permits adaptive responses to the dynamic forces imposed on the foot by weight-bearing and ambulation. On plain radiographs, the individual ligaments of the foot are not readily identified and are not commonly affected by pathology. For this reason individual description of the foot ligaments is not included here.

JOINT MOBILITY

The ankle joint functions as a hinge joint. A transverse axis through the talus allows for dorsiflexion and plantarflexion of the talus and foot in the sagittal plane. Foot motion is complex, and movements occurring here involve multiple joints and planes.

The basic motions of the foot and ankle are:

- *Plantarflexion and dorsiflexion:* Movement of the foot in a sagittal plane occurring through a transverse axis at the ankle joint
- *Abduction and adduction:* Movement of the forefoot away from or toward midline, occurring primarily at the transverse tarsal joints
- *Inversion and eversion:* Elevation of the medial or lateral borders of the foot occurring primarily at the subtalar joint
- *Supination and pronation:* Combined movements of inversion, adduction, and dorsiflexion, or the combined movements of eversion, abduction, and plantarflexion, respectively, occurring at multiple joints.

GROWTH AND DEVELOPMENT[5]

The foot is formed during the eighth week of gestation. At birth only the calcaneus, talus, and occasionally the cuboid are ossified. The ossification centers for the diaphyses of the metatarsals and phalanges are also present at birth. Ossification centers for the remaining tarsals, metatarsal and phalangeal heads and bases, and the distal tibia and fibula appear between 1 and 4 years of age (Figs. 9–4 through 9–7). The tarsals fuse at adolescence, and the remainder of the foot and ankle fuses by adulthood, at 18 to 20 years of age. Although the foot is composed of as much soft tissue as bone at birth, at maturity the foot is 90 percent bone.

In normal development, the lower extremities of the 3-month-old fetus are flexed, the hips are externally

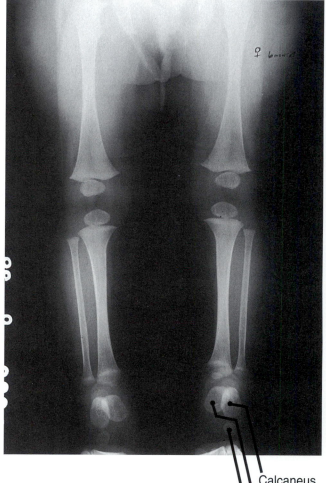

Calcaneus
Talus
Cuboid

FIGURE 9–5. Normal radiographic appearance of a 6-month-old female. At this age, the only ossified bones of the foot are the calcaneus, talus, and cuboid. At the ankle, the epiphysis of the distal tibia has just begun to ossify. Ossification centers for the remaining bones of the foot appear between 1 and 4 years of age. (The phalanges appearing at the bottom of the radiograph are those of an adult holding the feet of the infant to assist in positioning.)

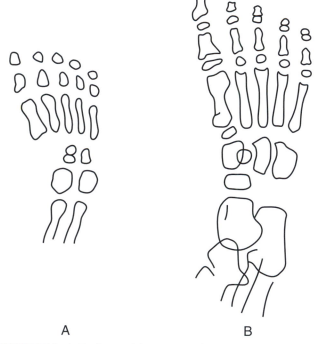

A   B

FIGURE 9–4. Radiographic tracings of the ossified portions of the foot (*A*) at birth and (*B*) at age 5. (Adapted from Meschan,[5] p. 219.)

rotated, and the legs are crossed with the feet plantarflexed and adducted, resting against the fetus's abdomen. By the second trimester the lower extremities uncross and "derotate," and the plantar surfaces of the feet come to rest on the mother's uterine wall. Failure of this postural change to occur may cause deformities of the feet to be present at birth.

The feet of newborns will normally appear flat owing to immature tarsal, muscular, and ligamentous development and the fat pad present on the sole of the foot. The longitudinal arch develops along with ambulatory skills, but persistence of pronated feet and genu valgus is not uncommon during early childhood and generally dissipates with further maturity.

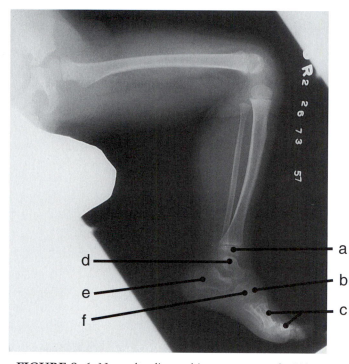

FIGURE 9–6. Normal radiographic appearance of a 2½-year-old male. At this age, the (a) distal tibial epiphysis, the (b) navicular, and the (c) shafts of the metatarsals and phalanges are ossified. The (d) tatus, (e) calcaneus, and (f) cuboid have been ossified since birth.

ROUTINE RADIOGRAPHIC EVALUATION[6–10]

Ankle

Basic: Anteroposterior (AP)
AP mortise
Lateral
Oblique
Optional: AP Inversion and Erosion Stress films

ANTEROPOSTERIOR (FIGS. 9–8, 9–9, 9–10)

The anteroposterior (AP) view of the ankle demonstrates the distal tibia and fibula, including the medial and lateral malleoli, and the head of the talus. The important observations are:

1. The lateral malleolus of the fibula extends below the medial malleolus. This anatomic feature provides joint stability.
2. The lateral malleolus is superimposed behind the lateral aspect of the tibia.
3. Only the upper and medial portions of the ankle mortise and its related radiographic joint space are visible.
4. The upper portion of the talar head is visible as it articulates in the ankle mortise.

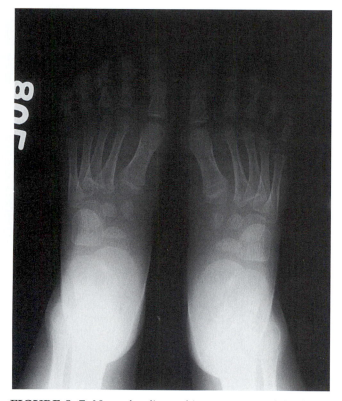

FIGURE 9–7. Normal radiographic appearance of the feet of a 3-year-old female. At this age, the ossification centers for all of the tarsals and for the majority of the metatarsal and phalangeal heads and bases are present.

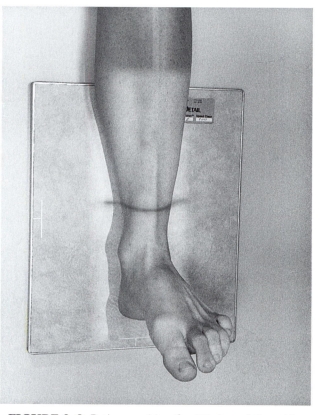

FIGURE 9–8. Patient position for AP view of the ankle.

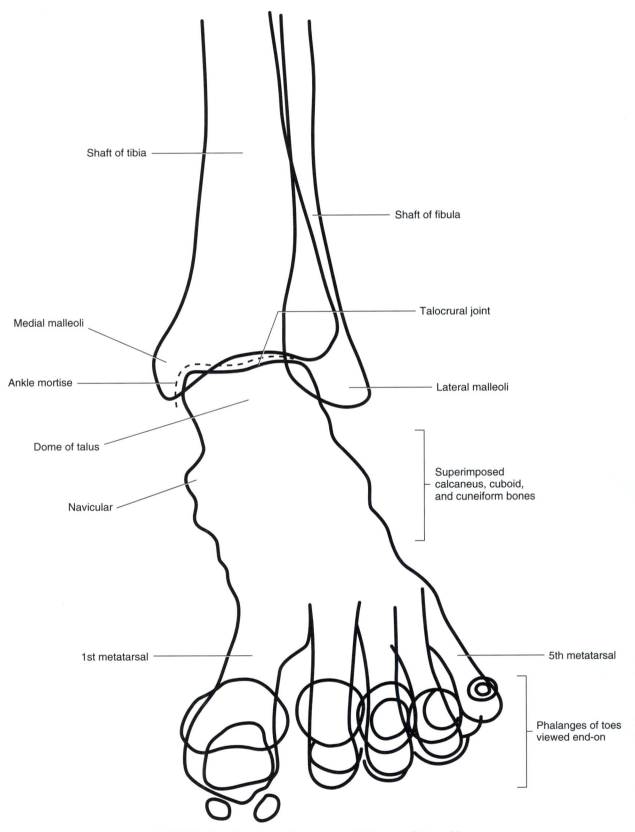

Shaft of tibia

Shaft of fibula

Talocrural joint

Medial malleoli

Ankle mortise

Lateral malleoli

Dome of talus

Superimposed
calcaneus, cuboid,
and cuneiform bones

Navicular

1st metatarsal

5th metatarsal

Phalanges of toes
viewed end-on

FIGURE 9–9. Radiographic tracing of AP view of the ankle.

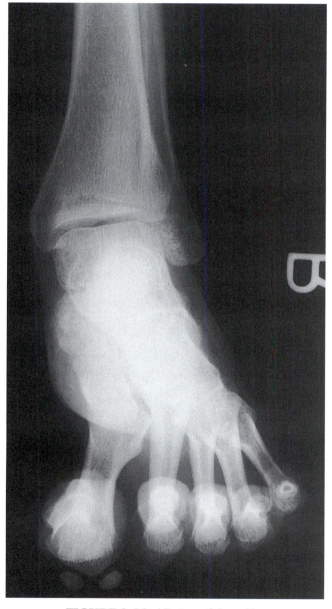

FIGURE 9–10. AP view of the ankle.

5. Medial or lateral shift or displacement of the talus within the mortise may indicate the presence of laxity, instability, or fracture at the ankle.

CLINICAL OBJECTIVES

1. Trace the distal tibia.
2. Trace the distal fibula.
3. Trace the proximal talus or talar dome.
4. Trace the ankle mortise.

ANTEROPOSTERIOR MORTISE VIEW (FIGS. 9–11, 9–12, 9–13)

This view demonstrates the entire ankle mortise. This variation of the AP view is achieved by rotating the leg and foot approximately 15 degrees to place both malleoli in the same plane, avoiding superimposition of the lateral aspect of the tibia over the fibula. The important observations are:

1. The entire radiographic joint space of the ankle proper, the ankle mortise, is visible.
2. Abnormal widening of one side of the mortise or displacement of the talus indicates the presence of ligamentous injury or fracture.

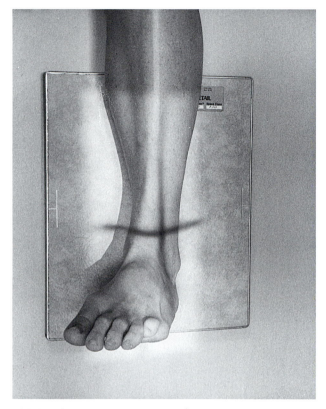

FIGURE 9–11. Patient position for AP mortise view of the ankle.

3. The tibiofibular joint articulation is not well demonstrated in this plane, as the lateral aspect of the tibia is slightly superimposed over the distal fibula.

CLINICAL OBJECTIVES

1. Trace the distal tibia.
2. Trace the distal fibula.
3. Trace the proximal talus or talar dome.
4. Trace the entire ankle mortise.

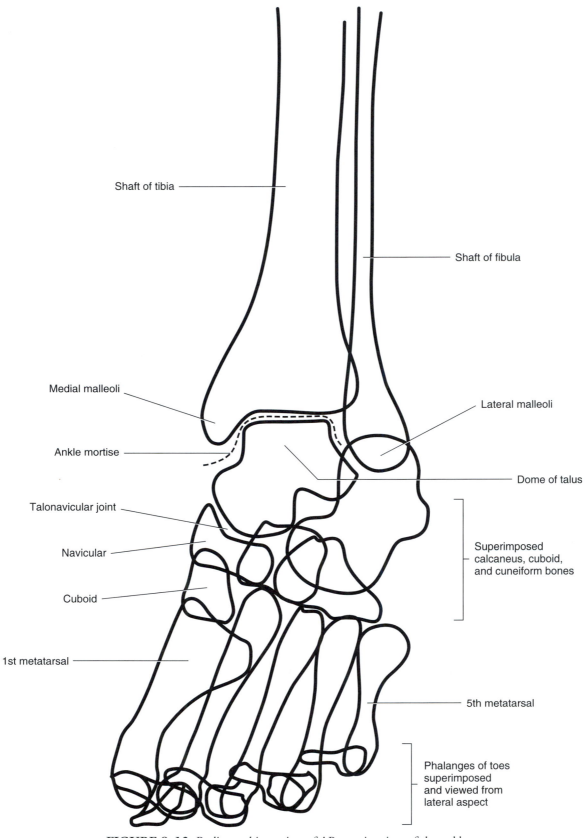

FIGURE 9-12. Radiographic tracing of AP mortise view of the ankle.

LATERAL (FIGS. 9–14, 9–15, 9–16)

This view demonstrates the anterior and posterior aspects of the distal tibia, the lateral relationship of the tibiotalar and subtalar articulation, the talus, and the calcaneus. The important observations are:

1. The fibula is superimposed behind the posterior tibia and talus.
2. The anterior tubercle and posterior malleolus of the tibia are well demonstrated.
3. The talocalcaneonavicular, or subtalar joint, is well demonstrated.
4. The talus and calcaneus are seen in their entirety, as well as their articulations with the navicular and cuboid bones.

CLINICAL OBJECTIVES

1. Trace the distal tibia, identifying the anterior tubercle and the posterior malleolus.
2. Trace the distal fibula as it lies superimposed behind the tibia and talus.
3. Trace the tarsal bones. Identify the talus, calcaneus, navicular, and cuboid.
4. Identify these joints: tibiotalar, talocalcaneonavicular or subtalar, calcaneocuboid, and talonavicular.

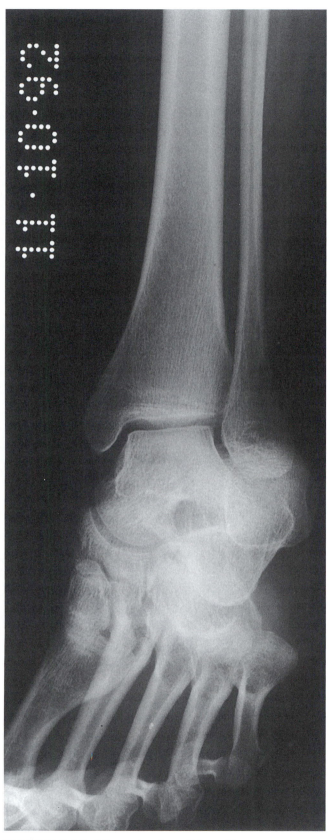

FIGURE 9–13. AP mortise view of the ankle.

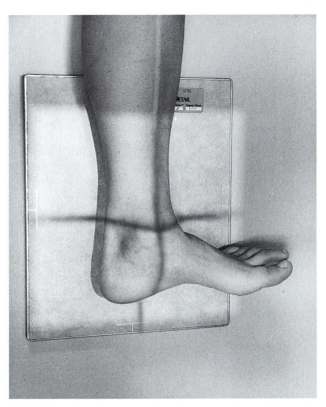

FIGURE 9–14. Patient position for lateral view of the ankle.

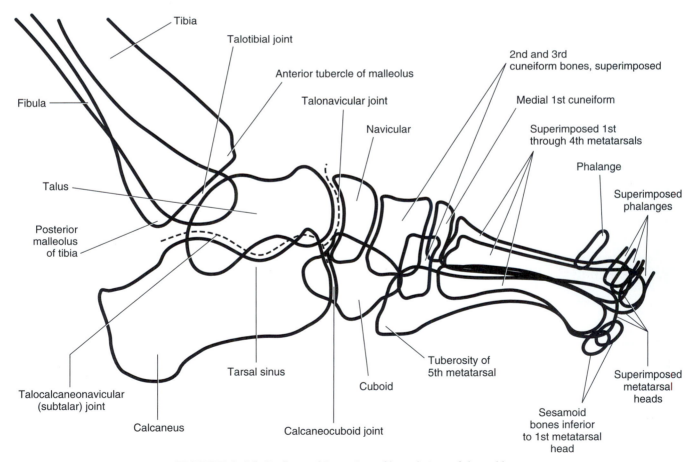

FIGURE 9–15. Radiographic tracing of lateral view of the ankle.

OBLIQUE (FIGS. 9–17, 9–18, 9–19)

This view demonstrates the distal tibiofibular syndesmosis, the talofibular joint, and the distal fibula and lateral malleolus. The important observations are:

1. The entire leg and foot have been rotated approximately 45 degrees from the AP view position.
2. The distal portion of the fibular shaft and the lateral malleolus is well visualized. The normal articulating relationships between the fibula and tibia and between the fibula and talus are noted. Abnormal widening of these joint spaces indicates instability of the ankle mortise.
3. The tarsals are not evaluated in this view, owing to multiple superimpositions. An exception is the dome of the talus that is clearly seen.

CLINICAL OBJECTIVES

1. Trace the fibula and tibia.
2. Trace the talus.
3. Identify the tibiofibular syndesmosis.
4. Identify the ankle mortise.

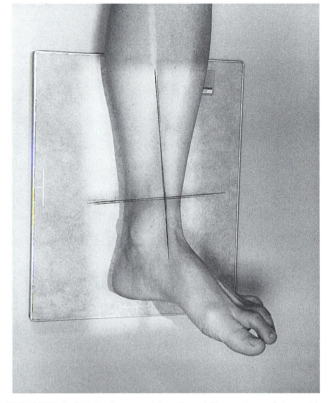

FIGURE 9–17. Patient position for oblique view of the ankle.

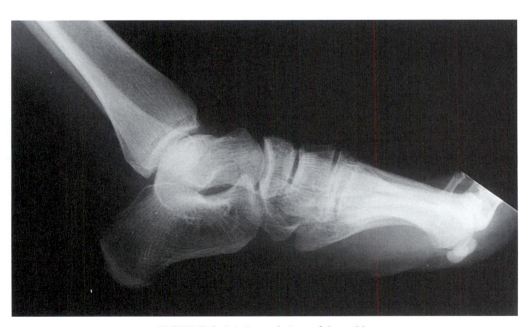

FIGURE 9–16. Lateral view of the ankle.

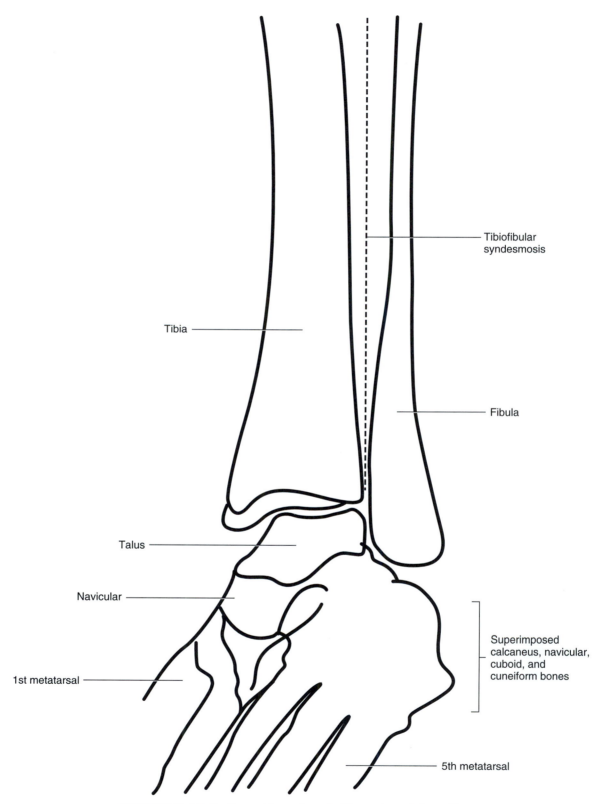

FIGURE 9–18. Radiographic tracing of oblique view of the ankle.

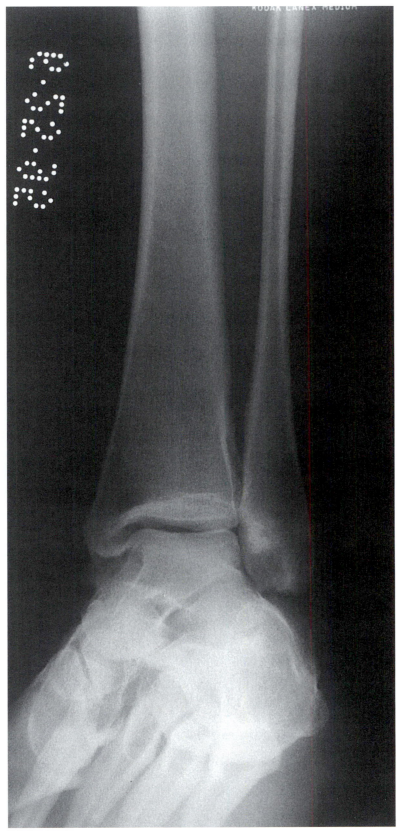

FIGURE 9–19. Oblique view of the ankle.

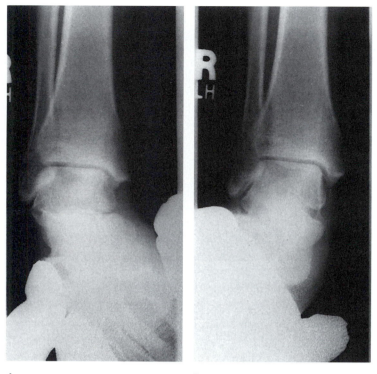

A   Inversion B   Eversion

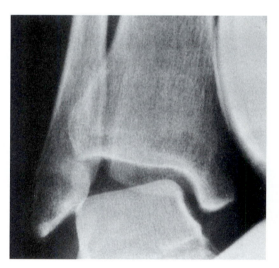

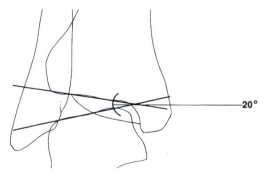

FIGURE 9–20. AP stress views. (*A*) Inversion. (*B*) Eversion. Because the ankle mortise joint space has remained relatively constant during both maneuvers; the ligaments are stable and inact. (From Bontrager,[8] p. 201, Figs. 6–99 and 6–100 with permission.)

AP INVERSION AND EVERSION STRESS PROJECTIONS (FIGS. 9–20, 9–21)

These views are done to demonstrate ankle mortise separation or ankle joint instability due to ligamentous tear, rupture, or avulsion. The important observations are:

1. The leg and ankle are positioned in a true AP manner and the foot is firmly fixed by a mechanism or manually held in neutral range. The plantar surface of the foot is turned medially for inversion and laterally for the eversion view.
2. The distal tibia, fibula, and talus are visible, similar to the routine AP view.
3. In a stable ankle with intact ligaments the joint space of the ankle mortise will remain relatively constant during the inversion and eversion maneuvers.
4. In an unstable ankle caused by ligamentous disruption, the ankle mortise will widen. An enlarged joint space will then be seen between the border of the talus and the malleolus that it is being gapped away from. For example:[11]
   - An abnormally wide space between the medial border of the talus and the medial malleolus on the eversion stress indicates a disruption of the medial collateral ligament
   - An abnormally wide space between the lateral border of the talus and the lateral malleolus indicates disruption of the lateral collateral ligament

FIGURE 9–21. Twenty degrees of talar tilt measured on an inversion stress film. This indicates disruption of the lateral collateral ligament. (From Greenspan,[1] p. 9.6, Fig. 9.9B, with permission.)

- An abnormally wide joint space between the distal tibia and fibula indicates disruption of the distal tibiofibular syndesmotic complex
5. Displacement of the talus is often referred to as talar "tilt" (see Fig. 9–21). An unstable ankle mortise allows abnormal positioning of the talus to occur during foot movement. The amount of talar tilt is measured as an angle determined by the intersection of lines drawn across the tibial plafond and the talar dome. The contralateral ankle is measured to establish a baseline of normal for that individual. Normal values may range from less than 5 degrees to 15 degrees of tilt during forced inversion, and up to 10 degrees during forced eversion. Values significantly greater than this are pathologic.

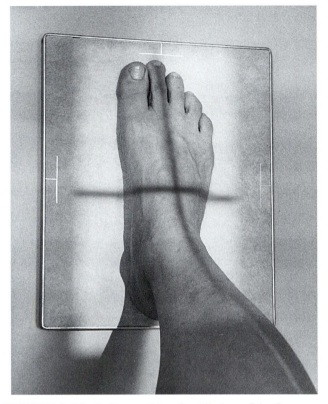

FIGURE 9–22. Patient position for AP view of the foot.

CLINICAL OBJECTIVES

1. Trace the distal tibia, fibula, and talus on Figure 9–20.
2. Identify the joint space representing the ankle mortise.
3. Inscribe the angle of talar tilt on both films.

Foot

Basic: AP
            Lateral
            Oblique

ANTEROPOSTERIOR OR DORSOPLANAR PROJECTION (FIGS. 9–22, 9–23, 9–24)

This view demonstrates the phalanges, metatarsals, cuneiforms, cuboid, and navicular. The important observations are:

1. This view is made with the sole of the foot on the film cassette and the x-rays projected through the top of the foot in a dorsal to plantar direction.
2. All of the bones of the forefoot and midfoot are well demonstrated. The talus, calcaneus, and distal tibia are superimposed over one another and not well visualized.
3. Note any sesamoid bones, commonly present at the first and sometimes the second or third metastarsal heads.

4. The *first intermetatarsal angle* is an important anatomic feature formed by the intersection of the lines bisecting the first and second metatarsal shafts.[12] This angle normally ranges from 5 to 15 degrees. The amount of angulation present in forefoot deformities can be quantified from this baseline.

CLINICAL OBJECTIVES

1. Trace each phalange and identify distal and proximal interphalangeal joints.
2. Trace each metatarsal bone and any sesamoids present. Identify the first intermetatarsal angle.
3. Trace and identify the tarsals of the midfoot.
4. Identify the transverse tarsal joint (Chopart's joint) and the tarsometatarsal joint (Lisfranc joint).

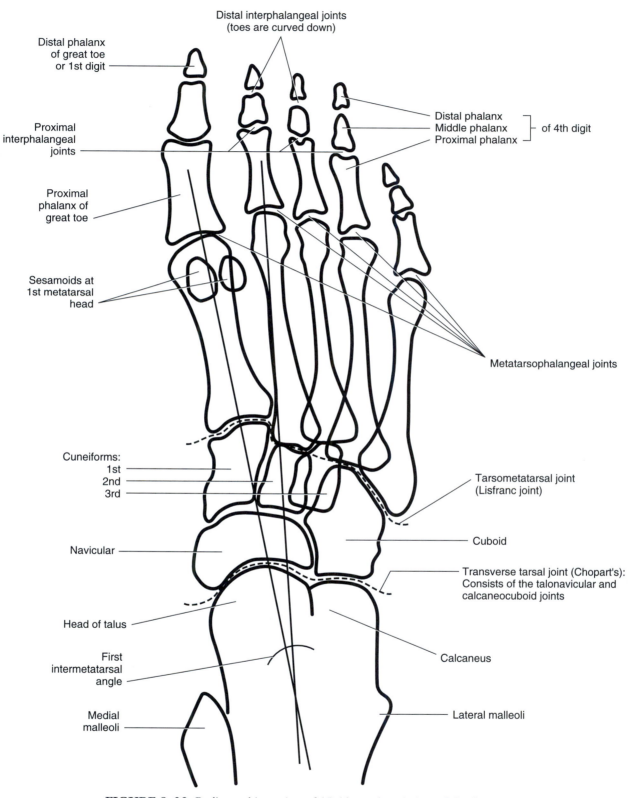

Distal interphalangeal joints
(toes are curved down)

Distal phalanx
of great toe
or 1st digit

Proximal
interphalangeal
joints

Distal phalanx
Middle phalanx   of 4th digit
Proximal phalanx

Proximal
phalanx of
great toe

Sesamoids at
1st metatarsal
head

Metatarsophalangeal joints

Cuneiforms:
1st
2nd
3rd

Tarsometatarsal joint
(Lisfranc joint)

Navicular

Cuboid

Transverse tarsal joint (Chopart's):
Consists of the talonavicular and
calcaneocuboid joints

Head of talus

First
intermetatarsal
angle

Calcaneus

Medial
malleoli

Lateral malleoli

FIGURE 9–23. Radiographic tracing of AP (dorsoplanar) view of the foot.

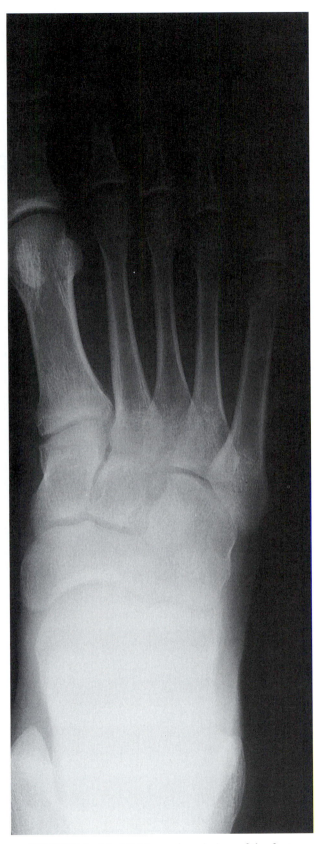

FIGURE 9–24. AP (dorsoplanar) view of the foot.

LATERAL (FIGS. 9–25, 9–26, 9–27)

This view demonstrates the calcaneus and talus, the subtalar joint, and the talonavicular and calcaneocuboid articulations. The important observations are:

1. This lateral profile of the foot visualizes the hindfoot and midfoot, but the metatarsals and phalanges of the forefoot are obscured by superimposition.
2. The transverse tarsal (Chopart) and tarsometatarsal (Lisfranc) joints dividing the midfoot from the hindfoot and forefoot are well demonstrated.
3. Note the articular relationship of the talus to the calcaneus. The anterior and middle facets of the subtalar joint are separated from the posterior facet by the radiolucent oval representing the tarsal sinus.
4. The *Boehler angle*, also known as the *tuberosity* or *salient angle*, is frequently used to evaluate the angular relationship of the talus and the calcaneus in the presence of trauma.[13] This angle is determined by the intersection of lines drawn (a) across the posterior superior margin of the calcaneus and (b) from the posterior aspect of the subtalar joint to the anterior process of the calcaneus. Normal values range from 20 to 40 degrees, and lesser values will be seen in the presence of calcaneal fractures.

CLINICAL OBJECTIVES

1. Trace the tibia and fibula. Note that the lateral malleolus is superimposed behind the talus.
2. Identify the transverse tarsal and tarsometatarsal joints.
3. Trace the talus and calcaneus. Identify the tarsal sinus and the subtalar joint.
4. Inscribe and measure the Boehler's angle.

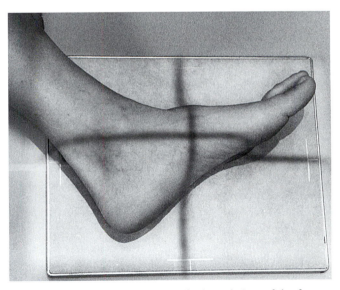

FIGURE 9–25. Patient position for lateral view of the foot.

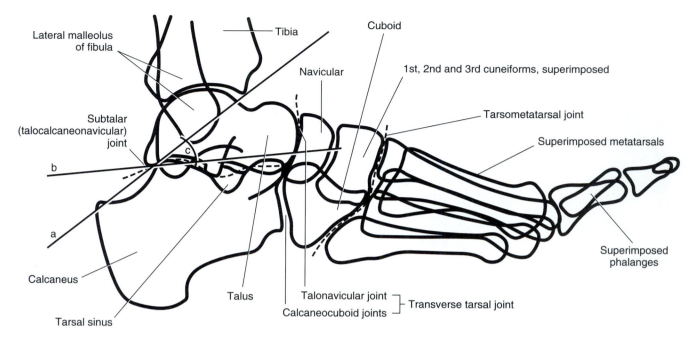

c = Boehler's angle

FIGURE 9–26. Radiographic tracing of lateral view of the foot.

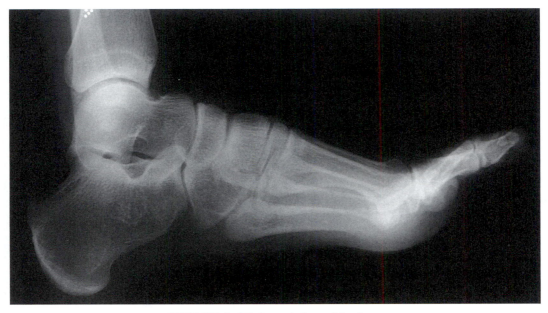

FIGURE 9–27. Lateral view of the foot.

OBLIQUE (FIGS. 9–28, 9–29, 9–30)

This view demonstrates the phalanges, the metatarsals, and the intermetatarsal joints. Also seen are the cuboid, the third cuneiform, the navicular, the anterior portions of the talus and the calcaneus, and the related midtarsal joints. The important observations are:

1. The foot has been rotated as a unit 45 degrees from the AP dorsoplanar view.
2. The shafts of the phalanges and metatarsals normally image with sharp, clearly defined cortical borders. Note any sesamoid bones present and superimposed at the metatarsal heads.
3. The distal phalanges of the second through fifth digits are normally quite small and may be difficult to identify.
4. Note the radiographic joint spaces seen at the intermetatarsal and midtarsal joint articulations.

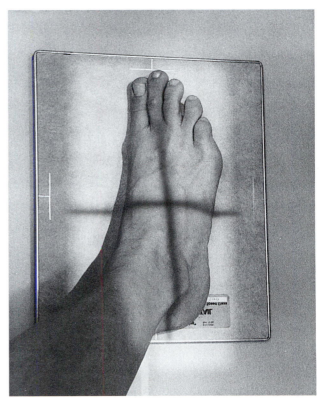

FIGURE 9–28. Patient position for oblique view of the foot.

CLINICAL OBJECTIVES

1. Trace and number the first through fifth digits or toes. Identify proximal, middle, and distal phalanges.
2. Trace and number the first through fifth metatarsals. Identify base, shaft, and head.
3. Trace the cuboid and third cuneiform.
4. Trace the talus, calcaneus, and navicular.

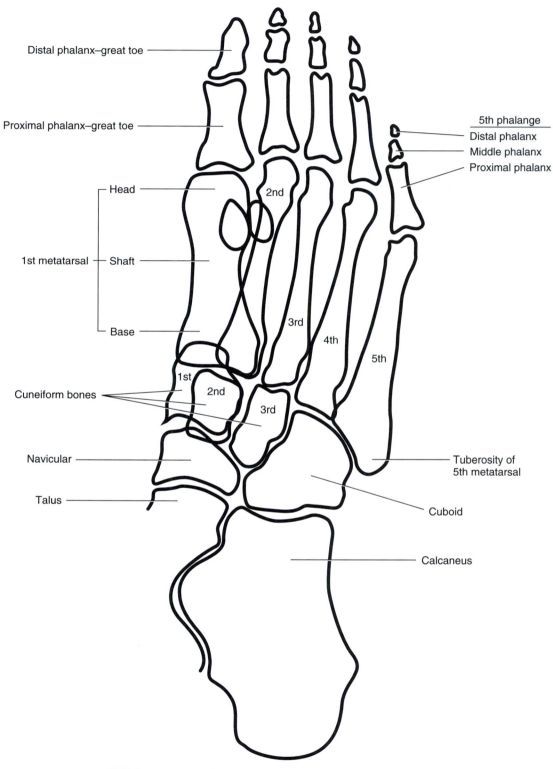

Distal phalanx–great toe

Proximal phalanx–great toe

5th phalange
Distal phalanx
Middle phalanx
Proximal phalanx

Head

2nd

1st metatarsal — Shaft

Base

3rd

4th

5th

1st

Cuneiform bones
2nd

3rd

Navicular

Tuberosity of
5th metatarsal

Talus

Cuboid

Calcaneus

FIGURE 9–29. Radiographic tracing of oblique view of the foot.

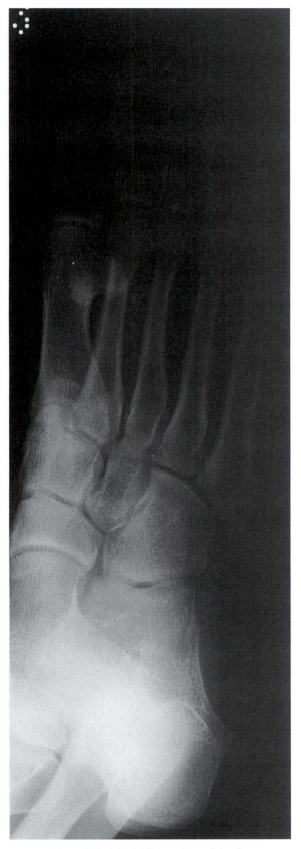

FIGURE 9–30. Oblique view of the foot.

TRAUMA[14-16]

Ankle

In adults, the ankle is the most frequently injured major joint in the body.[17] The precipitating force is usually an inversion stress, accounting for 85 percent of all traumatic conditions at the ankle.[18] The degree of damage caused is dependent on the direction and magnitude of the applied force. Injuries may thus range in severity from minor overstretching of ligaments affecting little functional loss to ligamentous rupture or avulsion, creating ankle joint instability and significant functional impairment. The most severe injuries involve ligamentous disruption with associated fracture or fracture-dislocation.

Diagnosis of most ankle fractures is made on the routine radiographic evaluation. Ankle sprains with resultant ligamentous tearing and joint instability are diagnosed by evaluating abnormal joint positioning on routine films and stress films. Many ancillary techniques are employed in addition to plain film radiography to assist in diagnosis. Conventional tomography and CT are used in evaluating intra-articular fractures, complex fractures, and the position of comminuted fragments. Arthrography and MRI are useful in the evaluation of ligamentous and cartilaginous injuries.

SPRAINS

The ankle is the most commonly sprained joint in the body. Various factors account for this. Anatomically, the talus and its variable surface articulations within the mortise predispose the joint to a degree of instability. The ankle joint is relatively stable in dorsiflexion, as the broader aspect of the talus is wedged in the mortise and little lateral motion is possible. In neutral and plantar flexion, however, the narrower aspect of the talus is within the mortise, and lateral motion is possible. These positions are considered unstable and render the ankle vulnerable to ligamentous sprain if abnormal inversion or eversion stresses are applied while the ankle is in these positions.

Sprains due to inversion stresses damage the lateral collateral ligament (Fig. 9–31). The anterior talofibular and calcaneofibular ligaments are the most frequently injured components of the lateral collateral ligament. Inversion sprains are the most common sprains, and the resultant damage is usually ligamentous without bony involvement (see Fig. 9–21).

Sprains due to eversion stresses damage the medial collateral ligament (MCL) (Fig. 9–32). Forceful eversion stresses are generally associated with bony damage due to the great tensile strength of the MCL. Avulsion fractures and other fractures will often occur before the MCL itself will structurally fail and sustain damage. Tearing of the distal tibiofibular syndesmotic complex is associated with either eversion or inversion stresses.

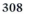

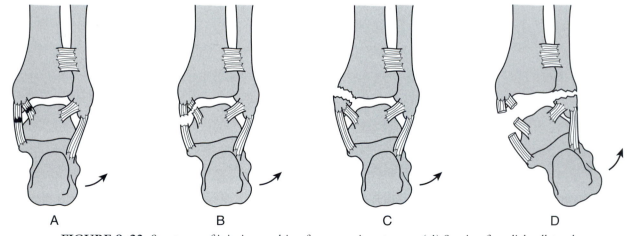

FIGURE 9–31. Spectrum of injuries resulting from inversion stresses. (*A*) Sprain of lateral collateral ligament; (*B*) rupture, or avulsion, of lateral collateral ligament; (*C*) transverse fracture of lateral malleolus; (*D*) fracture of medial malleolus with rupture, or avulsion, of lateral collateral ligament.

Avulsion fractures associated with sprains are due to the tearing of ligaments at their distal or proximal points of attachment.

Instability from sprains is due to tearing of one or more of the three principal stabilizing ligaments, which consequently allow the ankle mortise to widen. Without this anatomic architecture intact, the talus is free to "tilt" within the mortise during foot movement. Chronic instability usually leads to further trauma and degenerative joint changes. Treatment to restore the stability of the ankle mortise may be conservative cast immobilization, or surgical screw fixation followed by immobilization.

Diagnosis of ankle joint instability is made by viewing on routine radiographs and on the inversion and eversion stress radiographs (1) the position of the talus and (2) the width of the ankle mortise (Figs. 9–33, 9–34). Signs of instability are an abnormal amount of talar tilt during the stress views (see Fig. 9–21), or an abnormally wide ankle mortise indicated by an increased radiographic joint space.[19]

FRACTURES

Fractures and fracture-dislocations are common injuries at the ankle. The predisposing force mechanisms are often similar to those causing sprains, and fractures here are frequently seen to occur in combination with ligamentous ruptures, avulsions, and other fractures.

Numerous classification systems exist to classify ankle fractures via injury mechanisms and structural damage (Fig. 9–35). The most basic description in common usage describes the fracture site anatomically as either:

- A *unimalleolar fracture*, indicating fracture of either the lateral or medial malleolus (see Fig. 3–7B)

FIGURE 9–32. Spectrum of injuries resulting from eversion stresses. (*A*) Sprain of medial collateral ligament; (*B*) rupture, or avulsion, of medial collateral ligament; (*C*) fracture of medial malleoli; (*D*) fracture of lateral malleoli with rupture or avulsion of medial collateral ligament.

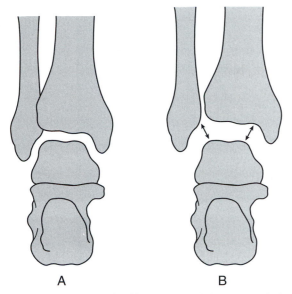

A   B

FIGURE 9-33. Signs of ankle joint instability may include the appearance of an abnormally wide ankle mortise, as seen on the AP view. (*A*) Normal mortise; (*B*) abnormally wide mortise.

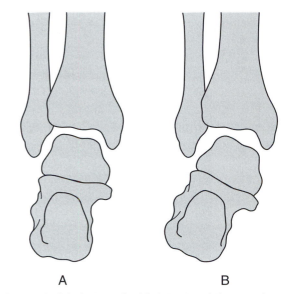

A   B

FIGURE 9-34. A sign of ankle joint instability may be an unusual degree of talar tilt seen on inversion or eversion stress films. Bilateral comparison is helpful in determining normal amount of tilt for the individual. (*A*) Normal talar tilt on eversion stress; (*B*) excessive talar tilt on eversion stress.

- A *bimalleolar fracture*, indicating fracture of both the lateral and medial malleoli
- A *trimalleolar fracture*, indicating fracture of both malleoli and the posterior rim of the tibia (Fig. 9–36).

Other fractures involving the ankle joint include *shaft* fractures of the fibula and tibia, *comminuted* fractures of the distal tibia, and *intra-articular* fractures of the tibial plafond or talar dome (Figs. 9–37 through 9–40).

Treatment of ankle fractures may be by closed reduction or by open reduction with surgical fixation. Re-establishing the architecture of the ankle mortise is always a treatment goal if possible. The amount of immobilization postreduction is usually lengthy if the mortise has been involved and extensive rehabilitation is necessary for recovery of function. The most common complications of ankle fractures are nonunion and degenerative joint changes associated with post-traumatic arthritis.

Foot Fractures

Foot fractures are generally described as being located at the hindfoot, midfoot, or forefoot. Fractures of the hindfoot's talus and calcaneus are common, with the calcaneus being the most frequently fractured tarsal.[20] Isolated fractures of the midfoot tarsals are uncommon, with the exception of the navicular, which is noted to sustain stress fractures and also avulsion fractures of its tuberosity. Fractures of the forefoot metatarsals and phalanges are quite common.

The radiographic evaluation of most foot fractures is complete on the routine series. Conventional and computed tomography is useful in diagnosing complex fractures and evaluating the extension of fracture lines. Radionuclide bone scans assist in diagnosing stress fractures earlier than possible on plain films.

FIGURE 9-35. Basic classification of ankle fractures. (*A*) Unimalleolar fracture, (*B*) bimalleolar fractures; (*C*) trimalleolar fracture (consisting of both malleoli and the posterior margin of the tibia.)

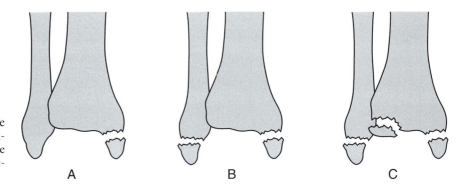

A   B   C

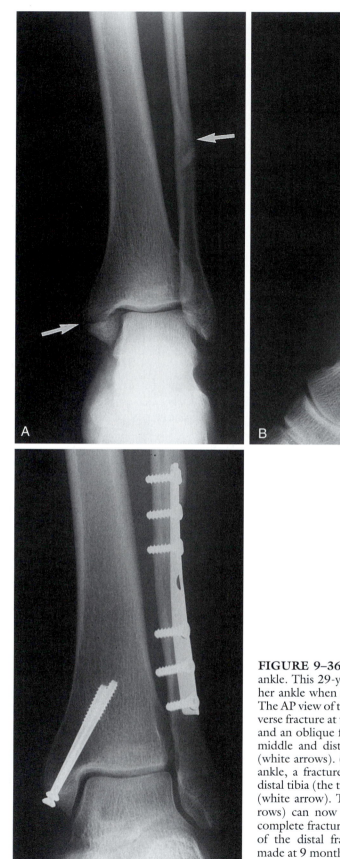

FIGURE 9–36. Trimalleolar fracture of the ankle. This 29-year-old female runner injured her ankle when she tripped in a pothole. (*A*) The AP view of the ankle demonstrates a transverse fracture at the medial malleoli of the tibia and an oblique fracture at the junction of the middle and distal thirds of the fibular shaft (white arrows). (*B*) On the lateral view of the ankle, a fracture of the posterior rim of the distal tibia (the third malleoli) is now apparent (white arrow). The fibular fracture (black arrows) can now be described as an oblique, complete fracture with posterior displacement of the distal fragment. (*C*) Follow-up film made at 9 months after surgical fixation shows successful healing and excellent remodeling of the both bones.

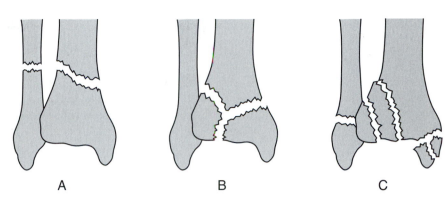

FIGURE 9–37. Other fractures involving the ankle joint include (*A*) shaft fractures of the tibia and fibula; (*B*) fractures of the distal tibia that have an intra-articular extension; and (*C*) comminuted fractures of the distal tibia.

A   B   C

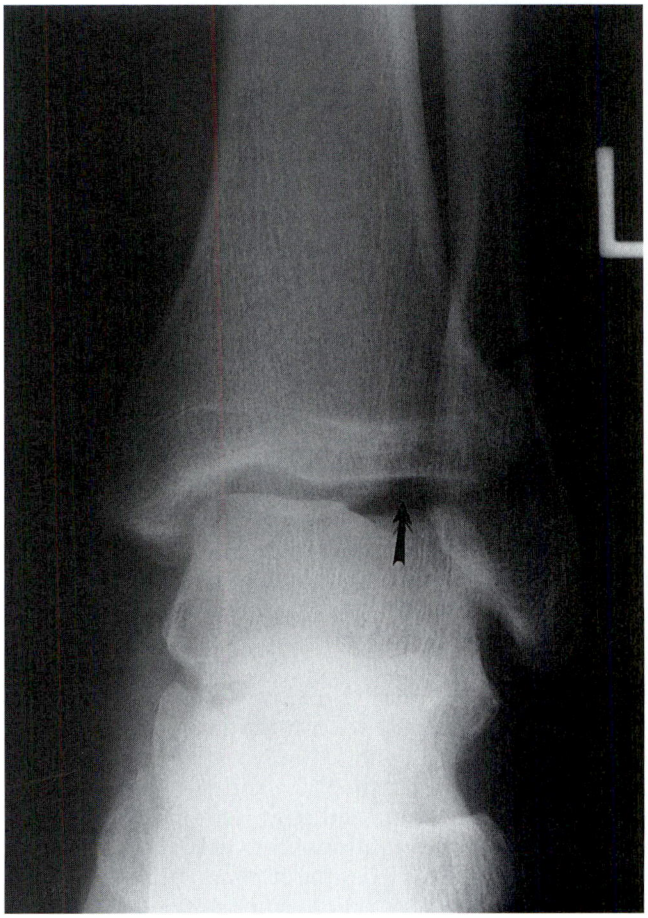

FIGURE 9–38. Impaction fracture of the tibial plafond and the talar dome. This 46-year-old male fell 20 feet out of a tree where he was hanging Christmas lights, and landed on his feet. The impaction at the ankle joint upon landing depressed the lateral aspect of the talar dome and impacted the lateral tibial plafond. A faint fracture line can be visualized extending from the articular surface of the tibia to the lateral tibial condyle (black arrows). This unfortunate man also sustained a burst fracture of the second lumbar vertebra (see Fig. 6–28). This combination of injuries is not uncommon with this type of fall, because the axial force that is sustained at landing is readily transmitted through the extremities to the spine. For this reason, patients who present with this type of history are routinely screened at both the ankle and spine, regardless of where their primary complaint may be.

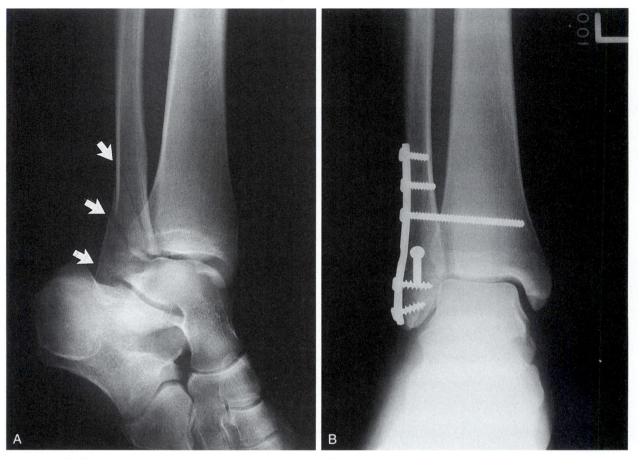

FIGURE 9–39. Comminuted fracture of the distal fibular shaft. This 24-year-old woman injured her ankle while skiing. (*A*) Lateral view of the ankle shows multiple fracture lines in the distal fibular shaft and lateral malleoli (white arrows). Note the posterior displacement of the entire fibula evidenced by the abnormally wide interosseous space and the subluxation of the distal fibula out of the fibular notch of the tibia. (*B*) AP view of the ankle made postoperatively demonstrates the side plate and multiple screw fixation device that has restored normal alignment of the joint. Note that the long screw that enters the tibia has successfully restored the position of the fibula in the fibular notch of the tibia, and consequently a normal ankle mortise has been re-established.

HINDFOOT FRACTURES

Calcaneal fractures are often sustained during falls from a height, in which the individual lands on his or her heels first. The injury is often bilateral, and is frequently associated with a vertebral compression fracture in the thoracolumbar spine due to the transmitted axial forces. Calcaneal fractures are broadly classified as *intra-articular*, involving the subtalar joint, or *extra-articular*, sparing the subtalar joint (Fig. 9–41). Intra-articular fractures occur with three times greater frequency than extra-articular fractures (Figs. 9–42, 9–43, 9–44). Treatment may be conservative or surgical. Long-term complications usually result from malunion, including posttraumatic arthritis at the subtalar or calcaneocuboid joints, and peroneal tendonitis from impingement of the tendons between the malpositioned calcaneus and tip of the fibula.[21]

Fractures of the talus occur second in frequency to calcaneal fractures (Figs. 9–45, 9–46, 9–47).[22] The injury mechanism is usually a large force applied through a dorsiflexed foot, such as a driver slamming on the brakes in an auto collision. Significant in these fractures is that because three-fifths of the bone is covered with articular cartilage, most all talar fractures are considered to be *intra-articular*. Additionally, the blood supply to the talus is tenuous, as no muscles attach to it and its cartilage-covered surface provides little area for vascular perforation. Thus the talus is predisposed to developing *avascular necrosis* post-fracture. Posttraumatic arthritis of the ankle and subtalar joints is also a common long-term complication, related to the articular surface damage, the prolonged immobilization necessary for bony union, and secondary to the presence of any necrotic changes.

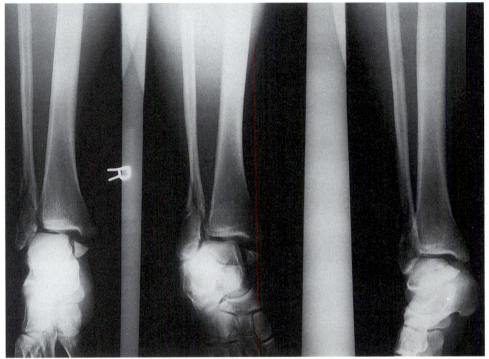

AP   Oblique   Lateral

FIGURE 9–40. Fracture of the medial malleolus and distal fibula. This 29-year-old female was injured when she stumbled after catching her heel in a moving escalator. Note the transverse fracture of the medial malleolus and a severely comminuted distal fibula. The abnormally wide ankle mortise and abnormally wide interosseous space is visible on both the AP and oblique views. On the lateral view, the anterior displacement of the fibula is the most striking feature.

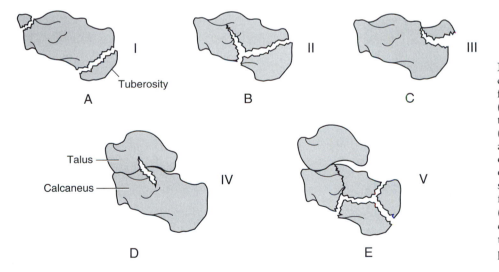

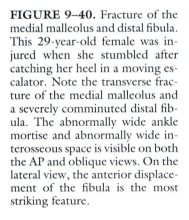

A   I   Tuberosity

B   II

C   III

Talus

Calcaneus

D   IV

E   V

FIGURE 9–41. The *Rowe* classification of calcaneal fractures defines five injury patterns. (*A*) Type I (21%), fractures of tuberosity, sustentaculum tali, or anterior process; (*B*) type II (3.8%), beak fractures and avulsion fractures of the Achilles tendon insertion; (*C*) type III (19.5%), oblique fractures not extending into subtalar joint; (*D*) type IV (24.7%), fractures involving the subtalar joint; (*E*) type V (31%), fractures with central depression and comminution. (Adapted from Greenspan,[1] p. 9.35.)

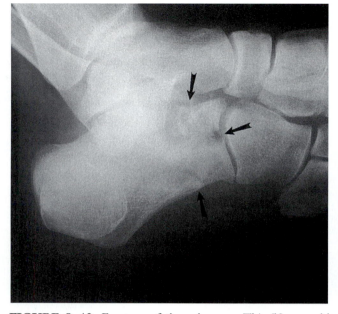

FIGURE 9–42. Fracture of the calcaneus. This 58-year-old woman was injured when she jumped down from a stepladder after losing her balance while washing windows. The fracture is comminuted and has an intra-articular extension into the subtalar joint and the calcaneo-cuboid joint (arrows).

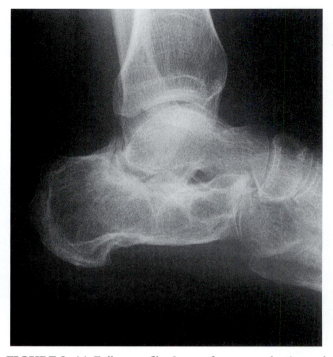

FIGURE 9–44. Follow-up film 1 year after open reduction and internal fixation with bone grafting shows fusion of the subtalar joint and the superior aspect of the calcaneo-cuboid joint. Functionally, these joints were stiff but painless, and motion at the talocrural joint was minimally limited. (See Figure 9–43 for acute stage film.)

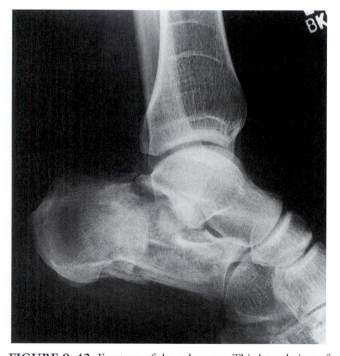

FIGURE 9–43. Fracture of the calcaneus. This lateral view of the foot demonstrates a severely comminuted calcaneal fracture with central depression of the calcaneal body, which has disrupted the subtalar articulation. This injury was sustained by a construction worker in a fall off a roof. (See Fig. 9–44 for follow-up film.)

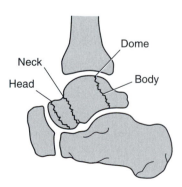

FIGURE 9–45. Fractures of the talus are described by their anatomic location at the body, dome, neck, or head. Because three-fifths of the talus is covered with articular cartilage, most fractures of the talus are considered to be intra-articular.

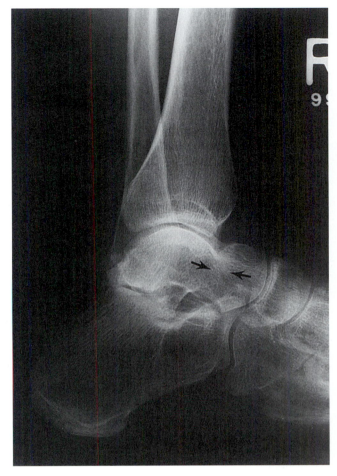

FIGURE 9–46. Nondisplaced and displaced fractures of the talar neck. The most common mechanism of talar neck fracture is hyperdorsiflexion of the foot on the leg, such as would occur in light aircraft accidents with the sole of the foot resting on the rudder bar at the point of impact, or in motor vehicle accidents when the driver slams on the brakes prior to impact. During the extreme dorsiflexion, the posterior capsular ligaments of the subtalar joint rupture and the neck of the talus impacts against the leading anterior edge of the distal tibia. A fracture line develops at this point and enters the nonarticular portion of the subtalar joint between the middle facet and the posterior facet. The lateral view of the foot demonstrates this nondisplaced fracture of the talar neck (between the arrows). If the adjacent joints are not disrupted, this fracture is usually treated with casts, immobilization, and non-weight-bearing for several weeks.

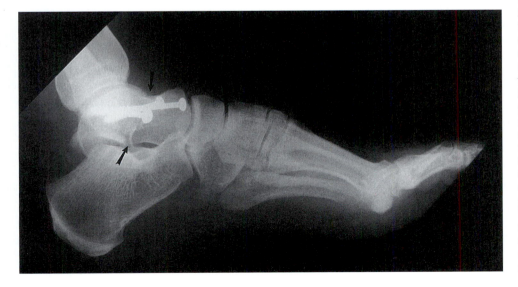

FIGURE 9–47. Nondisplaced and displaced fractures of the talar neck. The most common mechanism of talar neck fracture is hyperdorsiflexion of the foot on the leg, such as would occur in light aircraft accidents with the sole of the foot resting on the rudder bar at the point of impact, or in motor vehicle accidents when the driver slams on the brakes prior to impact. During the extreme dorsiflexion, the posterior capsular ligaments of the subtalar joint rupture and the neck of the talus impacts against the leading anterior edge of the distal tibia. A fracture line develops at this point and enters the nonarticular portion of the subtalar joint between the middle facet and the posterior facet. Displaced talar fractures such as this may be able to be treated with closed reduction and mobilization, but often require open reduction and internal fixation to achieve adequate anatomic reduction of the fracture and to preserve subtalar joint junction. The arrows mark the extent of the fracture line, and the multiaxis compression screws appear to have achieved satisfactory reduction.

315

MIDFOOT FRACTURES[23]

The relative immobility of the midfoot minimizes its susceptibility to isolated fractures. Fractures occurring in this region are often associated with other fracture or dislocation patterns. Sprains and *fracture-subluxations* or *fracture-dislocations* can occur at the transverse tarsal and tarsometatarsal joints, where the relatively rigid midfoot junctions with the more mobile hindfoot and forefoot. The tarsometatarsal (Lisfranc) joint is the most commonly dislocated joint in the foot (Fig. 9–48). In general, however, dislocations occur much less frequently than fractures. The mechanism of injury of a fracture-dislocation is usually a high-energy trauma. Surgical reduction is often necessary to restore alignment and function.

The navicular is one midfoot tarsal that is noted to sustain isolated injury. *Stress fractures* are seen primarily in young male athletes. Additionally, abnormal eversion forces at the foot may result in *avulsion fractures* at the dorsal lip or the tuberosity of the navicular. Treatment typically consists of cast immobilization.

FOREFOOT FRACTURES[24]

Metatarsal fractures result most commonly from direct injury, as when a heavy object is dropped on the foot. In these instances the fracture can occur at any location on the bone. Metatarsal shaft fractures usually result from indirect torque forces, as when the toe of the foot is abruptly caught and the foot twists (Fig. 9–49). *Stress fractures* due to excessive, repetitive forces, as in athletic activities, usually occur at the distal shafts of the second through fourth metatarsals, and at the proximal shaft of the fifth metatarsal. *Avulsion fractures* at the base of the fifth metatarsal result from a sudden inversion force as the peroneus brevis forcefully contracts. Treatment of metatarsal fractures is dependent on the amount of displacement. *Nondisplaced* fractures are typically treated with limited weight-bearing and immobilization, and *displaced* fractures usually require either closed or open reduction to restore function.

Phalangeal fractures result most commonly from objects being dropped on the toes, or "stubbing" injuries. Treatment generally consists of manual reduction, splinting or taping, and protected weight-bearing.

FOOT DEFORMITIES[25-27]

Abnormal foot positions may be congenital, developmental, or may result from traumatic conditions or neuromuscular impairment. The entire foot may exhibit structural or anatomic deformity, or the deformity may be confined to a segment of the foot, such as the fore, mid, or hindfoot.

Radiographically, the evaluation and description of foot deformities are derived from lines and angles drawn on the AP and lateral films. These measurements are used to describe anatomical deviations from

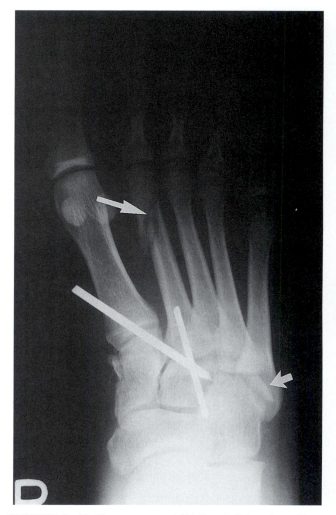

FIGURE 9–48. Tarsometatarsal (Lisfranc) dislocation with associated fractures. This 37-year-old man was injured when he fell off his horse and his foot remained caught in the stirrup. The forefoot was forcefully twisted and abducted laterally, resulting in a spiral fracture of the second metatarsal neck (long arrow), a shear fracture of the cuboid (small arrow), and a dislocation of the tarsometatarsal joint. This AP view of the foot shows the tarsometatarsal dislocation reduced and stabilized with two Steinmann pins.

the norm. Although lateral films are routinely taken in a non-weight-bearing position, additional weight-bearing lateral films provide further information regarding the flexibility, rigidity, or adaptability of a deformity to weight-bearing function.

Examples of some commonly seen foot deformities follow.

Hallux Valgus

Hallux valgus is a deformity of the forefoot in which the first metatarsal is deviated medially and the great toe is deviated laterally (Fig. 9–50). The etiology is var-

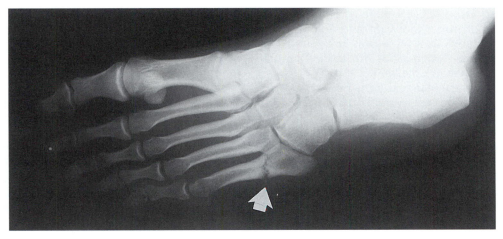

FIGURE 9–49. Fracture of the base of the fifth metatarsal. All fractures in this region have generally been referred to as "Jones fractures" after the original description put forth in 1902 by Sir Robert Jones, who personally sustained this fracture while dancing. Unfortunately, the persistence of this eponym has resulted in significant confusion in the management of these fractures, because at least two distinct fracture patterns occur at the base of the fifth metatarsal: avulsion fracture of the tuberosity at the attachment of the peroneus brevis, and transverse fracture of the proximal diaphysis, as seen above (arrow). The management of these two types of fractures is distinctly different because the healing potential of the diaphyseal fracture is diminished, and the rate of fibrous union or subsequent "refracture" is high. Inadequate initial treatment may contribute to delayed or nonunion of the diaphyseal fracture, and thus this fracture must be distinguished from the less complicated, more proximal avulsion fracture.

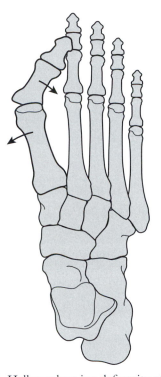

FIGURE 9–50. Hallux valgus is a deformity of the forefoot in which the first metatarsal is deviated medially and the great toe is deviated laterally.

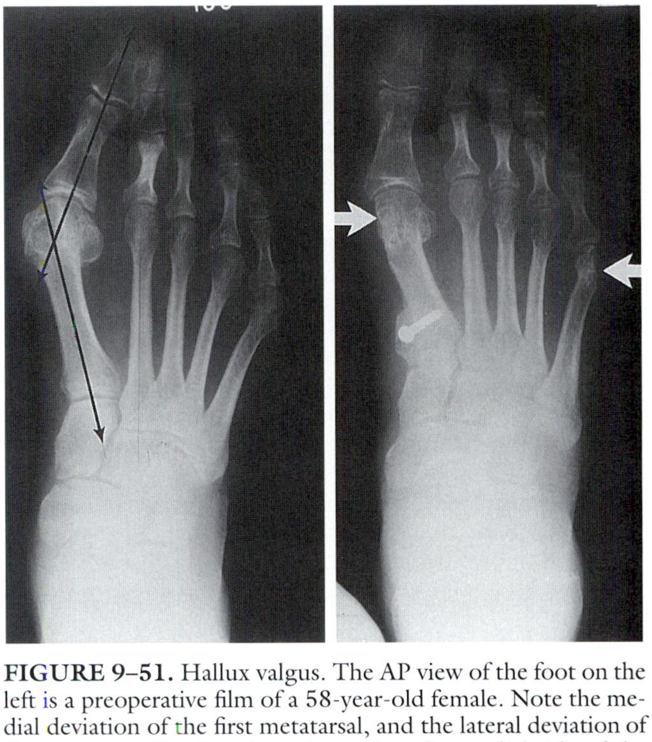

FIGURE 9–51. Hallux valgus. The AP view of the foot on the left is a preoperative film of a 58-year-old female. Note the medial deviation of the first metatarsal, and the lateral deviation of the great toe. Bunions have formed at the medial side of the first metatarsal head and the lateral side of the fifth metatarsal head. The AP film on the right is a postoperative film demonstrating an osteotomy with screw stabilization at the base of the first metatarsal and bunionectomies at the first and fifth metatarsal heads (white arrows).

ied, and associations have been made with biomechanical dysfunction, improper footwear, and predisposing congenital factors such as a wide first intermetatarsal angle and pes planus. Females are affected with much greater frequency than are males.[28]

The first metatarsophalangeal joint undergoes friction and stress in this deformity, and bunion formation on the medial side of the joint is a common occurrence. Although some patients may be asymptomatic, the more severe cases of hallux valgus significantly alter function and cause pain, especially if degenerative joint changes progress. Treatment may consist of corrective orthoses, bunionectomy, arthrodesis, or resection arthroplasty (Fig. 9–51).

The AP or dorsoplanar view of the foot demonstrates this deformity.

Pes Cavus and Pes Planus

Pes cavus and *pes planus* are terms used to describe abnormally high or abnormally low medial longitudinal arches, respectively (Fig. 9–52).The high fixed arch in pes cavus may be familial (Fig. 9–53). Athletes with excessively high arches may be predisposed to overuse injuries.[29,30] More severe cases are associated with neuromuscular disease, such as Charcot-Marie-Tooth disease.

The "flat foot" of pes planus is categorized as being either rigid or flexible (Fig. 9–54). A rigid pes planus demonstrates a low arch upon either weight-bearing or non-weight-bearing. Tarsal coalition, or an abnormal synostosis between the tarsals, may be one cause of rigid pes planus. A flexible pes planus demonstrates a low arch on weight-bearing and a return to a more normal arch when non-weight-bearing. Ligamentous laxity may be one cause of flexible pes planus. A flexible pes planus is considered normal in young children, but resolves with growth and maturity. Persistence of flexible pes planus into adulthood is usually treated with orthotic support.

The lateral views of the foot, taken in both weight-bearing and non-weight-bearing positions, are used to evaluate these conditions. Various anatomic relationships are measured to help define and describe the configuration of normal, high, or low arches.[31] The angle inscribed by the intersection of lines drawn through the talus and the first metatarsal shaft, the *talometatarsal angle*, is an example of one such angle.

Clubfoot[32]

The congenital deformity of the ankle and foot known as clubfoot is termed *"talipes equinovarus"* (*tali*, plural of talus; *pes*, foot) (Fig. 9–55). The hallmarks of

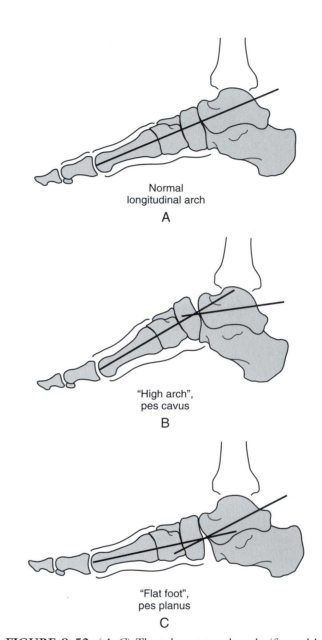

Normal
longitudinal arch

A

"High arch",
pes cavus

B

"Flat foot",
pes planus

C

FIGURE 9–52. (*A–C*) The talometatarsal angle (formed by the intersection of a line drawn along the midshaft of the first metatarsal and a line bisecting the talus on the lateral view of the foot) has been used to define (*B*) pes cavus and (*C*) pes planus. The determination of flexible versus rigid arches requires comparison of weight-bearing and non-weight-bearing views. (Adapted from Richardson, p. 536.)

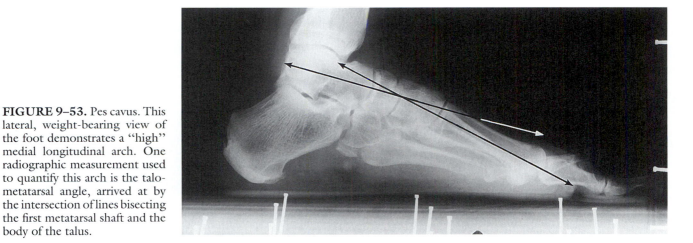

FIGURE 9–53. Pes cavus. This lateral, weight-bearing view of the foot demonstrates a "high" medial longitudinal arch. One radiographic measurement used to quantify this arch is the talometatarsal angle, arrived at by the intersection of lines bisecting the first metatarsal shaft and the body of the talus.

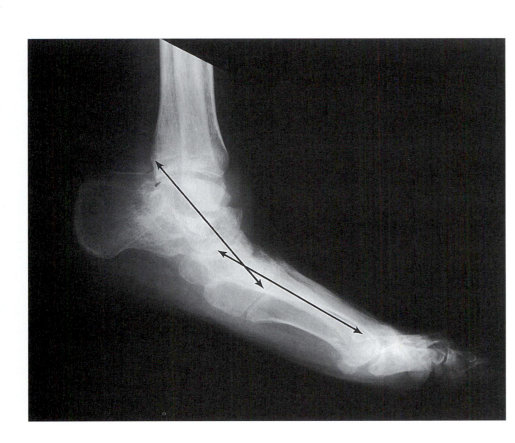

FIGURE 9–54. Pes planus. The "low" medial longitudinal arch of the foot is quantified on this lateral view by measuring the talometatarsal angle, an intersection of the lines inscribed across the body of the talus and through the midshaft of the first metatarsal.

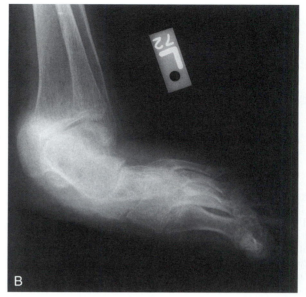

FIGURE 9–55. (*A*) The hallmarks of *talipes equinavarus* ("clubfoot") include a plantar-flexed position of the heel, inversion of the subtalar joint with varus position of the hindfoot, metatarsal adduction with varus position of the forefoot, and in severe deformities, dislocation of the subtalar joint. (*B*) *Talipes equinavarus.* This congenital deformity of the ankle and foot is commonly known as clubfoot. A severe degree of the deformity exists in this 25-year-old man who suffers from osteogenesis imperfecta. The hindfoot is in an extreme varus position and the subtalar joint has inverted and subluxed. There is a reversal of the medial longitudinal arch and the forefoot is extremely adducted.

this deformity include (1) an equinus or plantarflexed position of the heel; (2) inversion of the subtalar joint with a varus position of the hindfoot; (3) metatarsal adduction with varus position of the forefoot; and, in the most severe cases, (4) subluxation or dislocation of the subtalar or talocalcaneonavicular joint. Until the navicular ossifies by age 2 or 3, however, this element cannot be evaluated on radiograph.

The etiology of clubfoot during fetal development appears to be multifactorial. The less severe forms of

the deformity, known as postural clubfoot, are associated with abnormal intrauterine positioning. Treatment of clubfoot depends on the flexibility of the deformity. Mild conditions respond favorably to stretching, splinting, or cast immobilization. Severe conditions involving contractures and joint subluxations usually require open reduction surgery and prolonged immobilization. Radiographic evaluation is essential in order to monitor the effects of treatment as the foot continues to mature.

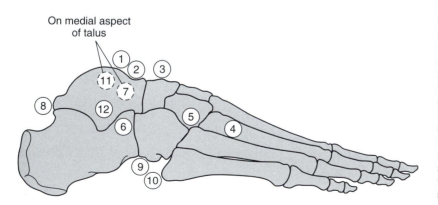

FIGURE 9–56. Names and locations of accessory bones seen in the foot. The * indicates those that occur with frequency. 1, talotibial ossicle (os talotibiale); 2, supratalar ossicle (os supratalare); 3, supranavicular ossicle (os supranaviculare); 4*, intermetatarsal ossicle (os intermetatarsale); 5, secondary cuboid (cuboides secundarium); 6, secondary calcaneus (calcaneus secundarius); 7*, external tibial ossicle (os tibiale externum); 8*, trigone ossicle (os trigonum); 9, peroneal ossicle (os peronaeum); 10, vesalian ossicle (os vesalianum); 11, accessory talus (talus accessorius); 12, secondary talus (talus secundarius). (Adapted from Greenspan,[1] p. 9.14.)

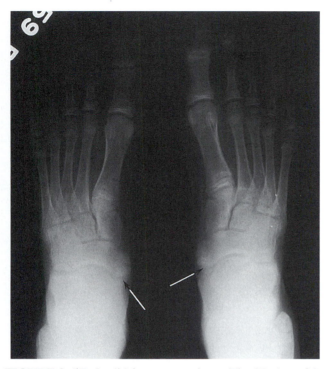

FIGURE 9–57. Os tibiale, accessory bone. The AP view of the feet of this 13-year-old female demonstrates bilateral os tibiale externum. The arrows mark the oval densities that represent these bilaterally symmetric accessory bones. At present, these accessory bones lie within the tendons of the posterior tibial muscles; however, they may eventually grow out of the tendons and coalesce with the contiguous navicular bone and lose their sesamoid status.

ANOMALIES

Accessory Bones[33]

Accessory bones are anomalous bones that usually form because of a failure of one or more ossification centers to unite with the main mass of bone. Accessory bones appear with some frequency at the foot. Studies have reported as high as 30 percent incidence in adults.[34] Accessory bones may be seen radiographically at various locations in the foot, and the locations and names of these are presented in Figure 9–56. The most commonly occurring accessory bones of the foot are the *os trigonum*, the *os intermetatarseum*, and the *os tibiale* or accessory navicular (Figs. 9–57, 9–58).[35]

Accessory bones can complicate the evaluation of foot injuries if they are present in the area of a suspected fracture.[36] Comparison films are not always helpful, as accessory and sesamoid bones are not always bilaterally symmetrical. In general, accessory bones are differentiated from acute fractures by the presence of an intact, smooth cortical shell with an underlying line of increased density. In contrast, acute fractures will have an irregular cortical surface and no appearance of increased density beneath the surface.

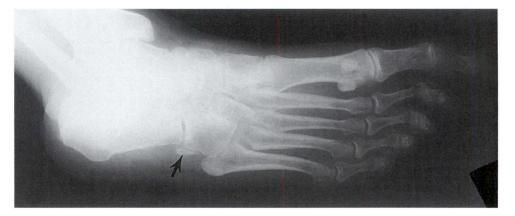

FIGURE 9–58. Os peroneum, accessory bone. On the oblique view of this foot, a large os peroneum is visible (arrow) imbedded within the tendon of the peroneus brevis muscle.

SUMMARY OF KEY POINTS

1. The routine radiographic evaluation of the ankle includes four projections:
   - **Anteroposterior view:** Demonstrates the distal tibia and fibula and head of the talus.
   - **Anteroposterior mortise view:** Is taken with the leg slightly rotated so that the entire joint space of the ankle mortise is visible.
   - **Lateral:** Demonstrates the anterior and posterior aspects of the tibia, the tibiotalar joint, and the subtalar joint.
   - **Oblique:** Demonstrates the tibiofibular syndesmosis and talofibular joint.
2. The AP inversion and eversion stress projections are optional views done to demonstrate ankle joint stability or instability by evaluating the relationship of the talus in the ankle mortise during forced inversion and eversion of the foot.
3. The routine evaluation of the foot includes three projections:
   - **Anteroposterior or dorsoplanar view:** Demonstrates all the bones of the forefoot and midfoot and their associated articulations
   - **Lateral:** Demonstrates the bones of the hindfoot and midfoot and their associated articulations
   - **Oblique:** Demonstrates the shafts of the metatarsal bones and the intermetatarsal joints
4. The ankle is the most frequently sprained joint in the body. The majority of injuries are precipitated by an inversion force. Damage may range in severity from minor sprains to ligamentous rupture, bony avulsions, and joint instability.
5. Numerous classification systems exist to describe ankle fractures. The most basic system divided fractures into:
   - **Unimalleolar fracture:** Involving either the lateral or medial malleoli
   - **Bimalleolar fracture:** Involving both the lateral and medial malleoli
   - **Trimalleolar fracture:** Involving both the lateral and medial malleoli and the posterior rim of the tibia
6. Fractures of the foot are generally described by anatomic location as fractures of the hindfoot, midfoot, or forefoot.
7. The calcaneus is the most frequently fractured bone in the hindfoot. The injury is usually sustained by landing on the heels in a fall from a great height. A frequently associated fracture in this scenario is a vertebral compression fracture in the thoracolumbar spine.
8. Most fractures of the talus are considered to be intra-articular. Complications of talar fractures include posttraumatic arthritis of the ankle and subtalar joints, and avascular necrosis.
9. Fractures at the midfoot rarely occur in isolation due to the relative immobility of this area. Sprains and fracture-dislocations occur at the transverse tarsal and tarsometatarsal joints, usually because of high-energy trauma.
10. Fractures of the forefoot metatarsals and phalanges are common injuries usually caused by direct blows. Stress fractures are also common injuries in the forefoot, usually appearing at the distal shafts of the second through fourth metatarsals, and the proximal shaft of the fifth metatarsal.
11. Some common foot deformities are hallux valgus, in which the first metatarsal is deviated medially while the great toe is deviated laterally, pes cavus, in which the longitudinal arch is abnormally high; and pes planus, in which the longitudinal arch is abnormally low.

REFERENCES

1. Greenspan, A: Orthopedic Radiology: A Practical Approach, ed 2. Raven Press, New York, 1992, p 9.1.
2. Netter, FH: The Ciba Collection of Medical Illustrations. Vol 8, Part I, Musculoskeletal System. Ciba-Geigy Corp, Summit, NJ, 1978, pp 106–110.
3. Ibid, p 110.
4. Richardson, JK and Iglarsh, ZA: Clinical Orthopaedic Physical Therapy. WB Saunders, Philadelphia, 1994, p 483.
5. Meschan, I: An Atlas of Normal Radiographic Anatomy. WB Saunders, Philadelphia, 1960, pp 218–219.
6. Weissman, B and Sledge, C: Orthopedic Radiology. WB Saunders, Philadelphia, 1986, pp 589–596, 625–633.
7. Greenspan, pp 9.1–9.16.
8. Bontrager, KL: Textbook of Radiographic Positioning and Related Anatomy, ed 3. Mosby, St Louis, 1993, pp 169–216.
9. Fischer, HW: Radiographic Anatomy: A Working Atlas. McGraw-Hill, New York, 1988, pp 36–43.
10. Wicke, L: Atlas of Radiographic Anatomy, ed 5. Lea & Febiger, Malvern, PA, 1994, pp 62–66.
11. Greenspan, pp 9.5–9.6.
12. Ibid, p 9.10.
13. Ibid, p 9.11.
14. Rockwood, CA and Green, DP: Fractures in Adults, Vol 2, ed 2. JB Lippincott, Philadelphia, 1984, pp 1665–1820.
15. Salter, RB: Textbook of Disorders and Injuries of the Musculoskeletal System, ed 2. Williams & Wilkins, Baltimore, 1983, pp 519–529.
16. Greenspan, pp 9.16–9.38.
17. Salter, p 519.
18. Greenspan, p 9.16.
19. Ibid, p 9.6.
20. Rockwood, p 1760.
21. Ibid, pp 1760–1788.
22. Ibid, pp 1728–1750.
23. Ibid, pp 1789–1795.
24. Ibid, pp 1806–1813.
25. Greenspan, pp 9.10–9.13.
26. Richardson, pp 534–537.
27. Salter, pp 103, 117, 222.
28. Richardson, p 541.
29. Ibid, p 534.
30. Ibid, p 535.
31. Ibid, p 536.
32. Ibid, pp 535–536.
33. Rockwood, pp 1718–1719.
34. Ibid, p 1718.
35. Richardson, p 491.
36. Greenspan, p 9.14.

SELF-TEST

Chapter 9

REGARDING FILM A:

1. Identify this projection.
2. Name the deformity at the first digit.
3. Describe the bony changes seen at medial side of the first metatarsal head.
4. Describe the positional relationship of the first and second toes to each other.

REGARDING FILM B:

5. Identify this projection.
6. Describe the joint positions of the ankles and feet as possible from this one projection.

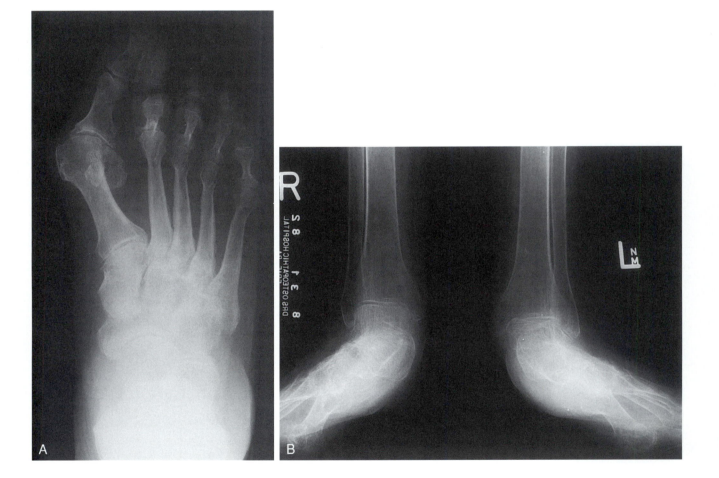

CHAPTER **10**

The Shoulder Joint Complex

The term *shoulder* requires elucidation. The glenohumeral joint is sometimes referred to as the *true* shoulder joint, but is only one of four articulations that comprise what is commonly called the *shoulder girdle* or *shoulder joint complex*. The combined and coordinated movements of the glenohumeral, acromioclavicular, and sternoclavicular joints, plus the scapulothoracic articulation, permit the arm to be positioned in space for efficient use of the hand. Impairment of a single articulation will inhibit normal functioning of the collective.

The routine radiographic evaluation of the shoulder includes basic anteroposterior (AP) views, which evaluate the glenohumeral and acromioclavicular joints. To provide a comprehensive radiographic look at the entire shoulder joint complex, radiographs of the scapulothoracic articulation are included herein, as are special stress views of the acromioclavicular joints. Radiographs of the sternoclavicular joints are presented in Chapter 5.

The goals of this chapter are first to present an overview of osseous radiographic anatomy. A brief description of ligamentous anatomy and joint mobility is presented to assist the reader in understanding the mechanisms of injury in this region. The routine radiographic evaluation of the shoulder joint complex follows. Here the reader has a chance to interact and learn radiographic anatomy by tracing a radiograph with a marker on a transparency sheet and then comparing the results with the radiographic tracing. Brief discussion, illustrations, and films of common trauma and abnormal soft tissue conditions conclude the chapter. The summary is organized into a list of practical points highlighting the clinical aspects of the chapter. A self-test challenges the reader's visual interpretation skills.

RADIOGRAPHIC ANATOMY

Osseous Anatomy[1]

The bones of the *shoulder joint* are the *proximal humerus*, the *scapula*, and the *clavicle*. The articulation between the humerus and the scapula is the *glenohumeral joint*, and the articulation between the scapula and the clavicle is the *acromioclavicular joint*.

The most proximal part of the humerus is the humeral *head*, which articulates in the scapular *glenoid fossa* (Fig. 10–1). The humeral *anatomic neck* is the slightly constricted region which lies just below the head. Inferior to the anatomical neck is the laterally projecting *greater tuberosity* and the anteriorly projecting *lesser tuberosity*. The tuberosities are separated by the *intertubercular* or *bicipital groove*. The narrowed region distal to the tuberosities is the *surgical neck*. Below the surgical neck is the humeral *shaft*.

The scapula is a flat, triangular bone with three borders, three angles, two surfaces, and prominent processes. The borders are identified as the *medial* or *ver-*

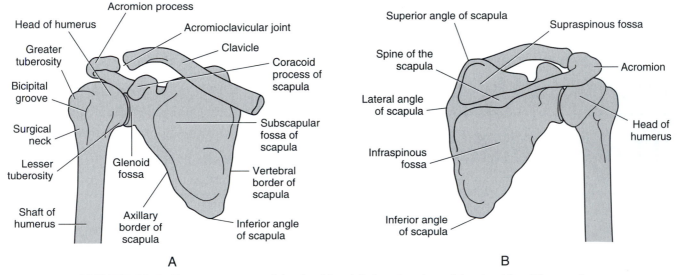

FIGURE 10–1. Osseous anatomy of the shoulder. (*A*) Anterior view of the shoulder; (*B*) posterior view of the shoulder.

tebral border, the *lateral* or *axillary border*, and the *superior border*. The angles or corners of the triangular scapula are named the *superior, inferior,* and *lateral angles*. The superior and inferior angles are at the ends of the medial border. The lateral angle and border give rise to the prominent process of the scapula and thus compose the greatest mass and weight of the scapula. The broadened end of the lateral angle supports the shallow *glenoid fossa*, which is deepened by the attachment of the fibrocartilaginous *glenoid labrum* and receives the humeral head. Medial to the glenoid fossa is the *coracoid process*, which projects superiorly and anteriorly.

The body of the scapula is thin and somewhat curved for greater strength.[2] The *costal surface* of the scapular body lies in close approximation to the thoracic ribs and this bone-muscle-bone articulation is referred to as the *scapulothoracic joint*. The costal surface of the body presents a shallow concave cavity, the *subscapular fossa*. The convex *dorsal surface* is divided into the *supraspinous fossa* and the *infraspinous fossa* separated by a bony ridge, the spine of the scapula. The spine of the scapula begins at the medial border and extends across most of the body of the scapula, forming at its end the large curving projection, the *acromion*.

The *clavicle* is a long bone with two curvatures. The lateral end of the clavicle articulates with the acromion, forming the *acromioclavicular joint*. The medial end of the clavicle articulates with the *sternal manubrium*, forming the *sternoclavicular joint*. The elongated portion of bone between the two ends is termed the *body* or *shaft* of the clavicle. In general, the clavicle in males is noted to be thicker and more curved than that in females.[2]

Ligamentous Anatomy

The glenohumeral joint is supported by various muscles, ligaments, and tendons reinforcing the joint capsule. The joint capsule attaches to the scapula at the glenoid fossa and to the humerus at the anatomic neck. The joint capsule is reinforced anteriorly by the *glenohumeral ligaments* and superiorly by the *coracohumeral ligament*. The *rotator cuff muscles* also reinforce the joint capsule (Fig. 10–2). These muscles are the *subscapularis, supraspinatus, infraspinatus,* and *teres minor*, located anteriorly, superiorly, posterosuperiorly, and posteriorly, respectively, enveloping the glenohumeral joint. The inferior aspect of the joint is the weakest structural area, as it is not directly reinforced by capsular ligaments or muscles.

The acromioclavicular joint is stabilized principally by the *coracoclavicular ligament* located medially to the joint, attaching the clavicle to the scapula via the coracoid process. The acromioclavicular joint capsule itself is rather weak and is reinforced by strong superior and inferior *acromioclavicular ligaments*.

JOINT MOBILITY[3]

Four articulations are involved in shoulder joint mobility. The glenohumeral, acromioclavicular, sternoclavicular, and scapulothoracic joints work in concert to afford the shoulder the greatest sum of functional mobility available at any single articulation in the body.

Arm elevation is possible in both the sagittal and frontal planes to 180 degrees or greater. Internal and external rotation are each accomplished to approxi-

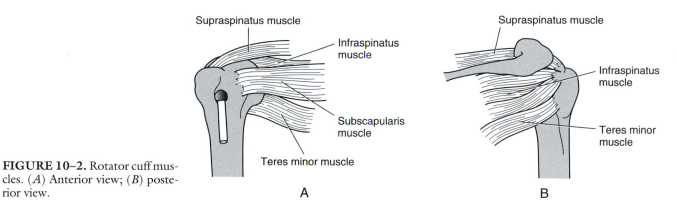

FIGURE 10–2. Rotator cuff muscles. (*A*) Anterior view; (*B*) posterior view.

mately 90 degrees, varying somewhat with the starting position of shoulder elevation. Backward extension in the sagittal plane is possible to 60 degrees. About 180 degrees of movement is possible in the horizontal plane. Other motions available at the shoulder include adduction and abduction. Circumduction, a combination of movement through these elemental planes, is freely available at the shoulder. Gliding of the articular surfaces occurs as component movements during all motions.

GROWTH AND DEVELOPMENT[4]

The clavicle, scapular body, and humeral shaft begin ossification at the seventh to eighth week of fetal life. The ossification center for the proximal humeral head appears at 36 weeks of fetal development. At birth only these structures are ossified and are readily visible on radiograph (Fig. 10–3).

The remainder of the scapula, including the acromion, coracoid process, glenoid fossa, vertebral border, and inferior angle, is largely cartilaginous at birth. Secondary centers of ossification appear at the coracoid process at about 1 year of age, and in most of the other structures of the scapula at puberty, fusing with the main body of the scapula at 18 to 25 years of age (Figs. 10–5*B*, *C*).

Secondary centers for the greater and lesser tuberosities of the humerus appear between 3 and 5 years of age and coalesce at about 6 years of age, forming one epiphysis. In many individuals the greater tuberosity may remain separated until it fuses with the humeral shaft at about age 16 (Figs. 10–4, 10–5*A*).

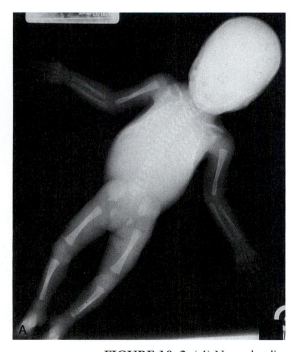

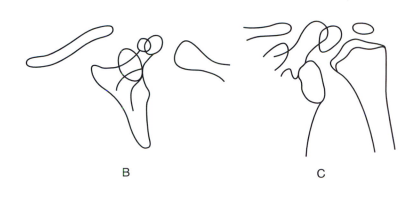

FIGURE 10–3. (*A*) Normal radiographic appearance of a healthy 6-month-old infant. Radiographic tracings of the ossified portions at the shoulder girdle (*B*) at birth and (*C*) at age 2 years. (Adapted from Meschan,[4] p 65.)

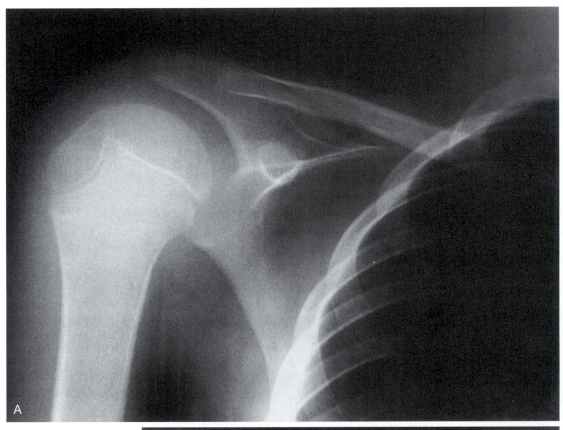

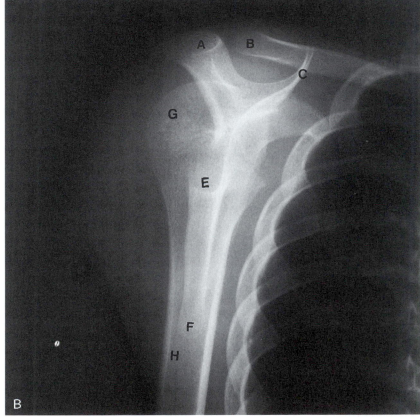

FIGURE 10–4. Normal radiographic appearance of the shoulder of a healthy 8-year-old. (*A*) AP view. By this age, the greater and lesser tuberosities of the humerus have coalesced and formed one epiphysis. (*B*) This oblique view of the shoulder demonstrates the relationship of the humeral head to the glenoid cavity and also demonstrates the parts of the scapula projected clear of the rib cage. *A*, acromion; *B*, distal end of the clavicle; *C*, superior border of the scapula; *D*, coracoid process; *E*, body of scapula; *F*, inferior angle of the scapula; *G*, humeral head; *H*, humeral shaft.

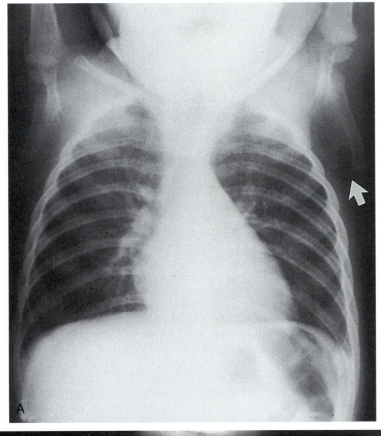

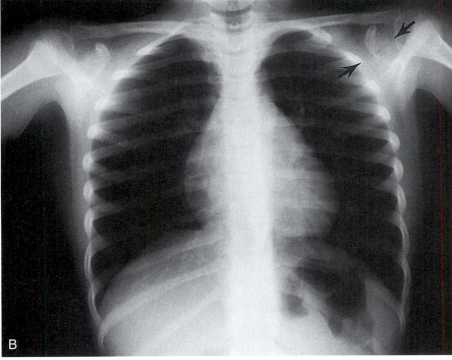

FIGURE 10–5. (*A*) Chest film of a 9-month-old boy, scapular anomaly demonstrated. The scapulae are easy to see on this view as they have been adducted during the positioning of the arms overhead and are no longer superimposed by the rib cage. An incidental finding on this chest film is an anomaly at the left scapula, which has been referred to as a "swallow tail" deformity. (*B*) Chest film of an 8-year-old boy, scapular anomaly demonstrated. A synchondrosis of the left scapular body was an incidental finding during evaluation of this chest film. Arrows mark the borders of the radiolucent line representing this defect. Note that at this age, the only ossified structures of the scapula are the body and the coracoid process.

ROUTINE RADIOGRAPHIC EVALUATION[5-9]

The routine radiologic evaluation of the shoulder for typical complaints and screening consists of two AP projections. The purpose of performing *two* AP projection rotations is to allow greater visualization of the various aspects of the humeral head and proximal third of the humeral shaft. The entire length of the humerus is radiographed in a separate evaluation, which includes the AP and lateral projections. In the presence of suspected fracture or dislocation, only one AP projection is made with the shoulder positioned in *neutral*.

The routine radiographic examination of the acromioclavicular joints is separate from the routine shoulder examination. The stability of the acromioclavicular joints is evaluated by performing *two* AP radiographs, one without weights and one with weights tied to the wrists. The purpose of the weights is to place a longitudinal pull through the arms that will stress the acromioclavicular joints. Instability is revealed by the amount of altered joint relationships on the weighted film versus the unweighted film.

The routine radiographic examination of the scapula is also separate from the routine shoulder examination. A certain portion of the scapula is well demonstrated on the shoulder AP radiograph, but much of the lateral border structures are superimposed by the humerus and ribs. For this reason, if the scapula is the area of interest, it will be filmed with special positioning to free it from as much superimposition as possible.

Shoulder

Basic: AP External Rotation
AP Internal Rotation

ANTEROPOSTERIOR EXTERNAL ROTATION (FIGS. 10–6, 10–7, 10–8)

This view is taken in the true AP *anatomic* position, which places the shoulder and arm in *external rotation*. This view demonstrates the *proximal third of the humerus*, the *lateral two-thirds of the clavicle*, the *acromioclavicular joint*, and the *upper and lateral portion of the scapula*. Any *calcium deposits* present in the muscles, tendons, or bursae of the shoulder may also be demonstrated. The important observations are:

1. The greater tuberosity is visualized in profile at the most lateral aspect of the humeral head.
2. The lesser tuberosity is superimposed at the mid area of the humeral head.
3. The medial portion of the humeral head is partially superimposed in the glenoid fossa. Thus, the glenohumeral joint space is not well visualized.
4. The crest of the spine of the scapula can be seen extending across the scapula and broadening into the glenoid fossa.
5. The vertebral and lateral borders of the scapula are superimposed behind the rib cage.
6. The coracoid process is visualized end-on.
7. The acromioclavicular joint is seen superior to the glenohumeral joint.

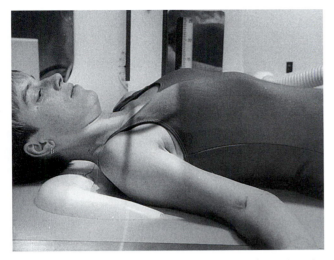

FIGURE 10–6. Patient position for AP external rotating view of the shoulder.

CLINICAL OBJECTIVES

1. Trace the proximal humerus and identify the greater and lesser tuberosities.
2. Identify the anatomic and surgical necks of the humerus.
3. Trace the borders of the scapula. Identify the crest of the spine of the scapula, coracoid process, glenoid fossa, and acromion.
4. Trace the clavicle. Identify the acromioclavicular joint.

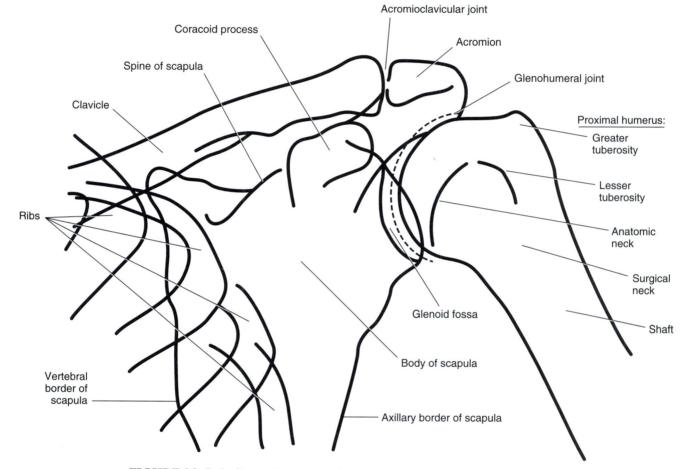

FIGURE 10–7. Radiographic tracing of AP external rotation view of the shoulder.

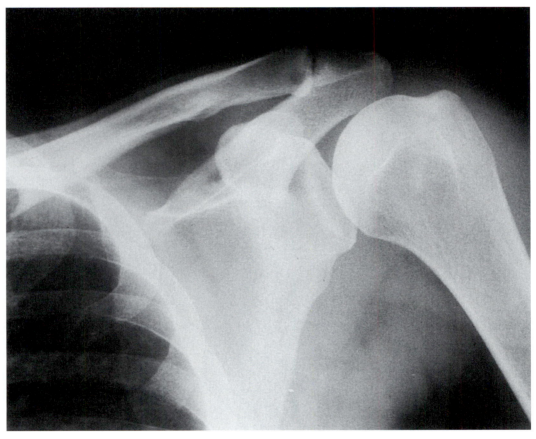

FIGURE 10–8. AP external rotation view of the shoulder.

ANTEROPOSTERIOR INTERNAL ROTATION (FIGS. 10–9, 10–10, 10–11)

This view is taken with the arm and shoulder positioned in *internal rotation*. This view demonstrates the *proximal third of the humerus*, the *lateral two-thirds of the clavicle*, the *acromioclavicular joint*, and the *upper and lateral portion of the scapula*. Any *calcium deposits* present in muscles, tendons, or bursae of the shoulder may also be demonstrated. The important observations are:

1. The greater tuberosity is now superimposed over the mid area of the humeral head.

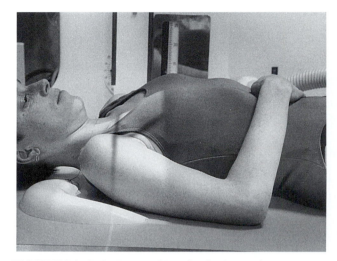

FIGURE 10–9. Patient position for AP internal rotation view of the shoulder.

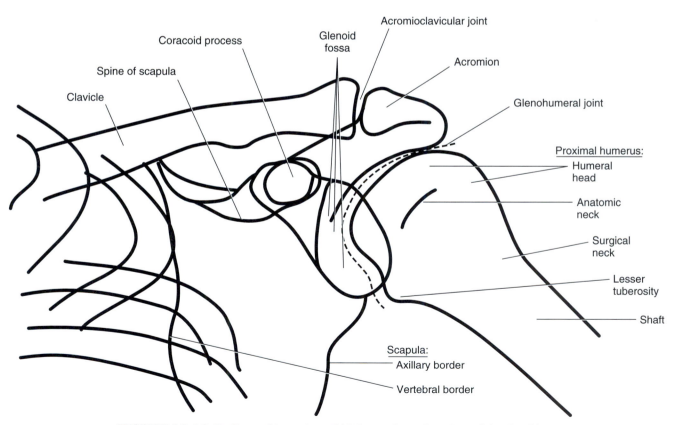

FIGURE 10–10. Radiographic tracing of AP internal rotation view of the shoulder.

2. The lesser tuberosity is now seen in profile on the medial aspect of the humeral head.
3. The medial portion of the humeral head is partially superimposed in the glenoid fossa. Thus the glenohumeral joint space is not well visualized.
4. The crest of the spinous process of the scapula can be seen extending across the scapula and broadening into the glenoid fossa.
5. The vertebral and lateral borders of the scapula are superimposed behind the rib cage.
6. The coracoid process is visualized end-on.
7. The acromioclavicular joint is seen superior to the glenohumeral joint.

CLINICAL OBJECTIVES

1. Trace the proximal humerus and identify the lesser tuberosities.
2. Identify the anatomic and surgical necks of the humerus.
3. Trace the borders of the scapula. Identify the crest of the spinous process, coracoid process, glenoid fossa, and acromion.
4. Trace the clavicle. Identify the acromioclavicular joint.

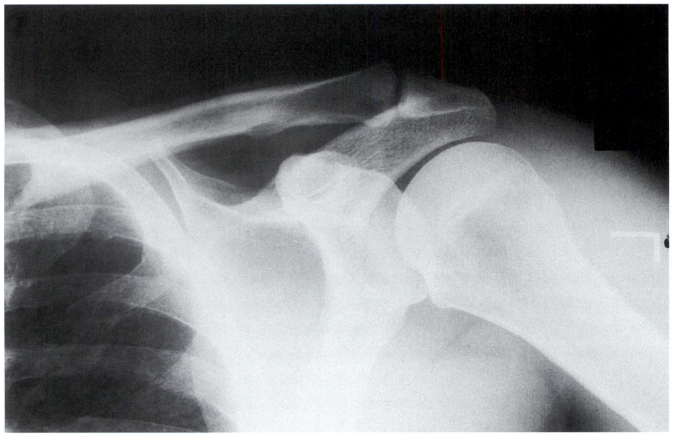

FIGURE 10–11. AP internal rotation view of the shoulder.

Acromioclavicular Joint

Basic: AP, Bilateral, Without Weights
              AP, Bilateral, With Weights

AP, BILATERAL, WITH AND WITHOUT WEIGHTS (FIGS. 10–12 THROUGH 10–16)

These two views demonstrate both *acromioclavicular (AC) joints* at once for comparison purposes. After the first radiograph is made without weights, a second radiograph is made with a minimum of 10- to 15-lb weights tied to each wrist. This second radiograph is considered a *stress view* done to determine possible *AC joint separation*. Other structures visible on either radiograph are the entire length of the *clavicles*, both *sternoclavicular joints*, and both *shoulders* as described in the AP views. The important observations are:

1. This AP radiograph is made with the arms at the patient's sides in *neutral* alignment. Thus the appearance of the greater and lesser tuberosities at the humeral head will be different from the internal and external AP shoulder views.
2. The AC joint is evaluated by examining the relationship of the acromion to the clavicle.[10] The normal joint space distance at this articulation ranges from 0.3 to 0.8 cm. Additionally, the relationship of the coracoid process to the clavicle is also examined. The normal distance between the inferior aspect of the clavicle and the coracoid process, the *coracoclavicular distance*, ranges from 1.0 to 1.3 cm (see Fig. 10–16). The amount of abnormal increases in these

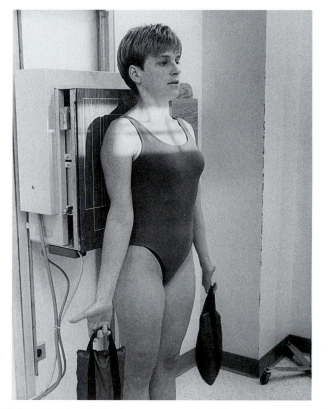

FIGURE 10–12. Patient position for bilateral AP view of acromioclavicular joints, with weights.

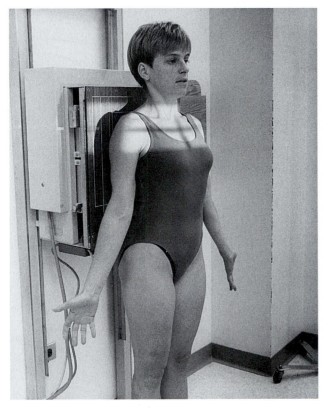

FIGURE 10–13. Patient position for bilateral AP view of acromioclavicular joints, without weights.

distances helps determine the severity of the ligamentous injury. Grading of AC separation can thus be quantified using these distances:

Grade I, mild sprain: Minimal widening of the acromioclavicular joint space with the coracoclavicular distance still within normal range.

Grade II, moderate sprain: Widening of the AC joint space to 1.0 to 1.5 cm with a 25 percent to 50 percent increase in the coracoclavicular distance.

Grade III, severe sprain: Widening of the acromioclavicular joint space 1.5 cm or greater with a 50 percent or more increase in the coracoclavicular distance. The AC joint is dislocated and the clavicle appears to be displaced superiorly.

CLINICAL OBJECTIVES

Identify these structures on both shoulders on both radiographs:
1. Trace the proximal humerus. Identify the greater and lesser tuberosities.
2. Trace the borders of the scapula, the spinous process, the coracoid process, the acromion, and the glenoid fossa.
3. Trace the clavicles.
4. Identify the acromioclavicular joint and the coracoclavicular distance.

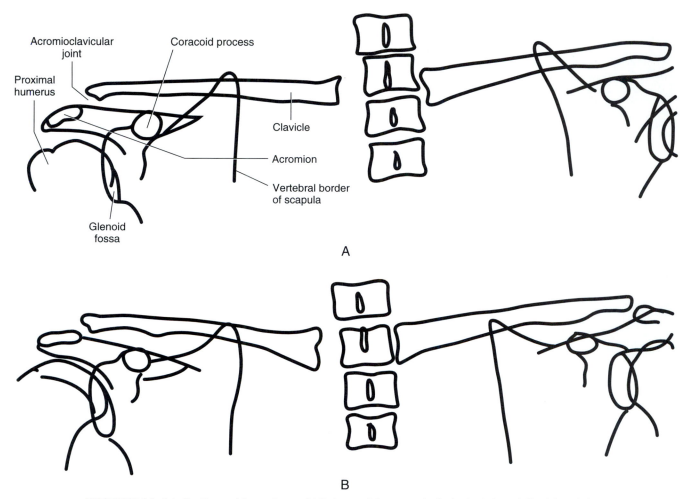

A

B

FIGURE 10–14. Radiographic tracings of AP views of the acromioclavicular joints. (*A*) with weights (*B*) without weights.

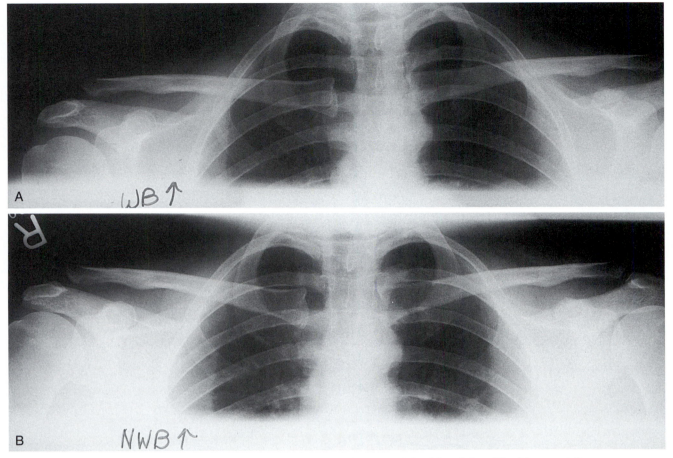

FIGURE 10–15. AP view of bilateral acromioclavicular joints. (*A*) with weights. (*B*) without weights.

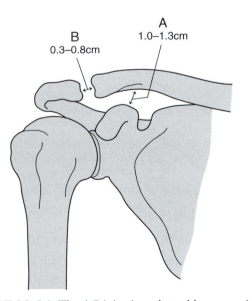

FIGURE 10–16. The AC joint is evaluated by measuring (*A*) the coracoclavicular distance, and (*B*) the joint space distance. Normal value range is given. (Adapted from Greenspan, p 5.23)

Scapula

Basic: AP
Lateral

ANTEROPOSTERIOR (FIGS. 10–17, 10–18, 10–19)

This view demonstrates the entire *scapula*. The lateral half of the scapula is seen free of superimposition of the ribs and lungs. The medial half of the scapula is seen through blurred thoracic structures. The important observations are:

1. The patient's arm has been abducted 90 degrees and externally rotated. This position has allowed the scapula to abduct and rotate upward so that the lateral half is now cleared of the rib cage and can be evaluated in more detail. A form positioning device is used to aid in positioning the shoulder girdle, and this is noted by the metallic chain of beads embedded within the form, visible on the top side of the radiograph.
2. All three borders and angles of the scapula are usually visible.

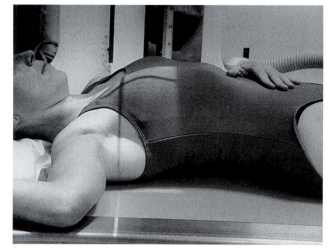

FIGURE 10–17. Patient position for AP view of the scapula.

CLINICAL OBJECTIVES

1. Trace the entire scapula. Identify the vertebral, lateral, and superior borders, the superior, inferior, and lateral angles, the coracoid process, the acromion, the spinous process, and the glenoid fossa.
2. Trace the humeral head. Identify the greater and lesser tuberosities.

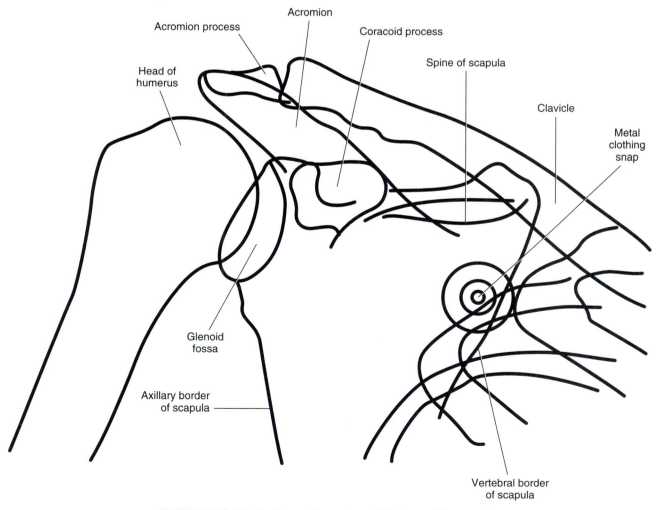

FIGURE 10–18. Radiographic tracing of AP view of the scapula.

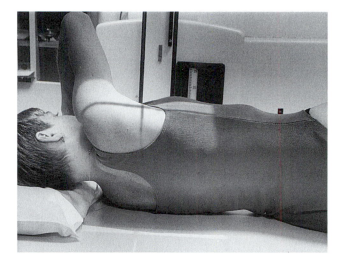

FIGURE 10–20. Patient position for lateral view of the scapula.

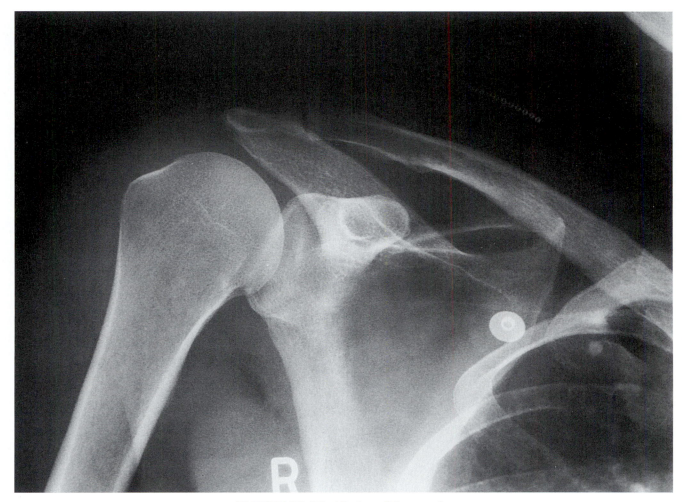

FIGURE 10–19. AP view of the scapula.

LATERAL (FIGS. 10–20, 10–21, 10–22)

This view demonstrates a lateral view of the **scapula**, as projected clear of the rib cage. The *body* of the scapula is best evaluated in this radiograph. The important observations are:

1. The patient's arm is positioned across the front of his or her chest to free the body of the scapula from superimposition of the humeral shaft, or the patient's arm may be positioned behind his or her back to free the acromion and coracoid process from superimposition of the humeral head.

2. The profile of the scapular body is clearly seen. Fractures of the scapular body are readily visible on this view.

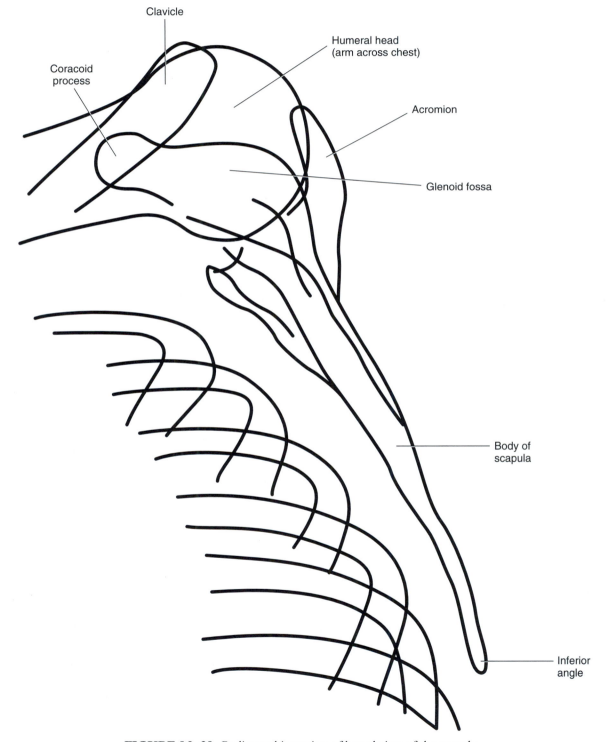

FIGURE 10–21. Radiographic tracing of lateral view of the scapula.

CLINICAL OBJECTIVES

1. Trace the proximal humerus superimposed behind the scapula.
2. Trace the body of the scapula, the acromion, coracoid process, and glenoid fossa.

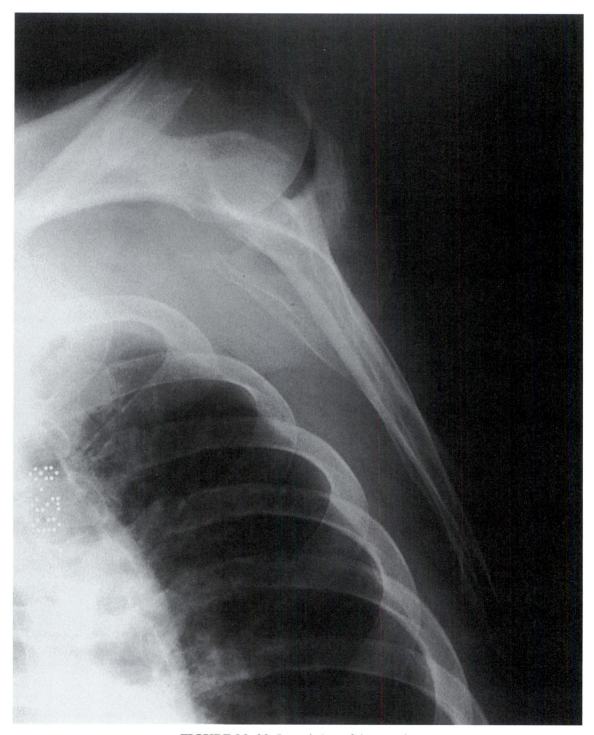

FIGURE 10–22. Lateral view of the scapula.

Additional Views

Numerous special projections exist to evaluate certain conditions at the shoulder. The length of the humerus itself is radiographed in a separate evaluation, which includes the AP and lateral projections (Figs. 10–23 through 10–26). The *axillary* view, done with the x-ray beam directed through the shoulder joint in an inferior-superior or superior-inferior direction, is helpful in determining the exact relationship of the humeral head to the glenoid fossa in evaluating glenohumeral dislocations (Fig. 10–27). An *oblique* view of the shoulder allows the glenohumeral joint space to be seen free of superimposition and is also useful in diagnosing dislocations. A *tangential* view of the bicipital groove is done to determine injury to this specific structure. Other various special projections are used in the presence of trauma to prevent undue movement at the shoulder. In general, however, the basic routine AP films are most commonly performed and usually sufficiently demonstrate the shoulder area.

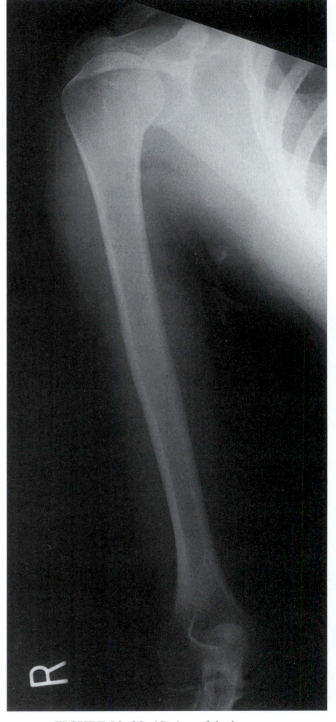

FIGURE 10–23. AP view of the humerus.

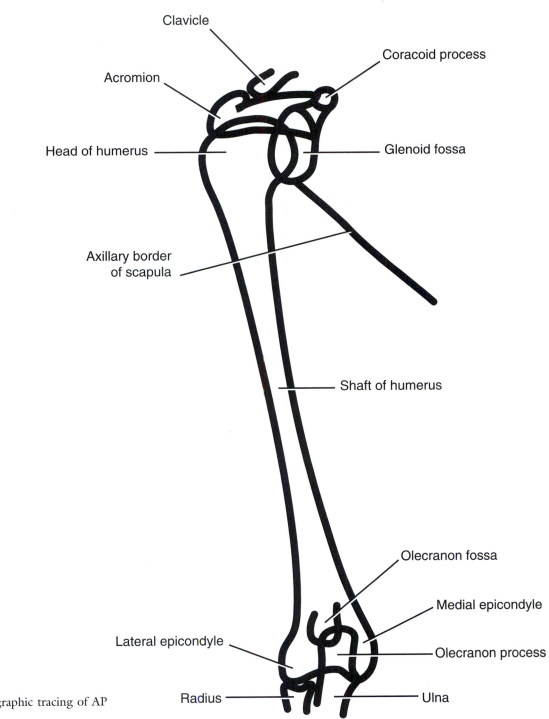

FIGURE 10–24. Radiographic tracing of AP view of the humerus.

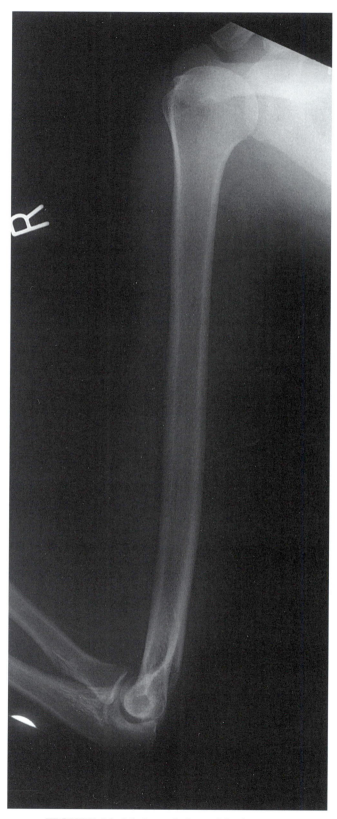

FIGURE 10–25. Lateral view of the humerus.

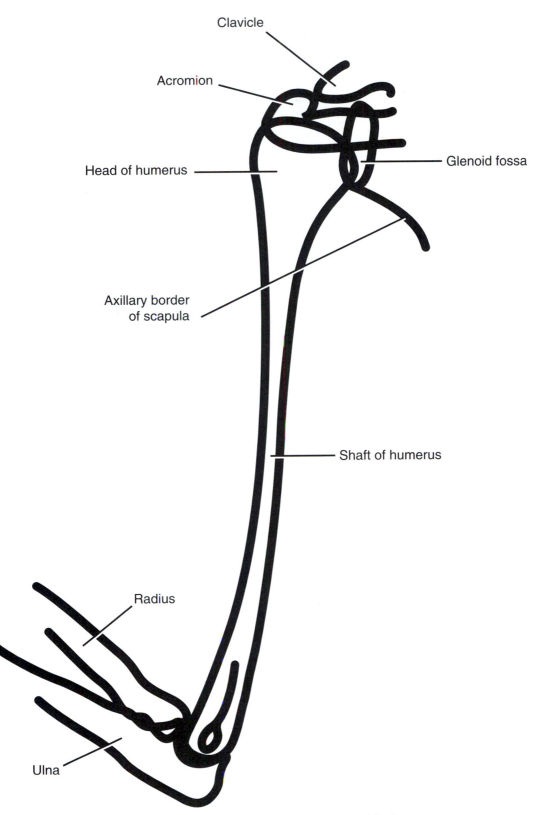

FIGURE 10–26. Radiographic tracing of lateral view of the humerus.

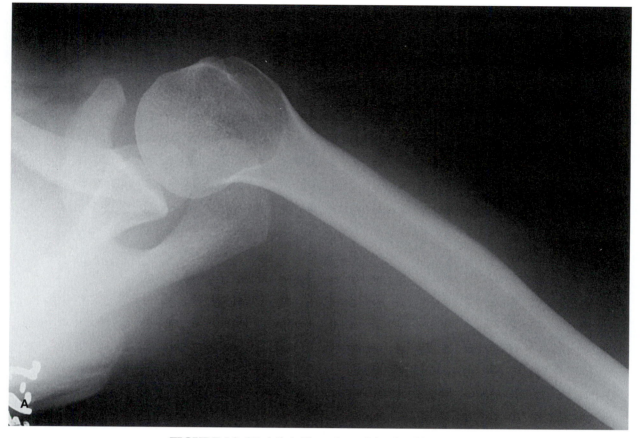

FIGURE 10–27. (*A*) Axillary view of the shoulder joint.

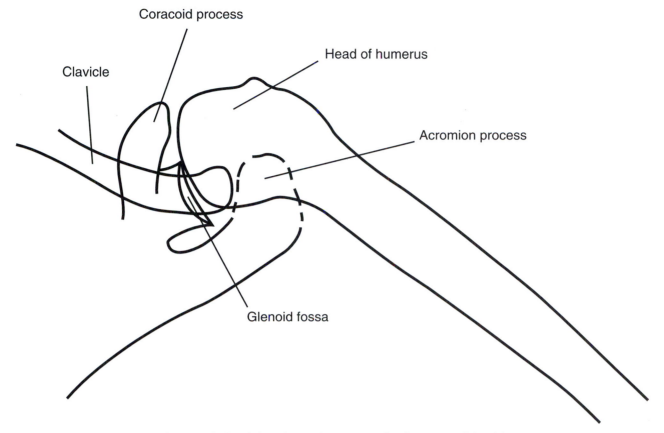

FIGURE 10–27. (*B*) Radiographic tracing of axillary view of shoulder.

TRAUMA[11-14]

The shoulder area possesses less mechanical protection and less bony stability than any other large joint in the body, rendering it susceptible to a variety of fractures, joint dislocations, and soft tissue and cartilage injuries.

The majority of shoulder fractures and dislocations are well demonstrated on plain films. Computed tomography (CT) is helpful in identifying fragment location in complex fractures. Soft tissue and cartilage injuries are evaluated by ancillary techniques including magnetic resonance imaging (MRI), CT, and contrast arthrography.[15]

Fractures of the Proximal Humerus

Fractures of the proximal humerus are commonly classified by their location within the boundaries of the four major anatomic segments (Fig. 10–28).[16,17]

1. The head, from the articular surface to the anatomic neck
2. The greater tuberosity
3. The lesser tuberosity
4. The shaft, at the level of the surgical neck

Fractures of the humeral head are rare and, when present, are often associated with dislocation. During the dislocation, a portion of humeral head may be sheared off against the glenoid labrum. This type of fracture may be considered an *osteochondral fracture*, as the fracture fragment would be partly composed of articular cartilage.[18] Fractures through the anatomic

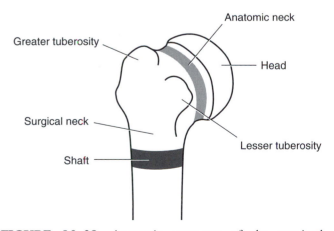

FIGURE 10–28. Anatomic segments of the proximal humerus.

neck, the constricted region just below the humeral head, are also rarely seen in isolation, more often present in combination with other fracture lines (Fig. 10–29).

Fractures of the greater tuberosity in middle-aged and older adults usually result from a fall directly on the point of the shoulder. These fractures are often undisplaced and treated conservatively with several weeks of sling immobilization (Fig. 10–30). Avulsion fractures of the greater tuberosity are more common in younger adults and usually occur by indirect injury, such as a fall with the arm adducted, combined with forceful contraction of the rotator cuff muscles attempting to limit excursion of the arm. The area of attachment of the rotator cuff muscles on the greater tuberosity is often greatly displaced, and maintenance of reduction requires immobilization in an abduction splint or shoulder spica cast for several weeks.[19]

Fractures of the lesser tuberosity are rare and usually occur due to avulsion forces resulting from forceful contraction of the subscapularis muscle.

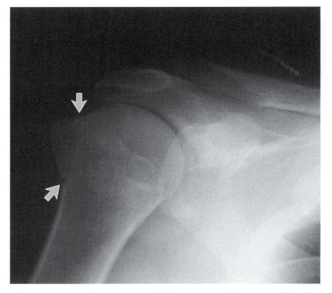

FIGURE 10–30. Fracture of the greater tuberosity of the humerus. This 37-year-old man injured his arm when he fell during an aggressive racquetball game. The AP view of the shoulder demonstrates a complete, vertical, minimally displaced fracture through the greater tuberosity (arrows).

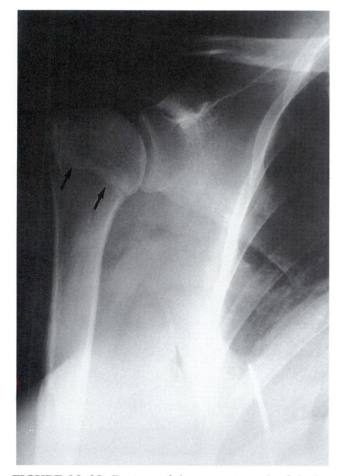

FIGURE 10–29. Fracture of the anatomic neck of the humerus. This 43-year-old woman injured her arm when she was tripped by her dog's leash and fell hard on an outstretched hand. This AP view of the shoulder demonstrates a complete, nondisplaced, and impacted fracture through the anatomic neck (arrows).

Fractures of the surgical neck of the humerus are common (Fig. 10–31). Fractures occurring here resulting from direct blows tend to be transverse and somewhat comminuted. Fractures resulting from an indirect injury, such as a fall on an outstretched hand whereby forces are transmitted up the arm, are more likely to produce a spiral fracture line and may extend to involve the tuberosities or anatomic neck. Impacted fractures at the surgical neck are common in the elderly, especially in osteoporotic women, often resulting from a relatively minor fall. Impacted fractures are treated conservatively with sling immobilization. The more severely displaced surgical neck fractures may require open reduction. The thick periosteum of the humeral shaft, related to the great amount of muscle surrounding the humerus, aids in rapid healing of fractures in this area.[20]

Pathologic Fractures of the Proximal Humerus[21]

Pathologic fractures occur through bone that has been abnormally weakened by either localized, disseminated, or generalized disease processes. The proximal humerus is a frequent site for pathologic fractures, usually presenting in the region of the surgical neck. These fractures are often the result of benign or malignant primary bone tumors, metastatic lesions, or related to radiation therapy.[21] The proximal humerus is also a common site of fracture in patients with generalized osteoporosis (see Fig. 2–56); the weakened ar-

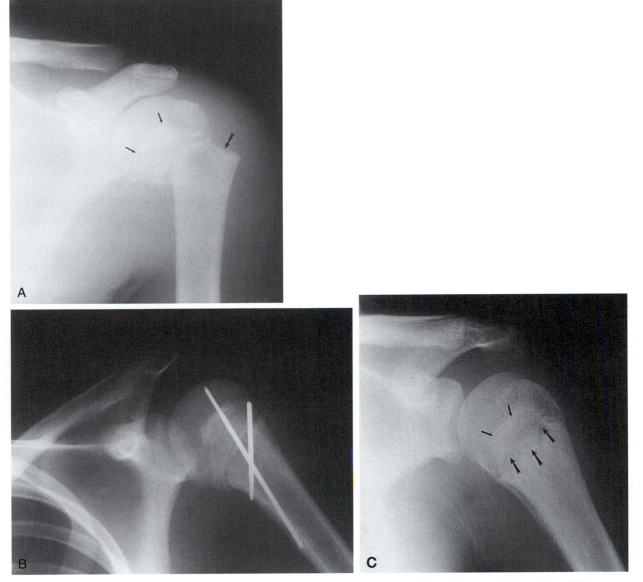

FIGURE 10–31. Fracture of the surgical neck of the humerus. This 15-year-old boy injured his shoulder in a motor vehicle accident. (*A*) This AP view of the left shoulder demonstrates a severely displaced surgical neck fracture. The distal fragment has displaced laterally and superiorly. The fracture line is transverse (large arrow). Note the epiphyseal plate of the humeral head (small arrows), which is distinguished from the fracture by smoothly rounded margins and increased density on the border of the epiphysis. (*B*) Follow-up films made 1 month after surgical fixation. Note good alignment and positioning at the fracture site and evidence of callus formation bridging the fracture gap. (*C*) 4½ months after injury. The metal fixation had been removed a few weeks prior. Large arrows point to the barely visible remnant of the fracture line, which is undergoing progressive remodeling. Small arrows point to the epiphyseal growth plate, which has also changed in appearance because of maturity after this length of time.

chitecture of osteoporotic bone is vulnerable to fracture from relatively minor trauma.

Fractures of the Clavicle[22]

Fractures of the clavicle are designated by their location at the *medial*, *middle*, or *lateral third* of the bone (Fig. 10–32). The middle third is the most frequent site of fracture. Clavicular fractures are common in children and are usually successfully treated with figure-8 bandage splinting of the shoulder girdles. Adults are similarly treated, although at times they may require open reduction (Fig. 10–33).

Fractures of the Scapula[23]

Fractures of the scapula are rare, and when present are usually the result of a direct blow. Fractures to the body and spinous process are usually minimally displaced due to the protection of the surrounding muscles (Fig. 10–34). Fractures at the lateral angle may require reduction to maintain the articular relationship of the glenohumeral joint. Fractures of the rim of the glenoid fossa are associated with glenohumeral dislocation.

Dislocations of the Glenohumeral Joint[24,25]

The glenohumeral joint is susceptible to subluxation and dislocation due to the relative lack of bony stabil-

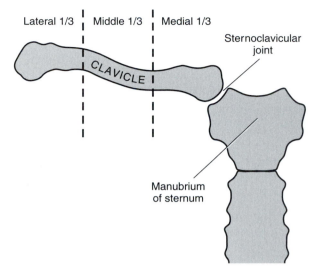

FIGURE 10–32. The location of trauma to the clavicle is designated by dividing the length of the clavicle into thirds.

ity and the large, redundant articular capsule. The displacement of the humeral head from its normal articulation to the glenoid fossa is probably the most common of all joint dislocations and may occur with or without associated fractures.[26]

Glenohumeral joint subluxation or dislocation can occur in different directions and is designated by the position of the humeral head to the glenoid fossa postdislocation. The humeral head may dislocate anterior, posterior, inferior, or superior to the fossa. The majority of glenohumeral dislocations, about 95 percent, are described as *anterior dislocations* (Fig. 10–35).[27] The hu-

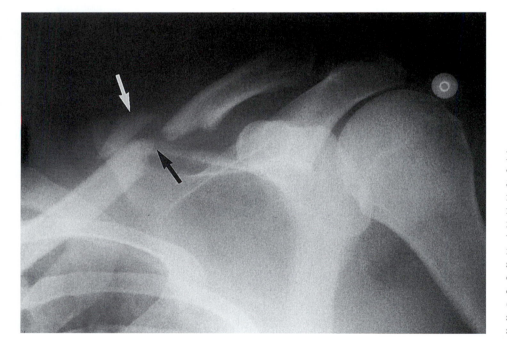

FIGURE 10–33. Fracture of the clavicle. Because the clavicle is an S-shaped bone, mechanical forces from the side cause a shearing effect on its middle third, where the majority of clavicle fractures such as this one occur. This 24-year-old male was injured as he fell to his side and was tackled during a game of touch football. The AP view demonstrates the fracture site (black arrow) and the large wedge-shaped fragment that has displaced superiorly (white arrow).

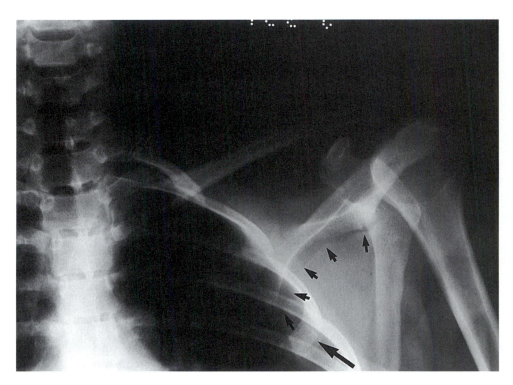

FIGURE 10–34. Fracture of the body of the scapula. This 33-year-old female was injured when she neglected to duck and was struck by the swinging boom on a sailboat. This AP view of the scapula demonstrates the transverse and minimally displaced fracture line through the body of the scapula (small arrows). Note an associated fracture of the rib (large arrow) sustained when the scapula impacted on the rib cage.

meral head comes to rest under the coracoid process or under the anterior aspect of the glenoid fossa. These may be referred to as subcoracoid or subglenoid dislocations, respectively.

The mechanism of anterior dislocation is usually forceful external rotation and extension while the arm is abducted. The greater tuberosity is levered against the acromion, and the humeral head is forced out of the glenoid fossa and through the restraint of the anterior ligaments and anterior capsule.[28] Associated fractures may include a compression fracture of the posterolateral aspect of the humeral head, known as the *Hill-Sachs lesion*, sustained as it strikes the glenoid rim during the dislocation (Fig. 10–36). Other associated fractures may occur at the greater tuberosity, surgical neck, or glenoid rim. A fracture of the anteroinferior rim of the glenoid, or detachment of the labrum from the rim, is known as a *Bankart fracture or lesion* and is indicative of recurrent dislocation (Fig. 10–37).[29,30]

Treatment after an initial dislocation is generally

nonsurgical and consists of reduction followed by immobilization and rehabilitation, allowing enough time for the anterior capsule to heal. Recurrent anterior subluxation or dislocation and chronic joint instability are common problems, and surgical repair is often necessary to establish stability and function in the joint.[31]

Radiographically, anterior glenohumeral joint dislocations are readily diagnosed on the AP view of the shoulder.[32] The Hill-Sachs lesion is visible on the AP view with the arm internally rotated. The Bankart fracture is also visible on the routine films, except if the defect is in the cartilaginous labrum. Labrum tears would be revealed on CT or MRI. *Posterior dislocations*, accounting for only 2 to 3 percent of glenohumeral dislocations, are problematic in diagnosing on the AP views. The abnormal position of the humeral head posterior to the glenoid fossa may be overlooked as normal superimposition. Special views, such as the *axillary* view, are required to ascertain the positional relationship of the humeral head to the glenoid fossa.

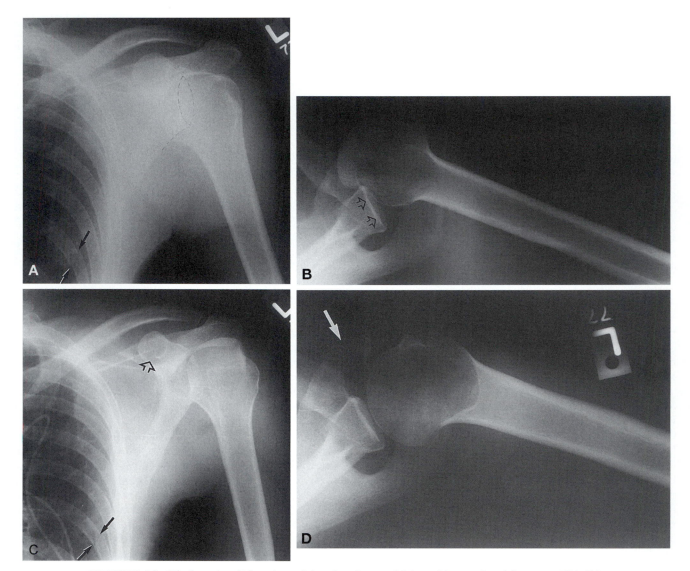

FIGURE 10–35. Anterior dislocation of the glenohumeral joint with associated fractures. This 56-year-old firefighter was injured during a rescue when the flooring in the second story of a house collapsed underneath him. (*A*) AP view of the shoulder demonstrates the displacement of the humeral head from the glenoid fossa (dotted line). Note the rib fracture (arrows). (*B*) Axillary view of the glenohumeral joint clearly demonstrates that the humeral head has displaced anteriorly from the glenoid fossa (fossa marked by open arrows). (*C*) AP film of the shoulder made after reduction. Note the fracture of the coracoid process now visible (open arrow). (*D*) Axillary view after reduction shows normal relationship of the humeral head to the glenoid fossa. The coracoid process fracture is more clearly demonstrated on this view and is now identified as a complete, transverse fracture of the tip of the coracoid process (white arrow).

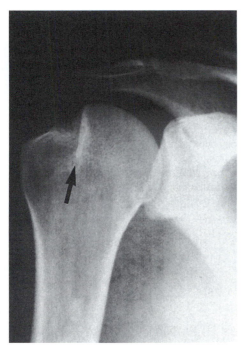

FIGURE 10–36. Hill-Sachs deformity associated with anterior humeral dislocation. The impaction of the angular surface of the interior glenoid rim produces the compression deformity of the articular surface, which has also been referred to as the "hatchet deformity" (arrow). (From Yochum, TR, and Rowe, LJ: Essentials of Skeletal Radiology, Williams & Wilkins, Baltimore, 1987, p 494, with permission.)

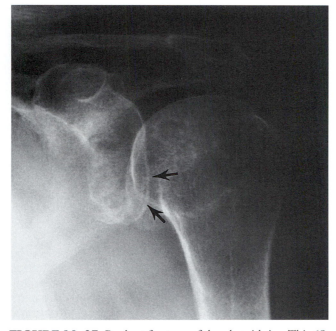

FIGURE 10–37. Bankart fracture of the glenoid rim. This 69-year-old woman presents with a chronic history of anterior glenohumeral instability, initiated by a traumatic anterior dislocation 10 years ago. This AP view of the shoulder demonstrates a fracture of the anterior-inferior rim of the glenoid, represented by the radiolucent line paralleling the margins of the fossa (arrows). The osteoarthritic changes in the joint, including sclerosis, spurring of the inferior joint surfaces, superior migration of the humeral head, and joint space narrowing, are likely to be secondary osteoarthritic changes related to the chronic instability of the joint.

Acromioclavicular Joint Separation[33–36]

Acromioclavicular separation, also commonly called *shoulder separation*, refers to various degrees of ligamentous sprain at the joint. The stability of this joint is achieved primarily by the coracoclavicular ligament, and additionally by the acromioclavicular ligament and joint capsule. Sprains are graded as mild, moderate, and severe in reference to the degree of disruption of these structures (Figs. 10–38, 10–39). See the routine radiographic examination of the acromioclavicular joints for the radiographic findings that define the specific grades of sprain.

The mechanism of injury is typically a downward force applied to the acromion process, from either a fall on the point of the shoulder or a direct blow. Various other forces may disrupt the joint such as traction on the arm, a fall on an outstretched hand, or a fall on a flexed elbow.

Treatment is controversial; management of all grades of sprain may be treated conservatively with varying lengths of immobilization, or surgical repair may be instituted in moderate and severe sprains. Several types of surgical repair exist, including wire or pin fixation of the acromioclavicular joint, reconstruction, repair, or fixation of the coracoclavicular ligament, excision of the distal clavicle, or dynamic muscle transfers. Complications identifiable on radiograph include arthritic changes in the joint, chronic subluxation, soft tissue calcification, and loosening or migration of metal fixation devices.

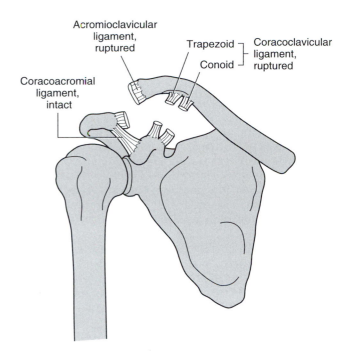

FIGURE 10–38. The stability of the acromioclavicular joint is achieved primarily by the coracoclavicular ligaments. Severe sprains or ruptures of these ligaments result in acromioclavicular joint separation.

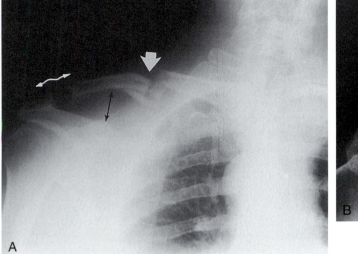

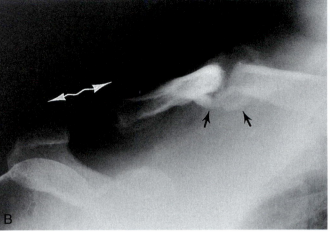

FIGURE 10–39. Acromioclavicular (AC) joint separation with clavicle fracture. (*A*) This 55-year-old farmer was injured when several sacks of grain fell down on him from the loft in his barn. This AP view of the AC joint demonstrates marked widening of both the acromioclavicular joint (white wavy arrow) and the coracoclavicular distance (black arrow), indicating a moderate to severe sprain of the AC joint. There is an associated comminuted fracture of the midshaft of the clavicle (large white arrow). (*B*) Management of this patient was complicated by the extremely slow union of the clavicular fracture. This AP film of the AC joint made 11 months later shows some callus (black arrows) uniting the fracture fragments, but the fracture is not united, as evidenced by the wide radiolucent gap at the fracture site. The disruption of the AC joint remains unchanged.

Rotator Cuff Tears[37,38]

The four muscles of the rotator cuff are the subscapularis, supraspinatus, infraspinatus, and teres minor. The tendons of these muscles converge and fuse with the fibrous capsule of the glenohumeral joint, inserting into the anatomic neck and tuberosities of the humerus. Underlying the rotator cuff is the synovial lining and joint space. Above the rotator cuff lies the subacromial bursa and its extension, the subdeltoid bursa.

Rotator cuff tears may result from an acute traumatic episode, such as during a glenohumeral dislocation, a fall on an outstretched hand, or from a forceful abduction movement of the arm.[22] Rotator cuff tears may also result from the progressive tendon irritation caused by repetitive trauma or impingement. Normal degenerative changes in the cuff seen most commonly in patients over 50 years of age predispose the structure to rupture from relatively minor trauma.

The most common tear involves the supraspinatus portion of the cuff 1 cm above its insertion on the greater tuberosity. All tears of the rotator cuff are generally classified as *complete* or *incomplete* tears. A complete tear of the rotator cuff, extending through the full thickness of the cuff, allows the joint space below the cuff to communicate with the subacromial-subdeltoid bursa located above the cuff.

The radiographic evaluation of suspected rotator cuff tears is usually complete with *contrast arthrography*. Contrast media is injected into the glenohumeral joint space and an AP radiograph is made (Fig. 10–40). An *intact* rotator cuff will confine the contrast medium to within the joint capsule itself and the structures that

normally communicate with the capsule—the sheath of the biceps tendon inferiorly and the subscapular bursa anteriorly. Only these structures will appear radiopaque if the rotator cuff is intact. A *complete tear* of the cuff will allow the contrast medium to travel up through the tear and fill the subacromial-subdeltoid bursa, causing the bursa to be radiopaque (Fig. 10–41). *Incomplete tears* may be identified by a collection of contrast medium at the tear site.

Recently, MRI has become more frequently used in the evaluation of rotator cuff tears (Fig. 10–42). The advantage of MRI over arthrography is that MRI is noninvasive and can provide the surgeon with specific information regarding the tendons involved; the location, size, and quality of the torn edges; and the amount of muscle atrophy and tendon retraction present.

Although plain film radiographs are surpassed by the aforementioned imaging studies in the evaluation of this soft tissue condition, there are numerous plain film findings associated with chronic tears of the rotator cuff that can be observed on the AP radiograph of the shoulder. These include (Figs. 10–43, 10–44):

1. **Irregularity of the greater tuberosity:** The tuberosity may appear flattened, atrophied, or sclerotic because of rupture of the supraspinatus tendon and lack of traction stress at the insertion site.
2. **Narrowing of the distance between the acromion and the humeral head:** This space is normally composed of the bursa and cuff muscles. Atrophy of the cuff muscles will decrease the thickness of the cuff, decreasing the space. Additionally, weak ro-

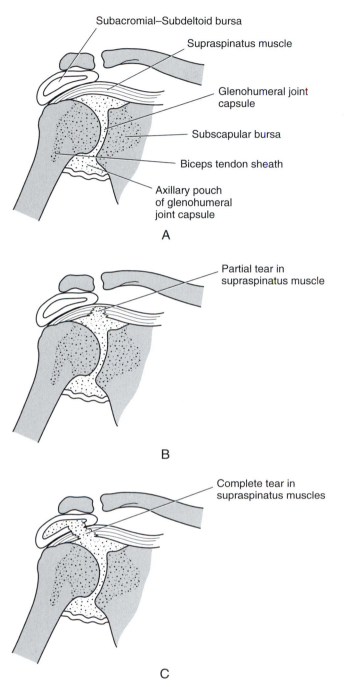

A

Subacromial–Subdeltoid bursa
Supraspinatus muscle
Glenohumeral joint capsule
Subscapular bursa
Biceps tendon sheath
Axillary pouch of glenohumeral joint capsule

B

Partial tear in supraspinatus muscle

C

Complete tear in supraspinatus muscles

FIGURE 10–40. Schematic diagrams of contrast arthrography in (A) a normal glenohumeral joint, where contrast medium is confined to the joint capsule and communicating structures (biceps tendon and subscapular bursa); (B) in a partial rotator cuff tear, where contrast medium leaks into the tear site; and (C) in a complete rotator cuff tear, where contrast medium travels up through the tear and fills the subacromial-subdeltoid bursa.

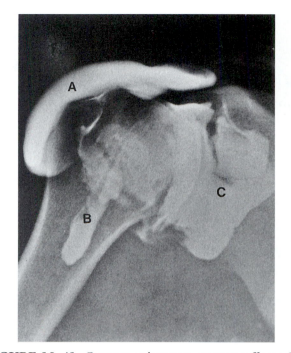

FIGURE 10–41. Contrast arthrogram, rotator cuff tear. Radiopaque contrast medium that was injected into the glenohumeral joint capsule has flowed upward through the tear in the rotator cuff and has filled the subacromial-subdeltoid bursae (A). This opacification of the bursa indicates abnormal communication between the bursa and the joint cavity, affirming the diagnosis of a tear in the rotator cuff. The other regions that demonstrate contrasts are (B) the sheath of the biceps tendon and (C) the subscapularis recess, both of which are normal extensions of the joint capsule and show filling of contrast under normal conditions. (From Greenspan,[6] p 5.20, Fig. 5–33 with permission.)

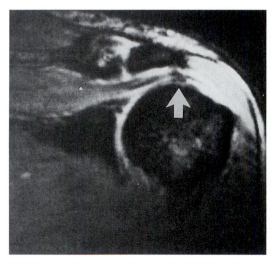

FIGURE 10–42. Rotator cuff tear, MRI. This oblique coronal MRI of the left shoulder demonstrates interruption of a supraspinatus tendon and fluid in the subacromial-subdeltoid bursae complex; diagnostic of complete rotator cuff tear. (From Greenspan[6] p 5.21, Fig. 5–35, with permission.)

tator cuff muscles will not oppose the pull of the deltoid muscle, and the humeral head will be pulled proximally, further decreasing the space.

3. **Erosion of the inferior aspect of the acromion:** The upward migration of the humeral head may cause changes at the acromion, including sclerosis, subchondral cyst formation, and loss of bone.

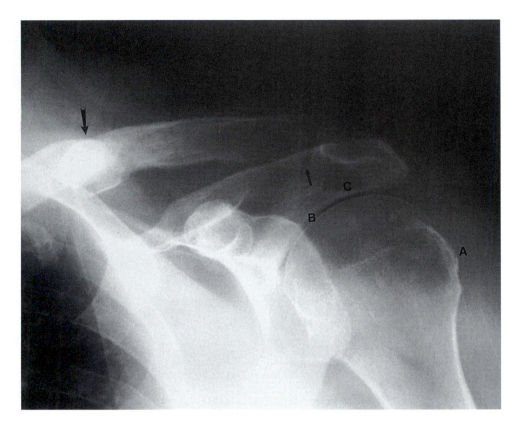

FIGURE 10–43. Rotator cuff tear, plain film findings. This 64-year-old male presents with complaints of progressive weakness in the muscles of his left shoulder. There was a history of trauma 2 years prior when he fractured his clavicle in a fall off his bicycle. This AP view of his shoulder demonstrates the classic plain film findings associated with chronic tears of the rotator cuff: (a) irregularity of the greater tuberosity, (b) narrowing of the distance between the acromion and the humeral head, (c) erosion or loss of bone in the inferior aspect of the acromion. The small arrow indicates early osteoarthritic changes present at the AC joint, and the large arrow indicates the site of the healed clavicle fracture.

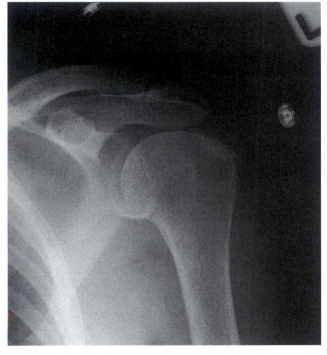

FIGURE 10–44. Rotator cuff tear, plain film findings. The shoulder of this 68-year-old man presents with a finding similar to that of the shoulder seen in Figure 10–44, including irregularity of the greater tuberosity, superior migration of the humerus with narrowing of the distance between the acromion and the humeral head, and erosion of the inferior aspect of the acromion. Additionally, a striking feature of this patient's shoulder is the flattening of the humeral head, a result of the abnormal positioning of the humerus against the acromion over time.

ABNORMAL CONDITIONS

Impingement Syndrome[39–41]

The *impingement syndrome* at the shoulder refers to the biomechanical trauma sustained to the rotator cuff tendons as they are entrapped between the humeral head inferiorly and the coracoacromial ligament and acromion superiorly during elevation of the arm. Chronic tendonitis, bursitis, and partial or complete tearing of the rotator cuff are lesions associated with this syndrome.

Neer described three progressive stages of impingement syndrome: stage I is characterized by edema and hemorrhage; stage II is characterized by fibrosis and thickening of the tendons and bursa with possibly a partial rotator cuff tear; and stage III is characterized by complete rupture of the rotator cuff.[42] Treatment in the earlier stages may be successful with conservative measures including rehabilitation and modalities to control inflammation. Surgical intervention designed to decompress the subacromial space and alleviate impingement of the soft tissues may be indicated when conservative treatment has failed. Resection of the coracoacromial ligament, anterior acromion, or distal clavicle and excision of acromioclavicular joint osteophytes are examples of such procedures.

Radiographic evidence of impingement syndrome

in the later stages includes subacromial proliferation of bone, osteophyte formation on the inferior surfaces of the acromion or acromioclavicular joint, and cysts or sclerosis of the greater tuberosity at the insertion of the rotator cuff tendons (Fig. 10–45). The earlier stages of impingement syndrome, particularly bursitis, edema, and tendonitis, are only accurately identified by the high soft tissue contrast resolution and multiplanar capabilities provided by MRI (Fig. 10–46).

Adhesive Capsulitis[43-45]

Adhesive capsulitis, commonly known as a *"frozen shoulder"* is defined as chronic inflammation and fibrosis of the glenohumeral joint capsule. The condition is characterized by pain and limited movement of the shoulder joint.

The etiology of adhesive capsulitis is unknown. Two categories are clinically apparent, however: *primary idiopathic* and *secondary*. Primary adhesive capsulitis ap-

pears spontaneously without identifiable stimulus. Secondary adhesive capsulitis is associated with a preexisting trauma to the shoulder or some other painful condition originating elsewhere in the body that results in prolonged voluntary or involuntary immobilization of the shoulder. Both categories exhibit similar clinical manifestations and histologic changes in the joint capsule. The condition tends to be self-limiting and may resolve spontaneously in several months.[44] The pain and functional disability usually require earlier active intervention, however, and analgesics and physical therapy represent the treatment approach of choice.

Plain film radiographs may only reveal localized osteoporosis at the shoulder owing to disuse atrophy. Contrast arthrography is the imaging study of choice in evaluation of suspected adhesive capsulitis (Fig. 10–47). Contrast medium injected into the glenohumeral joint capsule usually reveals the decreased volume capacity of the joint capsule. Loss of filling of the axillary and subscapular recesses of the capsule confirms a tight, thickened capsule.

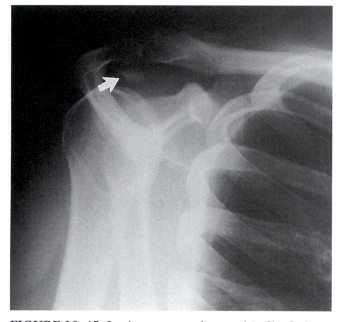

FIGURE 10–45. Impingement syndrome, plain film findings. This anterior oblique view of the shoulder (scapular Y position) is obtained by rotating the patient 30 degrees from a true lateral position. Structures best shown include an oblique lateral view of the proximal humerus superimposed over a lateral view of the scapula. The relationship of the humeral head to the glenoid cavity is well demonstrated. Additionally, the subacromial space is well visualized. Note that in the subacromial region of this shoulder of a 40-year-old man, a large calcification is seen in the tendon of the rotator cuff (arrow). This may represent a calcification of a partial rotator cuff tear, or fibrosis and calcification of frictioned tendons.

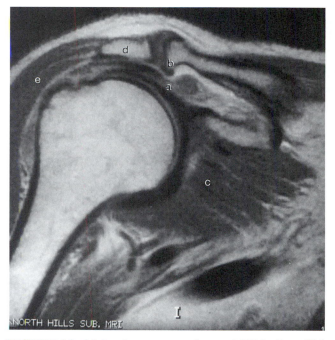

FIGURE 10–46. Impingement syndrome, MRI findings. This coronal MRI of the shoulder demonstrates a large osteophyte (b) on the inferior aspect of the distal clavicle impinging the supraspinatus muscle (a). Other structures noted are: (c) subscapularis muscle, (d) acromion, (e) deltoid muscle.

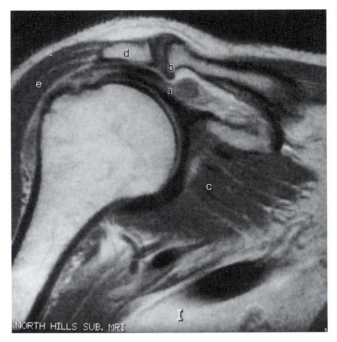

FIGURE 10–47. Adhesive capsulitis of the glenohumeral joint. This double-contrast arthrogram of the shoulder demonstrates the characteristic findings of a frozen shoulder. The capacity of the axillary pouch is markedly decreased and a subscapularis recess remains unopacified, while the lymphatic channels are filled with contrast medium secondary to increased intercapsular pressure. (From Greenspan,[6] p 6.21, Fig. 5.36 with permission.)

SUMMARY OF KEY POINTS

1. The routine radiographic evaluation of the shoulder includes two anteroposterior projections demonstrating the proximal humerus and portions of the clavicle and scapula. The purpose of two anterior views is to allow greater visualization of various aspects of the humeral head:
   - AP view with the arm externally rotated demonstrates the greater tuberosity of the proximal humerus in profile. The lesser tuberosity is superimposed over the humeral head.
   - AP view with the arm internally rotated demonstrates the lesser tuberosity in profile, and the greater tuberosity is superimposed behind the humeral head.
2. The routine radiographic evaluation of the acromioclavicular joints includes two bilateral AP projections. One projection is done without weights and the other with weights, providing traction through the patient's arms. The purpose of these views is to evaluate the stability of the acromioclavicular joints in cases of suspected ligamentous injury.
3. The routine radiographic evaluation of the scapula includes the AP and lateral projections. The AP demonstrates the lateral half of the scapula while the medial half is seen through blurred thoracic structures. The lateral projection evaluates the body of the scapula in profile.
4. Fractures of the proximal humerus are commonly classified by their location within the four major anatomic segments:
   - head (extending from the articular surface to the anatomic neck)
   - greater tuberosity
   - lesser tuberosity
   - shaft (at the level of the surgical neck)
5. The proximal humerus is a frequent site for pathologic fracture, usually presenting in the region of the surgical neck.
6. Fractures of the clavicle are designated by their location at the medial, middle, or distal thirds of the bone. The middle third is the most frequent site of fracture.
7. Fractures of the body of the scapula are rare, and when present are usually the result of a direct blow. Fractures of the rim of the glenoid fossa are associated with glenohumeral dislocation.
8. More than 95 percent of glenohumeral dislocations are anterior dislocations, whereby the humeral head comes to rest under the coracoid process or under the anterior aspect of the glenoid fossa. The Hill-Sachs lesion is a compression fracture of the posterolateral aspect of the humeral head sustained during dislocation. The Bankart lesion is a detachment of the labrum from the anterior inferior glenoid rim indicative of recurrent dislocations.
9. Acromioclavicular joint subluxations, commonly referred to as shoulder separation, refer to ligamentous sprain or rupture at the acromioclavicular joint and are graded as mild, moderate, or severe, in reference to the degree of instability.
10. The most common rotator cuff tear involves the supraspinatus portion of the cuff just proximal to its insertion on the greater tuberosity. Diagnosis is usually confirmed by arthrography or MRI. Plain film radiographic findings are evident in chronic cases.
11. The impingement syndrome at the shoulder refers to the biomechanical trauma sustained to the rotator cuff tendons as they are entrapped between the humeral head, the coracoclavicular ligament, and the acromion during shoulder elevation. Early diagnosis can be made by MRI. Degenerative bony changes associated with chronic later stages may be evident on plain films.
12. Adhesive capsulitis, also known as ''frozen shoulder,'' is a chronic inflammation and fibrosis of the glenohumeral joint capsule. Contrast arthrography is the imaging study of choice in the evaluation of this condition.

REFERENCES

1. Netter, FH: The Ciba Collection of Medical Illustrations, Vol 8, Part I, Musculoskeletal System. Ciba-Geigy Corp., Summit, NJ, 1978, pp 30–37.
2. Bontrager, KL: A Textbook of Radiographic Positioning and Related Anatomy, ed 3. CV Mosby, St Louis, 1993, p 147.
3. Nordin, M and Frankel, VH: Basic Biomechanics of the Musculoskeletal System, ed 2. Lea & Febiger, Malvern, PA, 1980, pp 225–248.
4. Meschan, I: An Atlas of Normal Radiograph Anatomy. WB Saunders, Philadelphia, 1960, p 64.
5. Weissman, B and Sledge, C: Orthopedic Radiology. WB Saunders, Philadelphia, 1986, pp 215–221.
6. Greenspan, A: Orthopedic Radiology: A Practical Approach, ed 2. Raven Press, New York, 1992, pp 5.1–5.22.
7. Bontrager, pp 145–167.
8. Fischer, HW: Radiographic Anatomy: A Working Atlas. McGraw-Hill, New York, 1988, pp 2–9.
9. Wicke, L: An Atlas of Radiographic Anatomy, ed 5. Lea & Febiger, Malvern, PA, 1994, p 76.
10. Greenspan, p 5.22.
11. Ibid, pp 5.1–5.22.
12. Schultz, RJ: The Language of Fractures, ed 2. Williams & Wilkins, Baltimore, 1990, pp 165–186.
13. Brashear, HR and Raney, RB: Shand's Handbook of Orthopaedic Surgery, ed 9. CV Mosby, St Louis, 1978, pp 436–447.
14. Rockwood, CA and Green, DP: Fractures in Adults, Vol 1, ed 2. JB Lippincott, Philadelphia, 1984, pp 653–674.
15. Greenspan, p 5.13.
16. Ibid, p 5.15.
17. Rockwood, p 678.
18. Schultz, p 175.
19. Ibid, p 171.
20. Rockwood, p 677.
21. Schultz, p 175.
22. Richardson, JK and Iglarsh, ZA: Clinical Orthopaedic Physical Therapy. WB Saunders, Philadelphia, 1994, pp 195, 203.
23. Richardson, p 199.
24. Richardson, p 197.
25. Rockwood, pp 722–860.
26. Schultz, p 175.
27. Weissman, p 250.
28. Richardson, p 198.
29. Greenspan, p 5.17.
30. Weissman, p 255.
31. Richardson, p 199.
32. Greenspan, p 5.17.
33. Rockwood, pp 860–910.
34. Greenspan, p 5.21.
35. Richardson, p 201.
36. Weissman, pp 270–274.
37. Ibid, pp 231–234.
38. Greenspan, pp 5.19–5.21.
39. Richardson, pp 194–195.
40. Greenspan, p 5.18.
41. Weissman, p 235.
42. Neer, CS II: Impingement lesions. Clin Orthopedics 173:70, 1983.
43. Greenspan, p 5.21.
44. Richardson, p 194.
45. Weissman, 237.

SELF-TEST

Chapter 10

REGARDING FILM A:

1. Identify the projection.
2. Identify three findings that infer an advanced pathological state exists. Hint—look at gross bony architecture, soft tissue shadows, and density changes.

REGARDING FILM B:

3. Identify the projection.
4. What joint is being stabilized by the internal fixation device.

REGARDING FILM C:

5. Identify the projection.
6. The great amount of internal fixation devices required to regain anatomic position leads you to believe that what type of fracture pattern existed?
7. What would you guess was the mechanism of this injury?

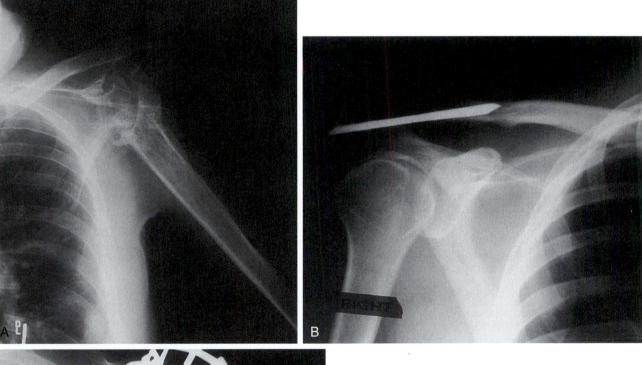

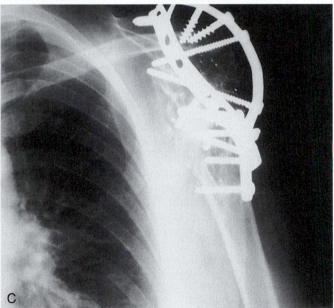

The Elbow

The elbow is the anatomic junction between the arm and forearm. Whereas the shoulder functions to place the upper extremity anywhere within the wide sphere of its range of motion, the elbow functions to adjust the extremity's height and length and functional position of the hand to accomplish prehensile tasks efficiently. The elbow's three separate synovial articulations housed within one joint capsule present unique challenges to clinicians involved in treating trauma and dysfunction at this joint.

The radiographic evaluation of the elbow is usually complete with the basic anteroposterior (AP), lateral, and oblique projections. Most fractures and dislocations are adequately demonstrated on basic projections. The irregularly shaped surfaces of the elbow sometimes require the additional imaging capabilities of conventional or computed tomography (CT). Ancillary imaging techniques commonly used in evaluation of the soft tissues and cartilage of the elbow include magnetic resonance imaging (MRI), arthrography, and arthrotomography.

The goals of this chapter are first to present an overview of osseous radiographic anatomy. Next, a brief review of ligamentous anatomy and joint mobility is presented to assist the reader in understanding the mechanisms of common joint injuries in this region. The routine radiographic evaluation of the elbow follows. Here the reader has an opportunity to learn radiographic anatomy by tracing a radiograph with a marker on a transparency sheet and then comparing results with the radiographic tracing. The chapter concludes with brief discussion and illustrations and films of common trauma at the elbow. The summary is or-

ganized into a list of practical points highlighting the clinical aspects of the chapter. A self-test challenges the reader's visual interpretation skills.

RADIOGRAPHIC ANATOMY

Osseous Anatomy[1]

The bones of the elbow are the distal *humerus*, the proximal *ulna*, and the proximal *radius* (Fig. 11–1). The articulation between the humerus and ulna is the *humeroulnar joint*. The articulation between the humerus and radius is the *humeroradial joint*. The articulation between the proximal portions of the ulna and radius is the *proximal radioulnar joint*. These three separate articulations are within a common joint capsule and together make up the *elbow joint*.

The humeral *shaft* expands at its distal end into *medial and lateral humeral condyles*. The articular portions of these condyles are the *trochlea* and *capitulum*. The spool-shaped trochlea is divided by a semicircular groove or *trochlear sulcus*. The trochlea is on the medial aspect of the distal humerus and articulates with the ulna. The rounded capitulum is on the lateral aspect and articulates with the radius. The *medial* and *lateral epicondyles* are projections located proximally to the trochlea and capitulum, respectively. The distal humerus is marked by three depressions or *fossae*. Anteriorly, the *coronoid fossa* and *radial fossa* receive the ulnar coronoid process and radial head at full elbow flexion. Posteriorly, the *olecranon fossa* receives the ulnar olecranon process at elbow extension.

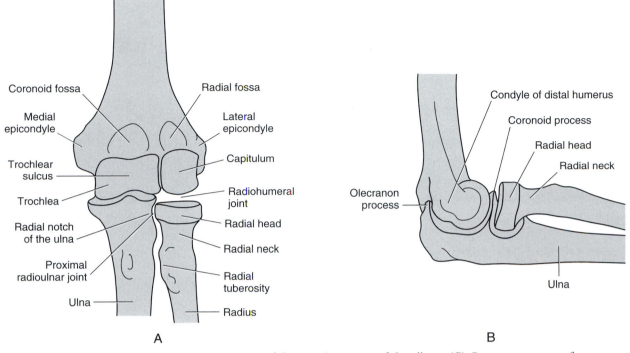

FIGURE 11–1. (*A*) Osseous anatomy of the anterior aspect of the elbow. (*B*) Osseous anatomy of the lateral aspect of the elbow.

The proximal ulna has two beaklike processes, the large *olecranon process* at its tip and the *coronoid process* on its anterior surface. Between these two processes lies the articular concave *trochlear notch*, which receives the trochlea. The shallow *radial notch* on the lateral side of the ulna articulates with the radial head.

The proximal radius is distinguished by a *head, neck,* and *tuberosity*. The radial head is disclike and cupped on its upper end, articulating with the capitulum above and the ulna medially. The neck is the constricted area below the head, and the tuberosity is an oval prominence distal to the neck.

The radial and ulnar bones together are referred to as the bones of the *forearm*. These bones are articulated proximally, as noted earlier, and through their shafts via the strong *interosseous membrane*, and distally, at the *distal radioulnar joint*, a pivot joint formed between the head of the ulna and ulnar notch of the radius. The forearm articulates to the wrist at the *radiocarpal joint*, formed by the distal radius, the *articular disc* of the distal radioulnar joint, and the proximal row of carpal bones.

Ligamentous Anatomy

Approximately half of elbow stability is provided by the bony configuration of the joint, and the remainder of stability results primarily from the joint capsule and its medial and lateral ligamentous reinforcements (Fig. 11–2).[2] The *ulnar (medial) collateral ligament* attaches to the medial humeral epicondyle and extends in a broad triangular expanse to the olecranon. The *radial (lateral) collateral ligament* attaches to the lateral humeral epicondyle and extends to the annular ligament and radial notch of the ulna.

The *annular ligament* of the radius is an oval band enclosing the head of the radius and attaching to the anterior and posterior margins of the radial notch of the ulna. The radial head is able to rotate within this ligamentous sling that provides its articular stability to the ulna.

The main muscles acting on the elbow joint are the triceps, biceps, and brachialis. They also are potentially important factors in joint stability.

JOINT MOBILITY[3]

The humeroulnar and humeroradial joints of the elbow function as hinge joints, permitting extension and flexion through a range from 0 to 135 degrees or greater. The proximal radioulnar joint is a trochoid joint, allowing approximately 90 degrees each of forearm pronation and supination.

GROWTH AND DEVELOPMENT[4]

Ossification of the elbow begins in the shafts of the humerus, ulna, and radius in the eighth week of fetal life. At birth only these structures are ossified and vis-

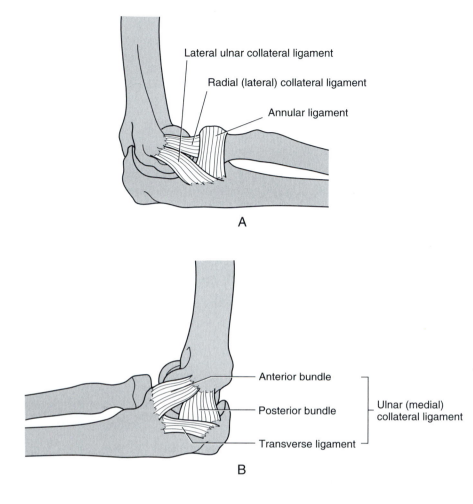

FIGURE 11–2. Ligaments of the elbow joint, from (A) the lateral aspect and (B) the medial aspect.

ible on radiograph (Fig. 11–3). The remaining architecture of the elbow is formed by seven secondary ossification centers. Four secondary ossification centers belong to the humerus: the center for the capitulum and the lateral portion of the trochlea appear in infancy, the center for the medial epicondyle appears after age 5, the center for the medial trochlea appears around age 10, and the center for the lateral epicondyle appears around age 14 (Fig. 11–4). The capitulum and trochlea coalesce to form one epiphysis at puberty. Three secondary ossification centers belong to the forearm: the center for the radial head appears about age 5, the center for the proximal ulna appears around age 11, and occasionally a separate center for the radial

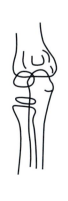

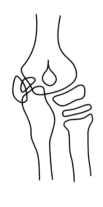

FIGURE 11–3. Radiographic tracings of the ossified portions of the elbow (A) at birth, (B) at age 5 years, and (C) at age 11 years.

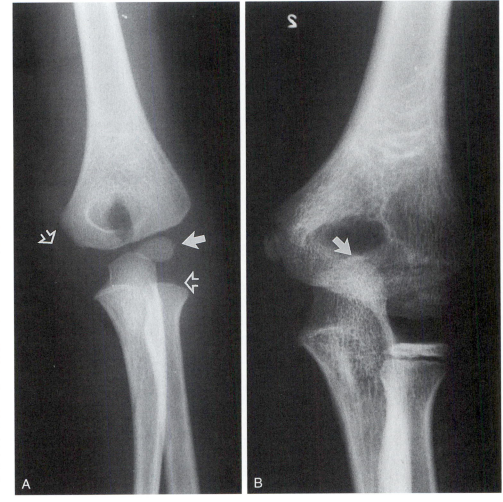

FIGURE 11–4. (*A*) Normal radiographic appearance of the elbow in a 5-year-old male. At this stage of maturity, the secondary ossification center for the capitulum is easily visible (solid arrow). The secondary ossification centers for the medial epicondyle of the humerus and the radial head are just beginning to ossify and are difficult to identify (open arrows). (*B*) Normal radiographic appearance of the elbow in a healthy 11-year-old male. At this stage of development, the capitulum and the trochlea have coalesced to form one epiphysis. The epiphysis of the radial head and medial epicondyle are also visible. The secondary ossification center for the proximal ulna (arrow) has just begun to ossify and is visible superimposed in the olecranon fossa.

tuberosity appears around puberty. All of these secondary centers complete fusion in the mid- to late-teenage years, with women showing earlier bone maturity than men.

ROUTINE RADIOGRAPHIC EVALUATION[5–9]

Routine radiographic evaluation of the elbow usually consists of AP, lateral, and oblique views. As with any complex joint, numerous special projections exist to demonstrate different perspectives sought on specific structures. For most screening purposes and typical complaints, however, these standard views suffice.

The radiographic evaluation of trauma at the elbow necessitates the additional evaluation of the forearm. Fracture or dislocation at the proximal radius and ulna is sometimes accompanied by associated trauma at the distal aspects or distal articulations of these bones. Thus in evaluating trauma cases, the radiographic evaluation of the elbow is not complete without evaluation of the entire forearm. For this reason, projections of the forearm are included here.

Elbow

Basic: AP
            Lateral
            Oblique, Internal or External

ANTEROPOSTERIOR (FIGS. 11–5, 11–6, 11–7)

This view demonstrates the *distal humerus* and *proximal radius* and *ulna*, seen in the anatomic position. The visible structures of the distal humerus include the lower third of the *shaft*, the *medial* and *lateral epicondyles*, the *olecranon fossa*, the *capitulum*, and the *trochlea*. The *humeroradial joint* space is visible, as is the *humeroulnar joint space*, superimposed by the *olecranon process*. The important observations are:

1. The patient's arm is in anatomic position, fully extended and externally rotated. The *carrying angle* of the elbow is revealed on this view. Normally the long axis of the forearm forms a valgus angle with the long axis of the humerus. Values for this angle are usually stated as being larger in females, although some researchers have noted no sex differ-

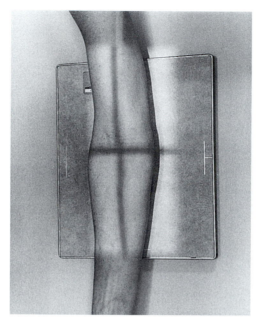

FIGURE 11–5. Patient position for AP view of the right elbow.

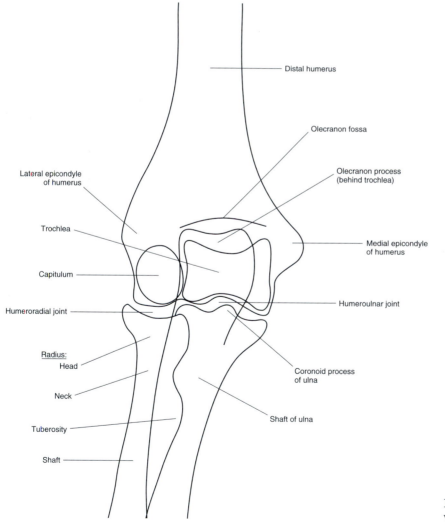

Distal humerus

Olecranon fossa

Olecranon process
(behind trochlea)

Lateral epicondyle
of humerus

Trochlea

Medial epicondyle
of humerus

Capitulum

Humeroradial joint

Humeroulnar joint

Radius:
  Head

Coronoid process
of ulna

Neck

Shaft of ulna

Tuberosity

Shaft

FIGURE 11–6. Radiographic tracing of AP
view of right elbow.

ence.[10] Average normal values range from approximately 5 to 15 degrees.[11] Abnormal increases or decreases in this angle may be a sign of fracture or posttraumatic deformity.

2. The olecranon process is articulated in the olecranon fossa in this position of elbow extension. The olecranon process can be visualized superimposed behind the trochlea of the humerus.

3. A portion of the radial head, neck, and tuberosity is superimposed by the ulna.

4. The humeroradial and humeroulnar joint spaces are well demonstrated.

CLINICAL OBJECTIVES

1. Trace the distal humerus. Identify the medial and lateral epicondyles, the capitulum, and the trochlea.
2. Trace the ulna. Identify the olecranon process and shaft.

3. Trace the radius. Identify the radial head, neck, and tuberosity.
4. Identify the humeroulnar and humeroradial joint spaces.
5. Measure the carrying angle of the elbow by noting the angle of intersection between a line connecting midpoints in the distal humeral shaft and a line connecting midpoints in the proximal ulnar shaft.[12]

LATERAL (FIGS. 11–8, 11–9, 11–10)

The lateral view, taken with the elbow flexed to 90 degrees, demonstrates the *distal humerus* and *proximal radius* and *ulna*. Visible structures include the *olecranon process*, the anterior portion of the *radial head*, and the *humeroradial joint*. The important observations are:

1. The olecranon process is seen in profile articulating in the olecranon fossa.
2. The coronoid process of the olecranon is superimposed by the posterior portion of the radial head.
3. Only the anterior portion of the radial head is viewed free of superimposition.
4. This true lateral projection superimposes structures of the distal humerus, causing distinct images to appear. The directly superimposed medial and lateral epicondyles form a large teardrop-shaped image. Below this image is a radiodense circle image, partially surrounded by concentric arcs. The circle image is produced by the trochlear sulcus. The inner concentric arcs are formed by the rims of the capitulum and trochlea. The outermost arc is formed by the trochlear notch.

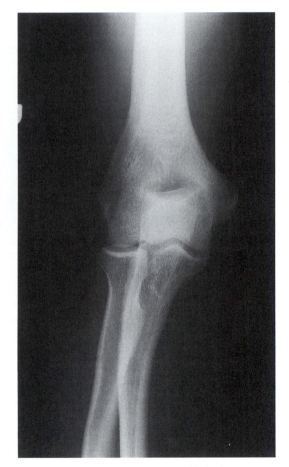

FIGURE 11–7. AP view of left elbow.

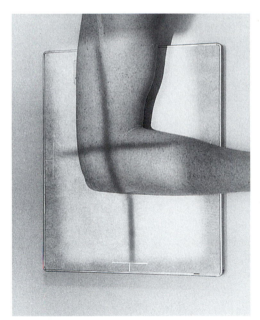

FIGURE 11–8. Patient position for lateral view of right elbow.

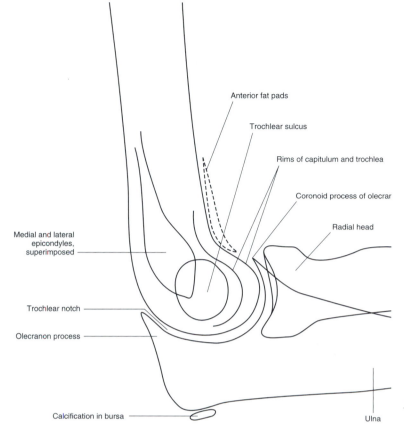

Anterior fat pads

Trochlear sulcus

Rims of capitulum and trochlea

Coronoid process of olecrar

Radial head

Medial and lateral
epicondyles,
superimposed

Trochlear notch

Olecranon process

Calcification in bursa

Ulna

FIGURE 11–9. Radiographic tracing of lateral view of right elbow.

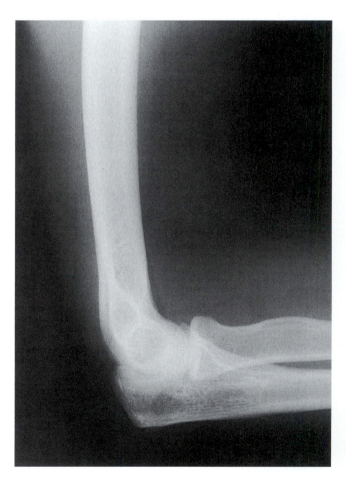

FIGURE 11–10. Lateral view of the elbow.

5. The *fat pads* of the coronoid and radial fossae are normally visualized superimposed together as a thin triangular lucency just anterior to the distal humerus. In the presence of joint effusion, the fat pads will displace further anteriorly.

CLINICAL OBJECTIVES

1. Trace the olecranon. Identify the olecranon process and the coronoid process.
2. Trace the radius. Identify the radial head, neck, and tuberosity.
3. Trace the distal humerus. Identify the epicondyles. Identify the concentric arc images of the (a) trochlear sulcus, (b) capitulum and trochlear rims, and (c) trochlear notch.
4. Trace the radiolucent image representing the *anterior fat pads*.

OBLIQUE

The oblique view of the elbow may be done as an *internal or external* projection. The choice of views is determined by the departmental routines, or by a specific area of interest. The elbow is in full extension for either projection.

Internal Oblique (Figs. 11–11, 11–12, 11–13)

The internal oblique view is done with the patient's extended arm and forearm internally rotated 90 de-

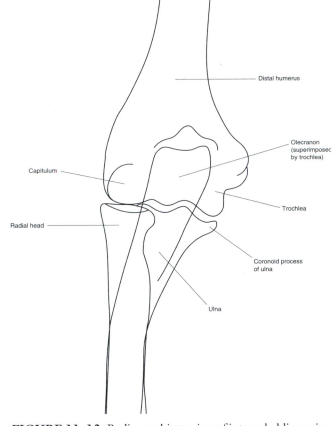

FIGURE 11–12. Radiographic tracing of internal oblique view of the right elbow.

grees from the anatomic position, or *pronated*. This position crosses the proximal radius over the ulna, superimposing most of these structures. The *coronoid process*, however, is visible without superimposition, and is best demonstrated on this view. The important observations are:

1. The coronoid process is visualized free of superimposition.
2. The olecranon process is articulated in the olecranon fossa.
3. The joint space between the trochlear notch and trochlea is visible.

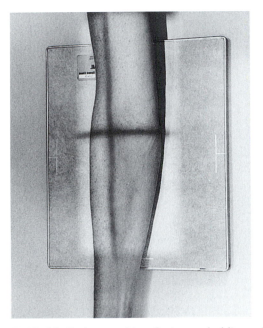

FIGURE 11–11. Patient position for internal oblique view of the right elbow.

CLINICAL OBJECTIVES

1. Trace the olecranon. Identify the olecranon process and the coronoid process.
2. Trace the radial head and neck superimposed by the ulna.
3. Trace the distal humerus. Identify the olecranon fossa.

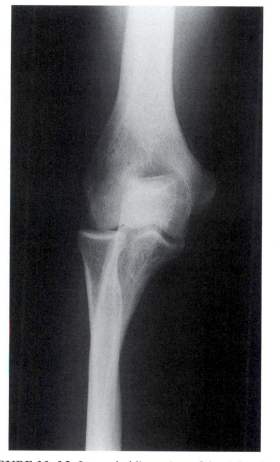

FIGURE 11–13. Internal oblique view of the right elbow.

External Oblique (Figs. 11–14, 11–15, 11–16)

The external oblique view is done with the patient's extended arm and forearm externally rotated 45 degrees from the anatomic position. This position best demonstrates the *radial head, neck, and tuberosity* viewed free of any superimposition. The important observations are:

1. The radial head, neck, and tuberosity are visualized free of superimposition.
2. The capitulum and lateral epicondyle are viewed in profile.
3. The humeroulnar and humeroradial joint spaces are visible.

CLINICAL OBJECTIVES

1. Trace the radius. Identify the head, neck, and tuberosity.
2. Trace the ulna.
3. Trace the humerus. Identify the capitulum and lateral epicondyle.

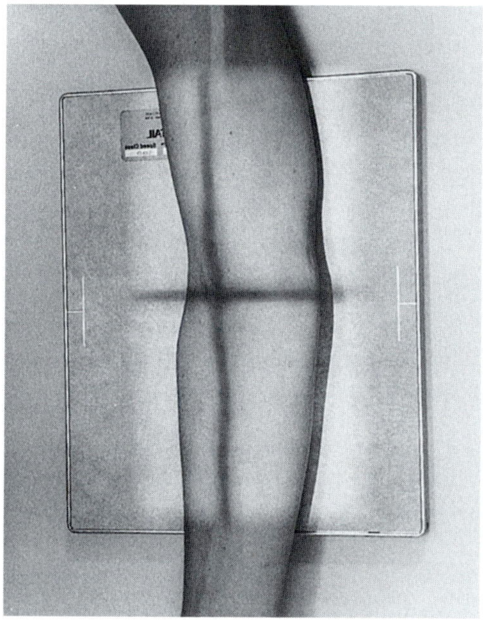

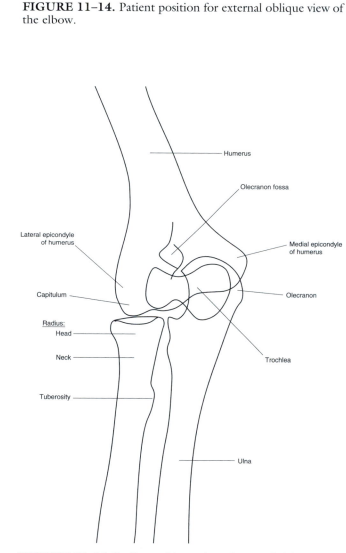

FIGURE 11–14. Patient position for external oblique view of the elbow.

FIGURE 11–15. Radiographic tracing of external oblique view of the right elbow.

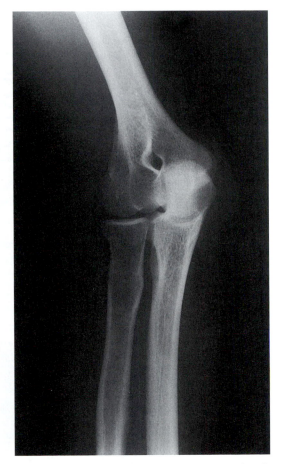

FIGURE 11-16. External oblique view of the right elbow.

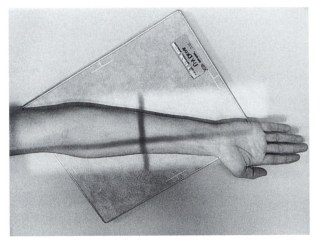

FIGURE 11-17. Patient position for AP view of the right forearm.

2. The entire length of the radius and ulna is visible. Note the normal bowing and contour of the shafts.
3. The olecranon is articulated in the olecranon fossa and is superimposed behind the trochlea.
4. Both the proximal and distal articulations of the forearm are visible. Elbow and wrist joint spaces will appear only partially open because of x-ray beam divergence over the length of the film. (Note that some facilities may include only the wrist articulation if the elbow has already been demonstrated on AP elbow projection.)

Forearm

Basic: AP
            Lateral

ANTEROPOSTERIOR (FIGS. 11-17, 11-18, 11-19)

This view demonstrates the elbow, the entire radius and ulna, and the wrist. The important observations follow:

1. The patient's elbow is extended, and the forearm is supinated in the anatomic position.

CLINICAL OBJECTIVES

1. Trace the entire radius.
2. Trace the entire ulna.
3. Identify the joints of the elbow: humeroulnar, humeroradial, and proximal radioulnar joints.
4. Identify the distal radioulnar joint.
5. Identify the radiocarpal joint.

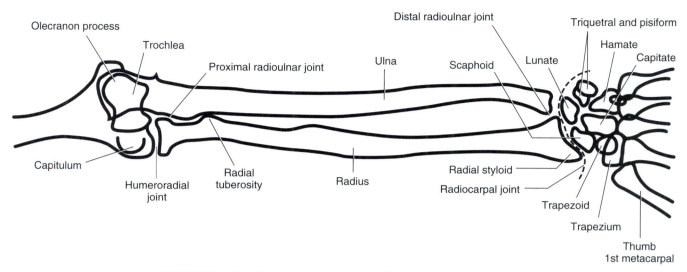

FIGURE 11–18. Radiographic tracing of AP view of the right forearm.

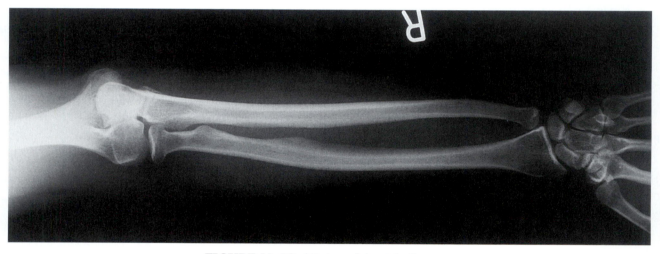

FIGURE 11–19. AP view of the right forearm.

LATERAL (FIGS. 11–20, 11–21, 11–22)

This view demonstrates the *elbow*, the entire length of the *radius* and *ulna*, and the *wrist*, seen in profile. The important observations are:

1. The patient's elbow is flexed 90 degrees, and the forearm is in neutral position.
2. Much of the radius and ulna are superimposed over each other. Note the normal bowing and contour of the shafts.
3. Elbow structures and the images they cast are similar to their appearances, as seen on the lateral view of the elbow (see Fig. 11–21).
4. The radial head superimposes the coronoid process.
5. Both the proximal and distal articulations of the

forearm are visible. Elbow and wrist joint spaces appear only partially open due to beam divergence.

CLINICAL OBJECTIVES

1. Trace the entire radius.
2. Trace the entire ulna.
3. Identify the humeroulnar and humeroradial joints.
4. Identify the radiocarpal joint.

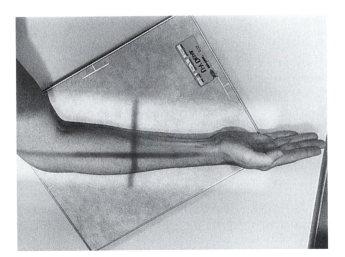

FIGURE 11–20. Patient position for lateral view of the right forearm.

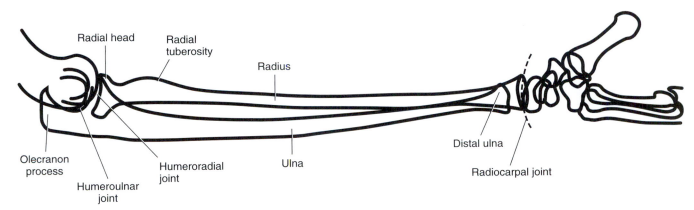

Radial head

Radial tuberosity

Radius

Olecranon process

Humeroulnar joint

Humeroradial joint

Ulna

Distal ulna

Radiocarpal joint

FIGURE 11–21. Radiographic tracing of lateral view of the right forearm.

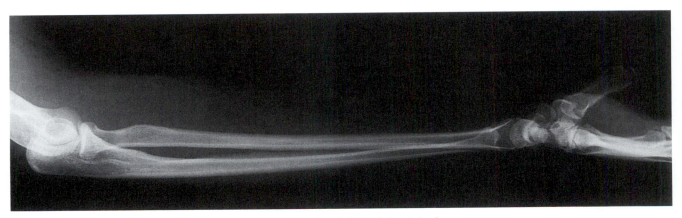

FIGURE 11–22. Lateral view of the right forearm.

TRAUMA[13-16]

Trauma to the elbow is common in all age groups. The protective reactions of the upper extremities as they reach out during falls often become the mechanisms of elbow or forearm injury as ground forces are transmitted up through the hand. Athletic endeavors also provide occasions for direct and indirect elbow trauma seen in adolescents and young adults. In general, trauma to the elbow joint is often poorly tolerated in adults. Residual pain, deformity, loss of motion, and posttraumatic arthritic joint changes are not uncommon following elbow fractures, dislocations, or subluxations. Children usually fare better than adults because of greater remodeling capacity. The surgical and postsurgical rehabilitation needs are often challenging to the orthopedist and the therapist who both strive to restore the functional abilities of the joint.

Radiographic evaluation of elbow trauma begins with the routine elbow and forearm projections. Most fractures, dislocations, and subluxations are adequately demonstrated on these views. Ancillary techniques that may be used in the diagnostic evaluation of complex, subtle, or osteochondral fractures include conventional tomography, CT, and arthrography. Soft tissue injuries or abnormalities of the tendons, ligaments, capsule, cartilage, or synovium may be evaluated by the use of contrast arthrography or MRI.

Plain film radiographs can reveal abnormal soft tissue signs that indicate underlying trauma.[17-19] The *positive fat pad sign* and the *abnormal supinator line* are indicators of joint effusion usually associated with fracture (see Fig. 2–18).

Fat pads are located anteriorly and posteriorly at the fossae of the distal humerus, overlying the joint capsule. The anterior fat pads of the coronoid and radial fossae are normally visualized on the lateral radiograph superimposed together as a thin, triangular lucency just anterior to the distal humerus. The posterior fat pad lies deep in the olecranon fossa and is normally not visible on the lateral radiograph. Distention of the joint capsule, owing to effusion, will cause the posterior fat pad to elevate out of the olecranon fossa and image as a semilunar lucency posterior to the fossa. Likewise, the anterior fat pads will displace farther anteriorly because of capsular pressure. This *positive fat pad sign* indicates to the radiologist that joint effusion has occurred and serves as a clue to the presence of fracture somewhere within the joint capsule. Note that a variety of conditions other than trauma may also cause elevation of the fat pads, including hemophilia, inflammatory arthritis, infection, intra-articular masses, and osteochondritis dissecans.

The fat plane overlying the supinator muscle, sometimes referred to as the *supinator line*, is seen as a thin, lucent line parallel to the anterior aspect of the proximal third of the radius.[20] It may normally be visible on the lateral radiograph approximately 1 cm from the anterior margin of the radius. In virtually all cases of acute radial head fracture, this line may become elevated, widened, or blurred. Conditions other than trauma causing this abnormal soft tissue sign include infection and inflammatory diseases.

Fractures of the Distal Humerus

Based on the anatomic site involved, fractures of the distal humerus are generally classified as (1) *supracondylar*, occurring above the condyles; (2) *transcondylar*, occurring across the condyles at the level of the olecranon fossa; (3) *intercondylar*, splitting the condyles apart in a Y or T shape or comminuted configuration; (4) *condylar*, involving either the medial or lateral condyle; (5) *articular*, involving the trochlea or capitulum; and (6) *epicondylar*, occurring at the medial or lateral epicondyles (Fig. 11–23).[21]

Supracondylar fractures are uncommon in adults but are the most common elbow fracture in children (Figs. 11–24, 11–25). This fracture is also the second most common of all extremity fractures in the pediatric age group, following fractures of the forearm.[22] Supracondylar fractures are divided into *extension* and *flexion* types. The extension type injury is due to a fall on an outstretched arm, displacing the distal fragment posterior to the humeral shaft. The flexion type injury, due to a fall on a flexed elbow, displaces the distal fragment anterior to the humeral shaft. The extension type is present in over 95 percent of cases and is more likely to be associated with neurovascular damage in the antecubital region.[23]

Treatment depends on the amount of displacement and associated neurovascular damage present. Choices include closed reduction with splinting, traction, percutaneous pinning, or open reduction with internal fixation.[24] Complications include malunion with resultant *cubitus varus* or *gunstock* deformity, peripheral nerve injury, and Volkmann's ischemia, a form of compartment syndrome due to occlusion of the brachial artery (see Fig. 11–25).

Radiographic identification of supracondylar fractures on the AP projection usually reveals a transverse fracture line above the origin of the joint capsule. The lateral projection reveals angulation of the distal fragment and oftentimes the displacement of the fat pads due to joint effusion.[25]

Transcondylar fractures share similar characteristics with supracondylar fractures (Fig. 11–26). Mechanisms of injury, radiographic evaluation, and treatment principles are basically the same. Major differences are that transcondylar fractures occur more commonly in falls by the elderly age group who are compromised by osteoporosis and that because this fracture is intracapsular, excessive callus formation in the olecranon or coronoid fossae can result in loss of joint motion[26] (see Fig. 11–26).

Intercondylar fractures result from direct force that causes the wedgelike olecranon to be driven into the distal humeral articular surface, splitting the condyles.

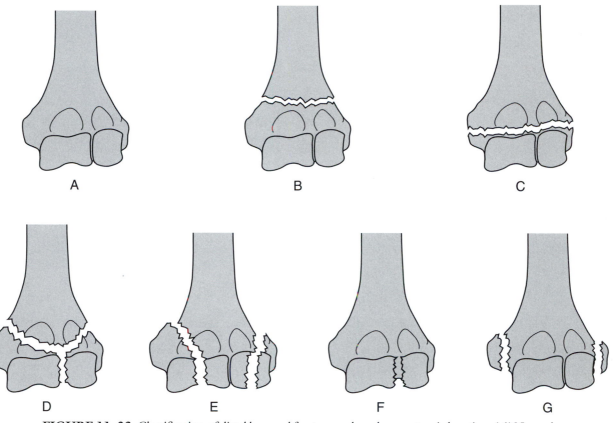

FIGURE 11–23. Classification of distal humeral fractures as based on anatomic location. (*A*) Normal; (*B*) supracondylar; (*C*) transcondylar; (*D*) intercondylar, T or Y shaped; (*E*) condylar; (*F*) articular; (*G*) epicondylar. (Adapted from Greenspan,[6] p 5.33.)

This fracture is seen in middle-aged adults but is relatively rare. Treatment is aimed at restoring functional joint surfaces, and the choice of reduction depends on the amount of displacement, ranging from conservative measures to resection arthroplasty or even prosthetic joint replacement. Weissman notes that after fracture healing, the final clinical result may not coincide with the final radiographic appearance. That is, "excellent function may coexist with distorted anatomy, and poor function may be present in spite of optimal radiographic appearances."[27]

Condylar fractures are uncommon in adults but are seen with some frequency in children. The oblique fracture line extends through both nonarticular and articular portions of the condyle. Fractures of the lateral condyle are most common, generally thought to occur as a result of a varus force avulsing the condyle.[28] Treatment again depends on the amount of displacement and disruption of the articular surfaces present. Many complications are associated with these fractures, including delayed union, malunion, nonunion, avascular necrosis, arrested growth, overgrowth, deformities, and myositis ossificans.

Articular fractures include fractures of the capitulum and trochlea. These fractures are rare in both children and adults. When present, the fracture line is usually in the coronal plane, parallel to the anterior surface of the humerus. These fractures are often sustained during falls whereby the radial head transmits a shearing force to the capitulum, or the olecranon transmits a compressive wedgelike force to the trochlea. As the fracture fragments are largely cartilaginous, radiographs may not always reveal their true size. Depending on the degree of displacement, treatment may be conservative or surgical, with the goal of preserving functional joint surfaces. A common complication is loss of motion and posttraumatic arthritic changes in the joint.[29]

Epicondylar fractures are uncommon in adults and, when present, are usually the result of a direct blow, with the prominent medial epicondyle more likely to be involved.[30] In children and adolescents, the medial epicondyle is more commonly injured from avulsion forces sustained through the physeal growth plate, or in association with elbow dislocations (see Fig. 3–17). Minimal displacement is treated by closed reduction; moderate or greater displacement often requires internal fixation. Complications include entrapment of possible fracture fragments within the joints, nonunion, and associated ulnar nerve injury.[31]

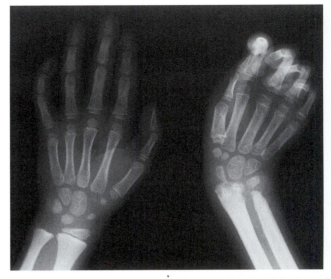

FIGURE 11–25. Volkmann's ischemia. This is a PA view of the hands of a 6-year-old boy. The left hand is normal. The child suffered a supracondylar fracture on the right at the age 2½. Healing was complicated by occlusion of the brachial artery and infection, which obliterated the biceps muscle, median nerve, and ulnar nerve. The hand is nonfunctional. Note the shortening of the forearm bones, deformity of the distal radius and ulna, diminished size of the carpals and metacarpal bones, contractures of the fingers, and diffuse muscle wasting.

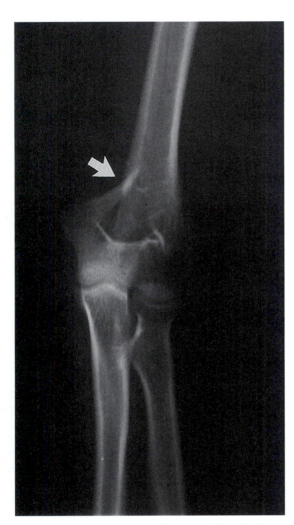

FIGURE 11–24. Supracondylar fracture of the distal humerus. The sharp angulation and area of increased radiodensity (arrow) represent an impaction fracture of the medial supracondylar region.

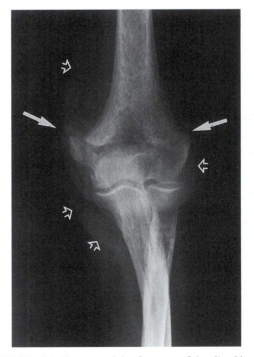

FIGURE 11–26. Transcondylar fracture of the distal humerus. This 82-year-old male was injured during a fall on his outstretched hand. The fracture is complete, extending transversely through both cortices at the transcondylar level (arrows). Note the excessive amount of joint effusion as seen confined by the extent of the joint capsule (open arrows).

Fractures of the Radial Head

Fractures of the radial head are common in adults, composing about one-third of all fractures about the elbow.[32] The mechanism of injury is usually a fall on an outstretched hand with the elbow partially flexed and supinated. Radial head fractures are divided into three types by the Mason classification system (Figs. 11–27, 11–28):

- *Type I:* Undisplaced fractures, typically treated with immobilization.
- *Type II:* Displaced fractures with separation, depression, or angulation of the fracture fragment, treated conservatively or by radial head excision if the articular surface is significantly displaced.
- *Type III:* Comminuted fractures, generally treated by radial head resection.[33,34]

Radial head fractures associated with elbow dislocations are designated as type IV fractures, and treatment of the fracture after reduction of the dislocation is based on the amount of displacement present.[35,36]

Radiographic evaluation of these fractures is adequately demonstrated on the AP and lateral views.[37]

Fractures of the Proximal Ulna

The trochlear notch, formed by the olecranon and coronoid processes, articulates with the humeral trochlea, providing both flexion-extension mobility and mediolateral stability at the elbow. Thus, fractures of the proximal ulna that disrupt the trochlear notch have the potential to disrupt function at the elbow (Fig. 11–29).[38]

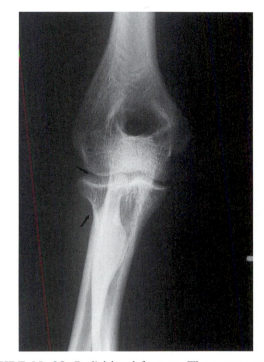

FIGURE 11–28. Radial head fracture. The arrows mark the ends of the fracture line, which extends longitudinally through the articular surface of the radial head. The fracture fragment shows minimal depression and displacement, probably classified as a type I fracture in the Mason classification system.

Fractures of the olecranon usually result from a fall on the point of a flexed elbow. Olecranon fractures are generally classified as undisplaced, displaced, or comminuted. The fracture line may be extra-articular, confined to the olecranon tip, or intra-articular, extending to the articular surface. Treatment is generally conservative for undisplaced fractures, and displaced fractures are most often treated by open reduction and internal fixation. Olecranon fractures are usually well demonstrated on the lateral radiograph of the elbow (Fig. 11–30).[39,40]

Fractures of the coronoid process rarely occur in isolation and are most often associated with posterior dislocations at the elbow. During a dislocation, the process is avulsed by the brachialis muscle as the elbow is hyperextended (see Fig. 3–18). Coronoid process fractures are usually occult or subtle fractures. An unrecognized coronoid process fracture that goes untreated may fail to unite, leading to chronic instability in the joint. Fractures of the coronoid process are not easily diagnosed on the AP or lateral radiographs, because of superimposition. The oblique view or other special views allow demonstration of the coronoid process free of superimposition. Complications of these fractures include the possibility of a fracture fragment loose within the joint, warranting surgical exploration.[41,42]

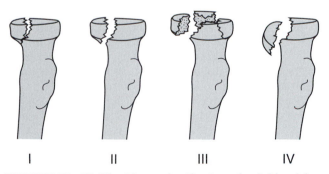

I   II   III   IV

FIGURE 11–27. The Mason classification of radial head fractures identifies three types of injury patterns: type I, undisplaced fractures; type II, marginal fractures with displacement; and type III, comminuted fractures. Type IV fractures were later suggested to encompass radial head fractures associated with dislocation. (Adapted from Greenspan,[6] p 5.37.)

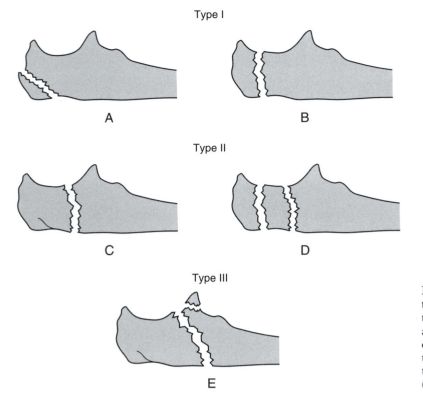

Type I

A   B

Type II

C   D

Type III

E

FIGURE 11–29. Classification of olecranon fractures. Type I are fractures of the proximal third of the olecranon, subdivided into (*A*) extra-articular and (*B*) intra-articular groups. Type II are fractures of the middle third, subdivided into (*C*) one or (*D*) two fracture lines. (*E*) Type III are fractures of the distal thrid. The most common is type II. (Adapted from Greenspan,[6] p 5.40.)

Fractures of the Radial and Ulnar Shafts

Fractures of the radial and ulnar shafts in adults are commonly caused by direct trauma, often associated with motor vehicle accidents, violent blows, or falls from heights. The force required to fracture both bones is generally more severe than the force required to fracture one of the single bones.[43,44] These *forearm fractures* are subdivided depending on which bones are involved. Radiographic evaluation of forearm fractures includes projections of the elbow and forearm, including the wrist. The additional projections are necessary as the anatomic relationships of the radius and ulna form a ringlike configuration, and fracture at one site may disrupt an adjacent articulation. Also, associated fractures may simultaneously occur at the wrist or distal humerus.[45]

Fractures of both the radial and ulnar shafts are usually displaced fractures, due to the severity of the force necessary to injure both bones. Open reduction and internal fixation are often required to correct angular and rotational deformities in order to regain normal supination and pronation mobility (Fig. 11–31).[46] Complications include delayed union, nonunion, and radioulnar synostosis.

Fractures of the radial shaft alone[47,48] are classified into two distinct groups, (1) those occurring in the proximal two-thirds of the bone and (2) those occurring in the distal one-third. *Fractures in the proximal two-thirds* are

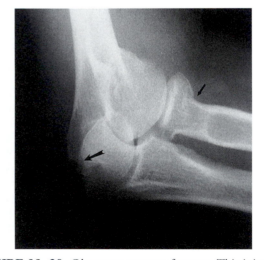

FIGURE 11–30. Olecranon process fracture. This injury was sustained during a fall on an outstretched hand while the elbow was in flexion. The large arrow indicates an avulsion fracture of the olecranon process caused by forceful contraction of the triceps. The small arrow indicates an impaction fracture of the radial head.

FIGURE 11–31. Fractures of the radial and ulnar shafts. This 14-year-old male was injured when he was thrown from a dirt bike. (*A*) This PA view of the wrist demonstrates complete, transverse, displaced fractures at the level of the metaphyses of both the radius and ulna. (*B*) This lateral view of the wrist demonstrates the great amount of displacement and overriding of the fracture fragments not appreciated on the PA view. Note the soft tissue outline paralleling the deformity. Despite the great amount of displacement, this fracture was successfully treated with closed reduction and cast immobilization. There was no residual deformity.

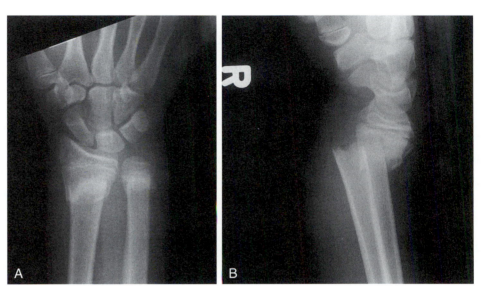

relatively uncommon, as the surrounding muscles provide protection to the area. Forces great enough to fracture the radius at this level will also usually fracture the ulna. Displaced fractures occurring in the proximal radial shaft generally require open reduction and internal fixation. Undisplaced fractures occurring *proximal* to the level of insertion of the pronator teres are treated by immobilization with the forearm in nearly full supination to prevent the unopposed pull of the supinator and biceps brachii from subsequently displacing the proximal fracture fragment. Fractures occurring *distal* to the insertion of the pronator teres do not require immobilization in this manner, as the pronator teres balances the pull of the supinators. *Fractures in the distal third* of the radial shaft are often associated with subluxation or dislocation of the distal radioulnar joint (Fig. 11–32). This fracture-dislocation pattern is known as *Galeazzi's fracture* (Fig. 11–33). The injury sustained at the distal radioulnar joint injury may be purely ligamentous tearing, or avulsion of the ligament at the ulnar styloid. Open reduction and internal fixation are usually necessary to regain supination and pronation mobility and avoid posttraumatic arthritic changes at the distal radioulnar joint.

In children, fractures of the radial shaft are the most common of all fractures in the body. The distal third of the radial shaft is involved in the majority of cases. The relative weakness of the metaphyseal region that has not yet remodeled is probably accountable for the susceptibility of this area to fracture. The typical mechanism of injury is a fall on an outstretched hand with the wrist in hyperextension. The common complications seen in the adult, including distal radioulnar dysfunction, loss of motion, and arthritic changes at the wrist, are rarely seen after children's distal radial fractures.[49]

Fractures of the ulnar shaft alone are fairly common.

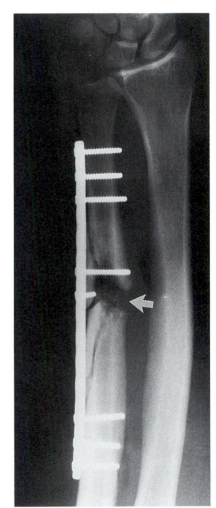

FIGURE 11–32. Fracture of the radial shaft. This 35-year-old male was injured when he was accidentally struck with a baseball bat. This severley comminuted midshaft fracture also demonstrates a segment of bone loss (arrow). This postoperative AP film of the forearm demonstrates a combination of side plate and screw fixation, which has successfully reduced the fragments and preserved the distal radioulnar joint.

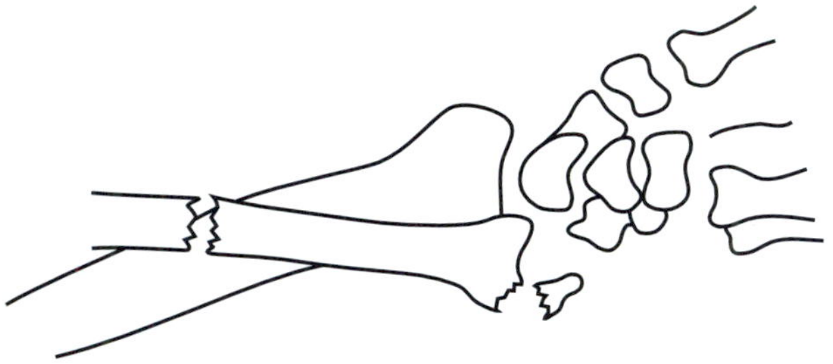

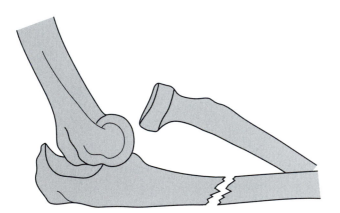

FIGURE 11–33. Galeazzi's fracture is a combination of fracture at the distal third of the radial shaft and subluxation or dislocation of the distal radioulnar joint.

The mechanism of injury is most often a direct blow, earning this fracture the name *nightstick fracture.* Undisplaced fractures are treated with immobilization, but displaced fractures generally require open reduction and internal fixation. A complication of fractures at the middle third and junction of the middle and distal thirds of the ulnar shaft is nonunion owing to poor blood supply at this region.[50]

A common fracture-dislocation injury involving the ulnar shaft is known by the eponym *Monteggia's fracture* (Fig. 11–34). This eponym refers to a fracture of the proximal third of the ulna combined with dislocation of the radial head. Adequate internal fixation of the fracture and proper postoperative positioning usually prevent the possible complications of radial head instability and nonunion. Damage to the radial nerve is not uncommon, but function nearly always returns with time.[51]

Dislocations of the Elbow

Dislocations of the elbow joint are described by the direction that the radius and ulna have displaced in relationship to the distal humerus (Fig. 11–35). Three main types of elbow dislocations are those involving (1) only the radius, (2) only the ulna, or (3) both the radius and ulna together. The most common type, accounting for 80 to 90 percent of all elbow dislocations, involves both the radius and the ulna, displaced in a posterior or posterolateral direction (see Fig. 3–18). The mechanism of injury is usually a fall on an outstretched hand or, less often, direct trauma or forces sustained in motor vehicle accidents. Conservative treatment via short-term sling immobilization is generally successful with minimal residual loss of motion and good preservation of functional stability.[52,53] Complications include calcification of the collateral ligaments and capsule; development of myositis ossificans, typically seen in an extensively damaged brachialis muscle; and ulnar or median nerve injury.[54] Radiographically, dislocations are easily diagnosed on the standard AP and lateral projections. The presence of dislocation signals the possibility of associated fractures of the radius or ulna; therefore, radiographs of the forearm are usually obtained to complete the evaluation of elbow joint dislocation.

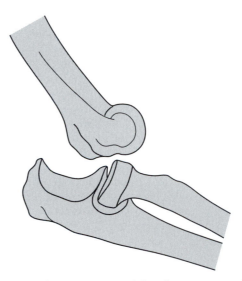

FIGURE 11–34. Monteggia's fracture is a combination of fracture of the proximal third of the ulna with dislocation of the radial head.

FIGURE 11–35. Dislocations of the elbow are named in reference to the position the radius and ulna have displaced in relationship to the distal humerus. Posterior, or posterolateral, dislocations are the most common.

SUMMARY OF KEY POINTS

1. The routine radiographic evaluation of the elbow includes three projections demonstrating the distal humerus, proximal ulna, proximal radius, and their associated articulations:
   - **Anteroposterior:** The elbow is demonstrated in anatomic position
   - **Lateral:** The elbow is flexed 90 degrees and the forearm is in neutral
   - **Oblique:** The elbow is extended and the forearm is either fully pronated or supinated
2. The radiographic evaluation in trauma cases includes the routine projections plus additional AP and lateral views of the forearm and the wrist. Trauma at the elbow is often associated with fracture or dislocation at these structures.
3. Two abnormal soft tissue signs indicative of joint trauma are visible on radiographs:
   - **The fat pad sign:** fat pads become displaced out of their fossae in response to increased capsular volume from effusion.
   - **Abnormal supinator line:** an elevation or blurring of the outline of the supinator muscle is seen in association with radial head fractures.
4. Fractures of the distal humerus are classified by location as supracondylar, transcondylar, intercondylar, articular, or epicondylar. The supracondylar fracture is the most common elbow fracture in children.
5. Fractures of the radial head compose about one-third of all elbow fractures in adults.
6. Fractures of the proximal ulna that disrupt the trochlear notch have the potential to seriously impair the stability and function of the elbow joint.
7. Fractures of the radial and ulnar shafts in adults require great force and are usually displaced fractures. Associated dislocations at the proximal and distal articulations are common.
8. In children, fractures of the distal radial shaft are the most common of all fractures in the body. The distal third of the shaft is involved in the majority of cases.
9. Elbow dislocations are described by the direction that the radius and ulna have displaced in relationship to the distal humerus. The majority of elbow dislocations involve both the radius and ulna displaced in a posterior or posterolateral direction.

REFERENCES

1. Netter, FH: The Ciba Collection of Medical Illustrations, Vol 8, Part I, Musculoskeletal System. Ciba-Geigy Corporation, Summit, NJ, 1978, pp 42, 66.
2. Richardson, JK and Iglarsh, ZA: Clinical Orthopaedic Physical Therapy. WB Saunders, Philadelphia, 1994, p 221.
3. Ibid, p 225.
4. Meschan, I: An Atlas of Normal Radiographic Anatomy. WB Saunders, Philadelphia, 1960, pp 97–99.
5. Weissman, B and Sledge, C: Orthopedic Radiology. WB Saunders, Philadelphia, 1986, pp 173–176.
6. Greenspan, A: Orthopedic Radiology: A Practical Approach, ed 2. Raven Press, New York, 1992, pp 5.22–5.30.
7. Bontrager, KL: A Textbook of Radiographic Positioning and Related Anatomy, ed 3. CV Mosby, St Louis, 1993, pp 99–145.
8. Fischer, HW: Radiographic Anatomy: A Working Atlas. McGraw-Hill, New York, 1988, pp 11–13.
9. Wicke, L: Atlas of Radiographic Anatomy, ed 5. Lea & Febiger, Malvern, PA, 1994, p 74.
10. Weissman, p 173.
11. Richardson, p 223.
12. Weissman, p 175.
13. Greenspan, pp 5.22–5.46.
14. Rockwood, CA, Wilkins, KE, and King, RE: Fractures in Children, Vol 3, ed 2. JB Lippincott, Philadelphia, 1984, pp 301–556.
15. Weissman, pp 169–214.
16. Richardson, pp 227–231.
17. Weissman, pp 179–180.
18. Greenspan, p 5.34.
19. Rockwood, Vol 3, p 374.
20. Weissman, pp 177–178, 180.
21. Ibid, p 185.
22. Rockwood, Vol 3, p 376.
23. Greenspan, p 5.34.

24. Richardson, p 230.
25. Weissman, p 185.
26. Rockwood, CA and Green, DP: Fractures in Adults, Vol. 1, ed 2. JB Lippincott, 1984, p 571.
27. Weissman, p 188.
28. Rockwood, Vol 3, p 437.
29. Ibid, Vol I, pp 590–595.
30. Weissman, p 185.
31. Rockwood, Vol 3, pp 489–495.
32. Richardson, p 228.
33. Ibid, p 228.
34. Weissman, p 161.
35. Richardson, p 228.
36. Weissman, p 161.
37. Greenspan, p 5.36.
38. Weissman, p 194.
39. Greenspan, p 5.38.
40. Weissman, p 194.
41. Ibid, p 194.
42. Greenspan, p 5.38.
43. Rockwood, Vol I, p 513.
44. Weissman, p 198.
45. Ibid.
46. Ibid, p 199.
47. Ibid.
48. Rockwood, Vol I, p 550.
49. Ibid, Vol 3, p 274.
50. Weissman, p 200.
51. Rockwood, Vol I, p 542.
52. Weissman, p 204.
53. Greenspan, p 5.42.
54. Rockwood, Vol I, p 613.

SELF-TEST

Chapter 11

REGARDING FILMS A, B, AND C:

1. Identify the <u>projections</u>.
2. All three films represent <u>normal findings</u> for different age groups. Identify which film belongs to the 5-year-old girl, the 10-year-old boy, and the 30-year-old man.
3. What <u>anatomic features</u> helped you determine the ages of the patients?

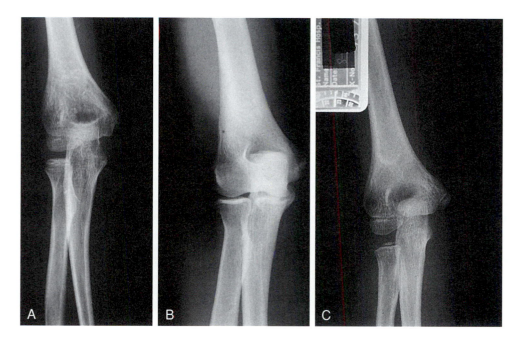

Hand and Wrist

The hand and wrist are one of the most frequently radiographed areas of the skeletal system in any age group. Various reasons account for this. The distal forearm is the most common site of fracture in children, and the hand is probably the most common site of fracture in adults. The exposed location of this most distal portion of the upper extremity predisposes the hand and wrist to a wide variety of other types of trauma. Additionally, the effects of microtrauma from normal repetitive prehensile actions are thought to contribute to the development of painful degenerative changes in the joints and soft tissues of the hand and wrist. Common disease processes such as the arthritides can cause hand and wrist joint deformities that seriously impair hand function. The physicians and therapists involved in diagnosis, treatment, and rehabilitation of the hand and wrist play crucial roles in restoring or preserving an individual's functional independence and occupational capabilities.

The radiographic evaluation of the majority of hand and wrist fractures and dislocations is complete on the standard plain film projections presented here. Evaluation of cartilaginous and soft tissue injuries requires ancillary imaging studies such as computed tomography (CT), arthrotomography, arthrography, and magnetic resonance imaging (MRI).

The goals of this chapter are first to present a review of osseous radiographic anatomy. A brief review of ligamentous anatomy and joint mobility is included to assist the reader in understanding the mechanisms of some common injury and deformity patterns. The routine radiographic evaluations of the hand and wrist follow. Here the reader has an opportunity to learn radiographic anatomy by tracing a radiograph with a marker on a transparency sheet and then comparing results with the radiographic tracing. Next, brief discussion and illustrations and films of common traumas, arthritides, and joint deformities are presented. The summary is organized into a list of practical points highlighting the clinical aspects of the chapter. A self-test challenges the reader's visual interpretation skills.

RADIOGRAPHIC ANATOMY

Osseous Anatomy[1]

The 27 bones that make up one hand and wrist are divided into three groups: the phalanges, the metacarpals, and the carpals (Figs. 12–1, 12–2).

The *phalanges* are the fingers and thumb, or digits, of the hand. They number 14, with a *proximal, middle,* and *distal phalanx* forming each finger, and a *proximal* and *distal phalanx* forming the thumb. Each phalanx is a miniature long bone characterized by the presence of a *base, shaft,* and *head,* most distal. The thumb is designated as the first digit, and the fingers are consecutively numbered as digits two through five.

Five *metacarpals* form the palm of the hand. They are numbered in the same manner as the digits, with the first metacarpal at the thumb and the fifth metacarpal at the little finger side of the hand. The metacarpals are also miniature long bones, each possessing a base, shaft, and head.

Eight *carpals* make up the wrist. They are divided

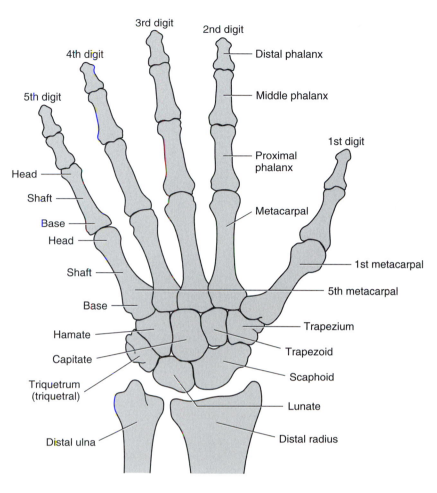

FIGURE 12–1. Osseous anatomy of the dorsal aspect of the hand.

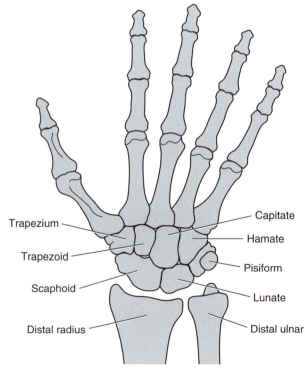

FIGURE 12–2. Osseous anatomy of the volar aspect of the hand.

into proximal and distal rows for ease of learning their positions. The proximal row, from the thumb side, consists of the *scaphoid, lunate, triquetrum,* and *pisiform* bones. The distal row, from the thumb side, consists of the *trapezium, trapezoid, capitate,* and *hamate* bones.

Joints and Ligaments of the Hand and Wrist (Fig. 12–3)

INTERPHALANGEAL JOINTS

These joints are located between the segments of each phalange. In the fingers they are designated as the *distal interphalangeal joints* and the *proximal interphalangeal joints.* The thumb possesses only one *interphalangeal joint.* Each joint is supported by an articular capsule and palmar and collateral ligaments. The dorsal aspect is reinforced by expansion of the extensor tendons.

METACARPOPHALANGEAL JOINTS

These joints are located between the bases of the proximal phalanges and the metacarpal heads. They are also each supported by articular capsules, palmar and collateral ligaments, and expansions of the exten-

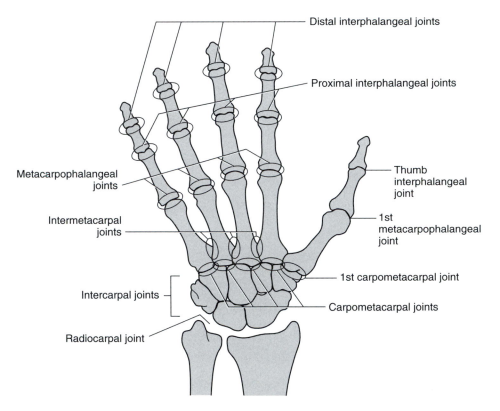

Distal interphalangeal joints

Proximal interphalangeal joints

Metacarpophalangeal joints

Intermetacarpal joints

Intercarpal joints

Radiocarpal joint

Thumb interphalangeal joint

1st metacarpophalangeal joint

1st carpometacarpal joint

Carpometacarpal joints

FIGURE 12–3. Joints of the hand and wrist.

sor tendons on their dorsal aspects. *Sesamoid bones,* small ossicles located within the tendons, are commonly present at these joints.

INTERMETACARPAL JOINTS

These joints are located between the adjacent bases of the four metacarpal bones of the fingers. Dorsal and palmar ligaments, as well as interosseous ligaments, support the intermetacarpal joints.

CARPOMETACARPAL JOINTS

These joints are located between the metacarpal bases and the distal row of carpal bones. The first carpometacarpal joint at the thumb is an independent articulation between the first metacarpal base and the trapezium, housed in its own strong articular capsule. The remaining carpometacarpal joints of the hand share the intercarpal synovial cavity. Dorsal and palmar carpometacarpal ligaments and interosseous ligaments support these articulations.

INTERCARPAL JOINTS

These joints refer to the articulations between the carpals themselves, contained within the intercarpal synovial cavity. This cavity also includes the intermetacarpal and second through fifth carpometacarpal joints. Dorsal and palmar intercarpal ligaments sup-

port the capsule, and within the capsule interosseous ligaments unite the individual carpal bones.

RADIOCARPAL JOINT

Referred to as the *wrist joint*, this joint is formed by the proximal row of carpal bones and their interosseous ligaments articulating with the distant radius and articular disc of the distal radioulnar joint. The articular capsule encloses the joint and is strengthened by the dorsal and palmar radiocarpal ligaments and the radial and ulnar collateral ligaments.

JOINT MOBILITY[2]

The varying articular surface shapes of the small joints of the hand permit many differences in range of motion between the individual fingers and the thumb. Amounts of range of motion can also greatly differ among individual persons, often relating to the amount of ligamentous laxity present. In general, the hand is extremely mobile and can coordinate between its components an infinite variety of movement.

The *interphalangeal joints* function as hinge joints permitting full extension or hyperextension and a great amount of flexion, ranging from 90 to 110 degrees or more. The *metacarpophalangeal joints* of the fingers are condyloid, allowing multiplanar motion and approximately 90 degrees of flexion. The *first metacarpophalangeal joint* at the thumb is a saddle joint allowing full or hyperextension and as much as 90 degrees of flexion. The *carpometacarpal joints* of the hand are gliding joints, permitting enough flexion and extension to allow cupping of the palm. The *first carpometacarpal joint* of the thumb is a saddle joint allowing a wide range of motion through a conical space, the most important of which is opposition to the fingers.

Motions at the *wrist joint complex*, consisting of the intercarpal joints, the radiocarpal joint, and the distal radioulnar joint, are intricately integrated, permitting motion in two planes and in combinations of those planes. The major motions are flexion-extension and abduction-adduction, also called radial and ulnar deviation. Varying widely among individuals, approximately 90 degrees of flexion, 80 degrees of extension, 20 degrees of radial deviation, and 30 degrees of ulnar deviation are possible. Forearm pronation and supination result from motion arising at the proximal and distal radioulnar joints, permitting the hand to axially rotate approximately 150 degrees.

GROWTH AND DEVELOPMENT[3]

The hand and wrist are often used as indicators of bone age in children (Figs. 12–4, 12–5, 12–6). The tim-

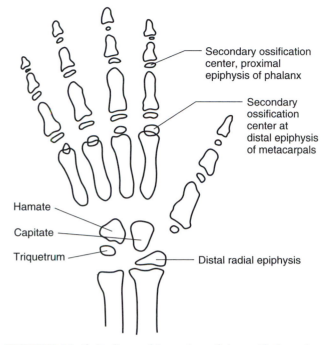

FIGURE 12–5. Radiographic tracing of the ossified portions of the hand at 2 years, 9 months (male). (Adapted from Meschan,[3] p 56.)

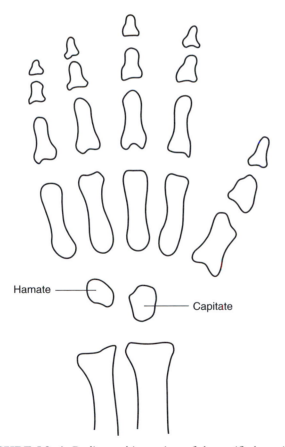

FIGURE 12–4. Radiographic tracing of the ossified portions of the hand at 6 months of age. (Adapted from Meschan,[3] p 55.)

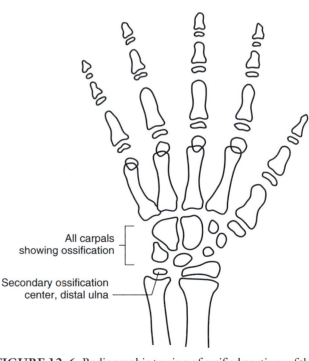

FIGURE 12–6. Radiographic tracing of ossified portions of the hand at 6 years, 9 months (male). (Adapted from Meschan,[3] p 56.)

ing of the appearances of ossification centers and configuration of the epiphyses has been radiographically demonstrated in large group studies of children and has become standardized.

Ossification of the shafts of the metacarpals and phalanges begins at 8 weeks of fetal life. At birth these structures are fairly well formed. The carpals are ordinarily cartilaginous at birth and are not visible on radiographs (Figs. 12–7, 12–8).

Ossification at the carpals takes place from a single center in each bone. First to appear are the centers for the capitate and hamate, usually by 6 months of age. The center for the triquetrum appears after age 2, followed by the centers for the lunate, trapezium, trapezoid, and scaphoid in yearly intervals to age 6. The pisiform begins ossification much later, after age 11.

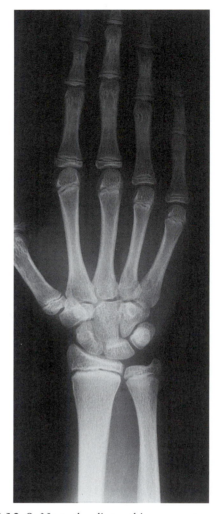

FIGURE 12–8. Normal radiographic appearance of the hand in an 11-year-old child. At this stage of development, all the carpals are visible, and all the secondary ossification centers in the forearm, metacarpal, and phalangeal shafts are well formed and easily visible. The epiphyseal plates appear "open" as radiolucent lines parallel to the ends of the epiphyses.

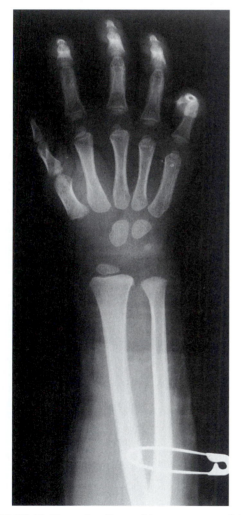

FIGURE 12–7. Normal radiographic appearance of the hand of a 3-year-old child. At this stage of development, the carpals showing ossification are the capitate, hamate, and triquetrum. The secondary center of ossification for the distal radial epiphysis is visible, as are the secondary centers for the heads of the metacarpals and the bases of the phalanges.

Ossification is usually complete at the carpals by ages 14 to 16, with girls maturing 1 or 2 years prior to boys.

At the metacarpals, secondary ossification centers appear in the distal epiphyses at age 2. Fusion of the metacarpals is complete by 16 to 18 years of age.

At the phalanges, secondary ossification centers appear in the proximal epiphyses at age 2, and their development parallels that of the metacarpals.

The radial and ulnar shafts begin ossification in the eighth week of fetal life and are well formed at birth. The secondary center of ossification for the distal radial epiphysis appears at the end of the first year, and for the distal ulnar epiphysis at 5 or 6 years of age. These epiphyses complete fusion to their respective shafts at 18 to 20 years of age.

ROUTINE RADIOGRAPHIC EVALUATION[4-7]

Radiographic positioning for the three basic projections (posteroanterior [PA], oblique, and lateral) of the hand and of the wrist are essentially the same, the difference being where the x-ray beam is centered. In a routine hand series, the beam is centered over the third metacarpophalangeal joint. In a routine wrist series the beam is centered over the midcarpal area.

If a single finger or the thumb is the area of interest, the three basic projections may be done individually for that specific digit.

For evaluation of trauma to the carpals, many optional projections are available to visualize specific anatomic sites. Two common optional projections, the ulnar and radial deviation views, are done similarly to the PA projections, with the wrist laterally flexed to either direction.

Radiographs of the hand and wrist are generally examined with the fingers pointing up. Consistent with this custom is the fact that metacarpal and phalangeal *heads* are then positioned *superiorly*, and their *bases inferiorly*, when viewed.

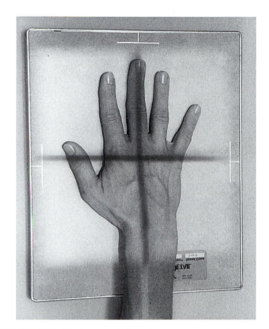

FIGURE 12–9. Patient position for posteroanterior view of the hand.

Hand

Basic: Posteroanterior
            Oblique
            Lateral

POSTEROANTERIOR (FIGS. 12–9, 12–10, 12–11)

This view demonstrates the *hand, wrist,* and *distal forearm*. Structures best shown are the *phalanges, metacarpals, carpals,* and all *joints* of the hand. The important observations are as follows:

1. The patient's palm and fingers are positioned flat on the film cassette. This results in a true PA view of the hand but an *oblique* view of the thumb.
2. Note the *symmetric* appearance of the concave sides of the shafts of each phalanx and metacarpal. The oblique perspective of the thumb is the exception.
3. Note the normal *tufted* appearance of the terminal ends of the distal phalanges.
4. Normally the long axis of the second metacarpal is in line with the long axis of the radius.
5. Normally there is slight ulnar deviation of the proximal phalanges of the fingers in respect to the metacarpals.
6. The interphalangeal and metacarpophalangeal joint spaces are visible.

7. Sesamoid bones are a frequent occurrence at the metacarpophangeal and interphalangeal joints of the thumb and at the metacarpophalangeal joint of the fifth finger.
8. The bases of the second through fifth metacarpals partially overlap.
9. At the wrist there is overlap of the trapezium and the trapezoid, as well as the pisiform and the triquetrum.

CLINICAL OBJECTIVES

1. Trace and number the phalanges. Identify proximal, middle, and distal segments. Identify the base, shaft, and head of a single phalanx.
2. Trace and number the metacarpals. Identify the base, shaft, and head of one metacarpal.
3. Trace any sesamoid bones present.
4. Trace the carpals. Identify in the distal row the trapezium, trapezoid, capitate, and hamate. Identify in the proximal row the scaphoid, lunate, triquetrum, and pisiform.
5. Identify the joints of the hand: the distal and proximal interphalangeal joints, the metacarpophalangeal joints, and the carpometacarpal joints.

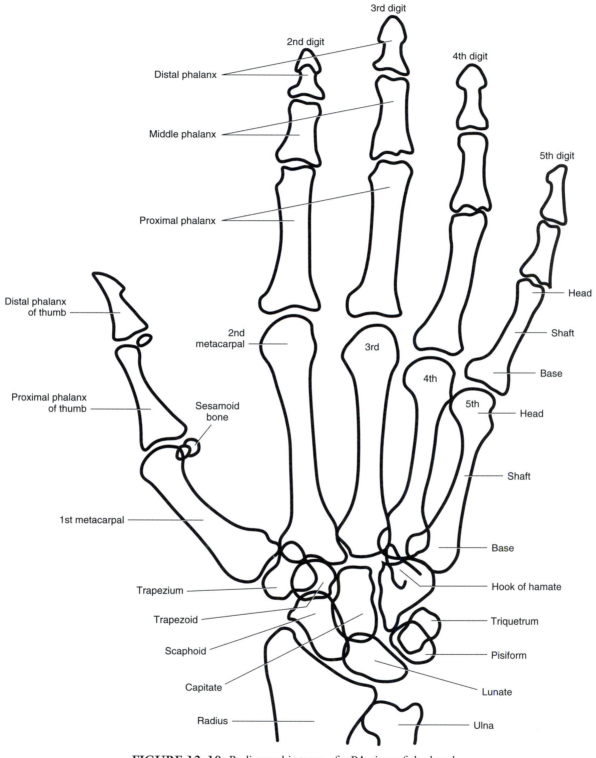

FIGURE 12–10. Radiographic trace of a PA view of the hand.

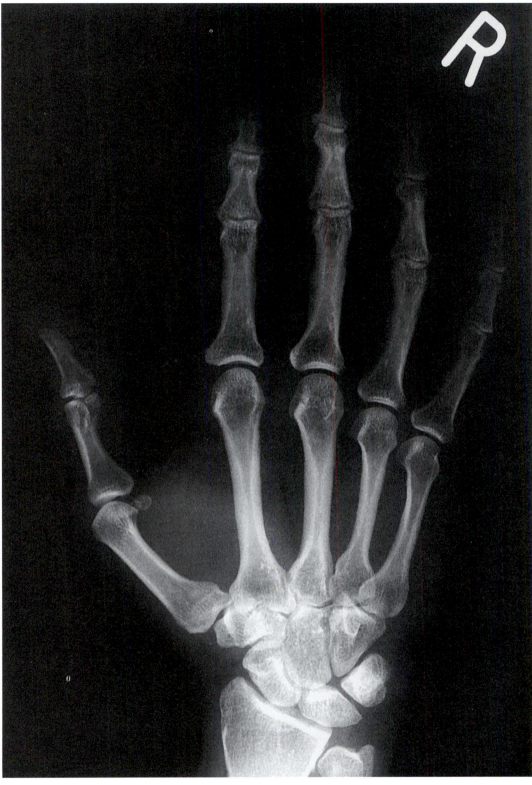

FIGURE 12–11. PA view of the hand.

OBLIQUE (FIGS. 12–12, 12–13, 12–14)

This view demonstrates the *phalanges, metacarpals, carpals,* and all *joints* of the hand in an oblique view. The important observations are:

1. The patient's hand and wrist have been placed flat on the film as for a PA projection and then the thumb side of the hand is lifted, rotating the hand and wrist 45 degrees from the PA position.

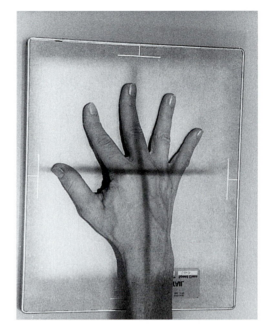

FIGURE 12–12. Patient position for oblique view of the hand.

2. The phalanges and metacarpals are demonstrated without superimposition. This lack of overlap of the long bones of the hand makes the *oblique view* advantageous over the direct *lateral view*, which superimposes many structures. The lateral view is necessary, however, to determine exact amounts of any displacements that may be present.
3. The interphalangeal and metacarpophalangeal joint spaces are visible.

CLINICAL OBJECTIVES

1. Trace and number the phalanges. Identify proximal, middle, and distal segments. Identify the base, shaft, and head of a single phalanx.
2. Trace and number the metacarpals. Identify the base, shaft, and head of one metacarpal.
3. Identify the joints of the hand: the distal and proximal interphalangeal joints, the metacarpophalangeal joints, and the carpometacarpal joints.
4. Trace any sesamoid bones present.

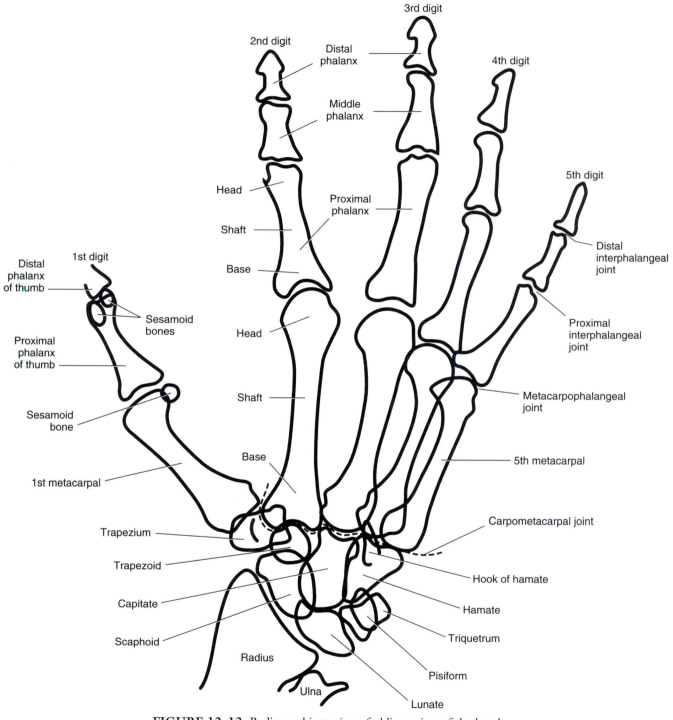

FIGURE 12–13. Radiographic tracing of oblique view of the hand.

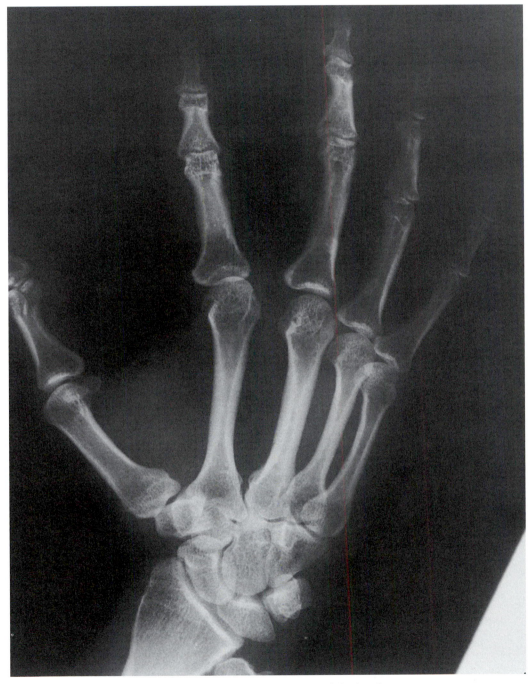

FIGURE 12–14. Oblique view of the hand.

LATERAL (FIGS. 12–15, 12–16, 12–17)

This view demonstrates the *hand* and *wrist* from a lateral perspective. The thumb, however, is seen in a true PA projection. Various *sesamoid bones* may be demonstrated on this view. The important observations follow:

1. The patient's ulnar side of the hand and wrist is positioned on the film cassette. This means the

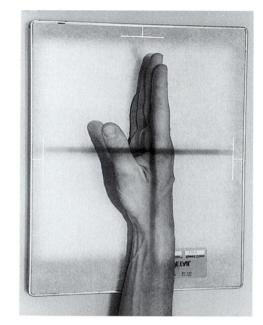

FIGURE 12–15. Patient position for lateral view of the hand.

thumb is farthest from the film and thus undergoes some magnification.

2. The phalanges and metacarpals are superimposed directly over each other, as are most of the carpals, as well as the distal radius and ulna.

3. Despite the superimposition of most of the bones of the hand and wrist, *displacement of a fracture fragment* is easily detected on this projection. Note that displacement will be described as being in a *dorsal* or *volar* direction.

CLINICAL OBJECTIVES

1. Trace the bones of the thumb: the first metacarpal, proximal phalanx, and distal phalanx.
2. Trace the phalanges that are visible. Identify the proximal, middle, and distal segments.
3. Trace the borders of the metacarpals.
4. Identify the joints of the hand: the distal and proximal interphalangeal joints, the metacarpophalangeal joints, and the carpometacarpophalangeal joints.

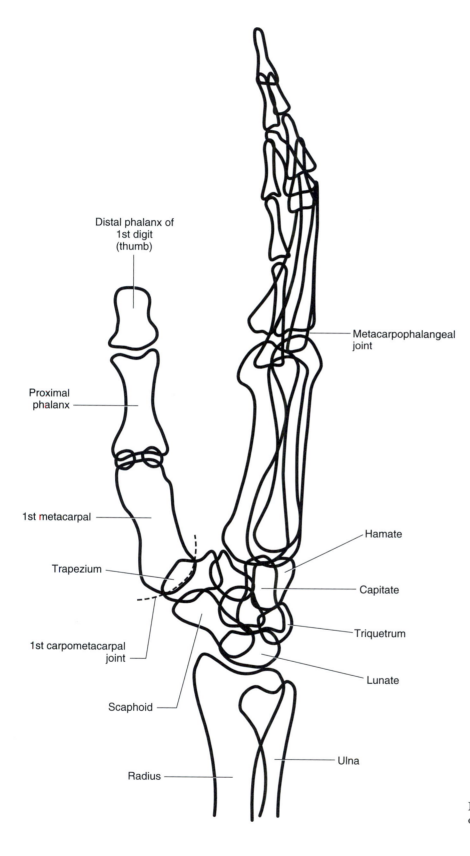

Distal phalanx of
1st digit
(thumb)

Proximal
phalanx

1st metacarpal

Trapezium

1st carpometacarpal
joint

Scaphoid

Radius

Metacarpophalangeal
joint

Hamate

Capitate

Triquetrum

Lunate

Ulna

FIGURE 12–16. Radiographic tracing of lateral view of the hand.

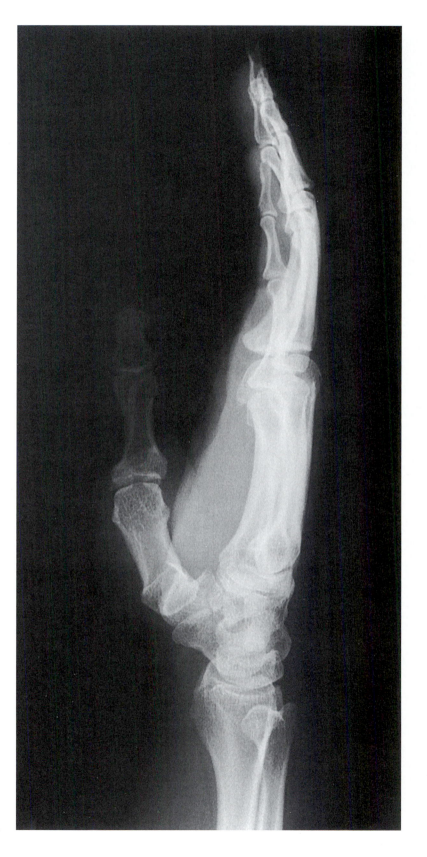

FIGURE 12–17. Lateral view of the hand.

Wrist

Basic: Posteroanterior
          Oblique
          Lateral
Optional: Ulnar Deviation
              Radial Deviation

POSTEROANTERIOR (FIGS. 12–18, 12–19, 12–20)

This view demonstrates the mid- and proximal portions of the *metacarpals*, the *carpals*, the *distal radius* and *ulna*, and all related *joints*. The important observations follow:

1. The patient's hand is placed palm down on the film cassette and the fingers are then slightly flexed to promote close contact between the wrist and the film cassette.
2. Three arcuate lines can normally be drawn along the articular surfaces of the carpals, outlining the proximal and distal rows (Fig. 12–21):
   • Arc I: Outlines the proximal convex surfaces of the scaphoid, lunate, and triquetrum
   • Arc II: Outlines the distal concave surfaces of the scaphoid, lunate, and triquetrum
   • Arc III: Outlines the proximal convex margins of the capitate and hamate.
   Distortions in these anatomic relationships may be diagnostic of carpal subluxations or dislocations.[7,8]
3. Note the carpals, which are demonstrated relatively free of superimposition: the scaphoid, lunate, capitate, and hamate. Note the oval image on the hamate representing the hook of the hamate.
4. Note which carpals are superimposed on this pro-

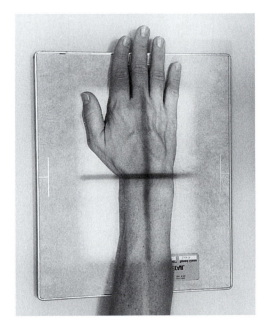

FIGURE 12–18. Patient position for posteroanterior view of the wrist.

jection: the trapezium and trapezoid, and the triquetrum and pisiform.
5. The relationship of the length of the ulna to the radius is termed *ulnar variance* (Figs. 12–22, 12–23, 12–24). Usually the articular surfaces of the ulna and radius, at the site of articulation with the lunate, are on the same level. This is referred to as *neutral ulnar variance*. In some individuals the ulna is shorter than the radius, and the term *negative ulnar variance* is applied. If the ulna is longer than the radius, the term *positive ulnar variance* is applied. The difference in length is measured in millimeters. This informa-

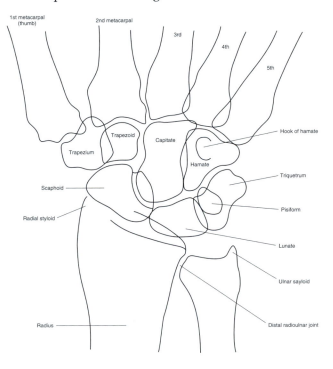

FIGURE 12–19. Radiographic tracing of PA view of the wrist.

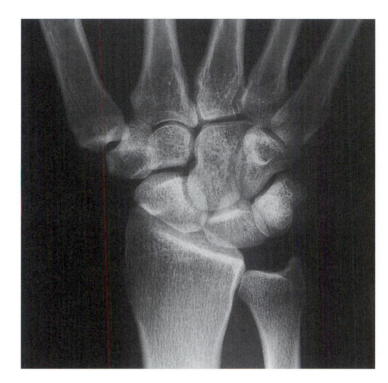

FIGURE 12–20. PA view of the wrist.

tion has practical importance for the orthopedist in assessing fracture displacement, choosing open or closed reduction treatment, and assisting in follow-up evaluation.[9,10]

6. The *radial angle* is another measurement that has significance for the orthopedist (Fig. 12–25). Sometimes referred to as the *ulnar slant of the articular surface of the radius*, an angle is formed by the intersection of two lines: (a) a line perpendicular to the long axis of the radius at the level of the radioulnar articular surface and (b) a line drawn across the radial articular surface. Normal values range from 15 to 25 degrees.[11]

CLINICAL OBJECTIVES

1. Trace and number the metacarpals.
2. Trace and identify the carpals.
3. Draw in the three arcuate lines at the carpals as described in the text.
4. Trace the distal radius and ulna.
5. Measure the ulnar variance.
6. Measure the radial angle.

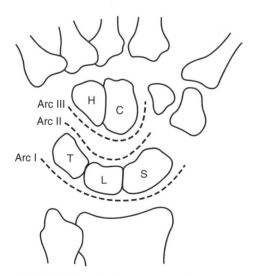

FIGURE 12–21. Three arcuate lines drawn along the articular surfaces of the carpals designate normal anatomic relationships.

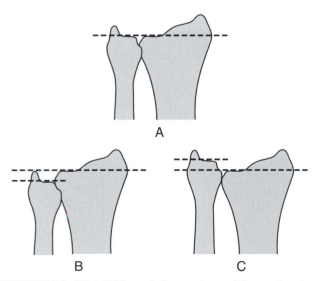

FIGURE 12–22. (*A*) Neutral ulnar variance, (*B*) negative ulnar variance, (*C*) positive ulnar variance.

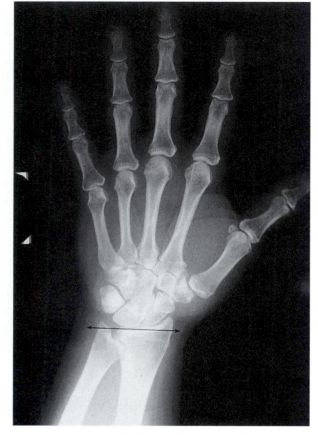

FIGURE 12–23. Negative ulnar variance.

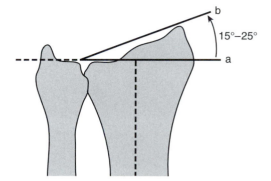

FIGURE 12–25. The radial angle, or ulnar slant of the articular surface of the radius, is measured as the angle formed by the intersection of the line perpendicular to the long axis (a) and the line drawn across the radial articular surface (b).

OBLIQUE (FIGS. 12–26, 12–27, 12–28)

This view demonstrates the mid and proximal *metacarpals*, the *carpals*, and the *distal radius* and *ulnar* in an oblique view. Structures best shown are the *trapezium*, the *scaphoid*, and the *first carpometacarpal joint* of the thumb. The important observations are:

1. The patient's hand and wrist are placed palm-down on the film cassette, and then the thumb side of the hand is lifted, rotating the hand and wrist 45 degrees from the PA position.
2. The first and second metacarpals are viewed with little superimposition.
3. The proximal portions of the third, fourth, and fifth metacarpals appear superimposed.
4. Certain aspects of the carpals are well demonstrated in this projection. Note:
    Hamate: The body of the hamate is visualized. The hook of the hamate is not superimposed as seen in the PA view.

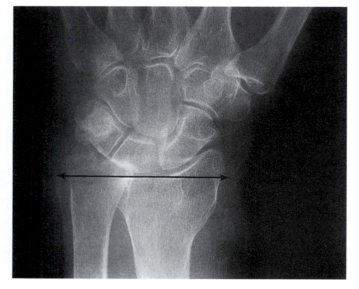

FIGURE 12–24. Positive ulnar variance.

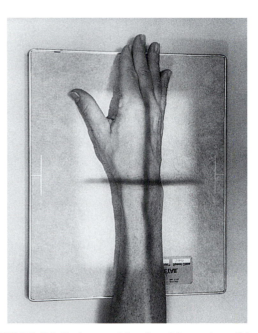

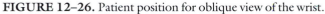

FIGURE 12-26. Patient position for oblique view of the wrist.

Triquetrum: The dorsal aspect of this bone is visualized.

Scaphoid: The medial aspect and volar aspect is visualized.

Trapezium: The trapezium itself and its articulations to the trapezoid, scaphoid, and first metacarpal are visualized.[12]

5. Note that the distal radius and ulna are slightly superimposed.

CLINICAL OBJECTIVES

1. Trace and number the metacarpals.
2. Trace the trapezium, trapezoid, and scaphoid.
3. Trace the triquetrum and hamate.
4. Trace the distal radius and ulna.

LATERAL (FIGS. 12-29, 12-30, 12-31)

This view demonstrates superimposed proximal *metacarpals*, *carpals*, *distal radius*, and *ulna* as seen from a lateral perspective. The important observations are:

1. The patient's ulnar side of the hand and wrist is positioned on the film cassette. The metacarpal of the thumb is farthest from the film and is somewhat magnified.

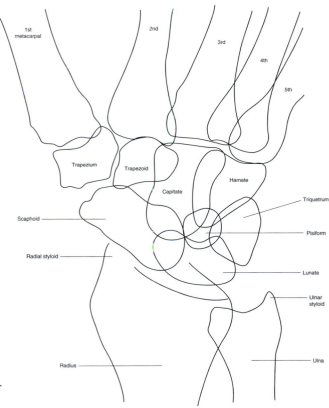

FIGURE 12-27. Radiographic tracing of oblique view of the wrist.

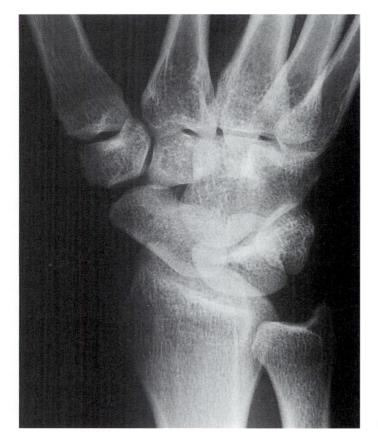

FIGURE 12–28. Oblique view of the wrist.

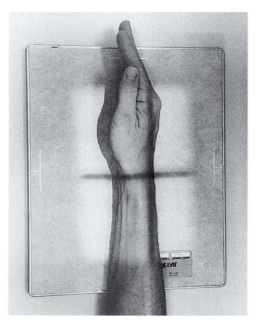

FIGURE 12–29. Patient position for lateral view of the wrist.

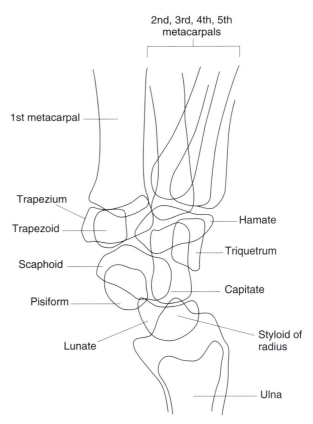

2nd, 3rd, 4th, 5th metacarpals

1st metacarpal

Trapezium

Trapezoid

Scaphoid

Pisiform

Lunate

Hamate

Triquetrum

Capitate

Styloid of radius

Ulna

FIGURE 12–30. Radiographic tracing of lateral view of the wrist.

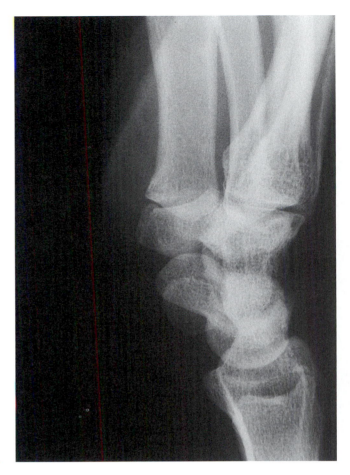

FIGURE 12–31. Lateral view of the wrist.

2. Despite the superimposition of the wrist and forearm, *displacement of a fracture fragment* is easily detected on this view. Displacement is described as being in a *dorsal or volar* direction.
3. The *volar tilt* of the radial articular surface normally ranges from 10 to 25 degrees. Also known as the *palmar inclination* (Fig. 12–32), this angle is determined by the intersection of (a) a line perpendicular to the midshaft of the radius and (b) a line drawn across the distal aspects of the radial articular surface. Like the anatomic relationships measured on the PA projection, this angle has practical importance to the orthopedist in assessing fracture displacement, choosing treatment, and assessing follow-up evaluations.[13,14]
4. Another significant anatomic relationship seen on the lateral view is the *alignment of the longitudinal axes of the radius, lunate, capitate, and third metacarpal bones* (Fig. 12–33). Variations of up to 10 degrees are considered normal, but major distortions may be diagnostic of fracture or dislocation.[15,16]

Note that the stacked arrangement of the normal radius-lunate-capitate relationship remains true in any degree of wrist flexion or extension.[17] That is, the radial articular surface will always contain the lunate, and the lunate will always cup the capitate in normal conditions.

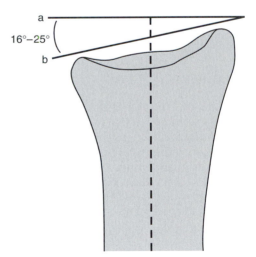

FIGURE 12–32. The *volar tilt*, or *palmar inclination*, is measured as the angle determined by the intersection of line (a), a line perpendicular to the midshaft of the radius, and (b), a line drawn across the distal radial articular surface.

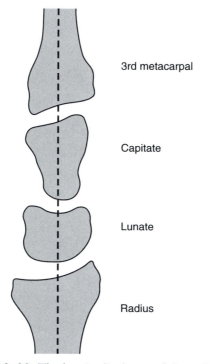

FIGURE 12–33. The longitudinal axes of the radius, lunate, capitate, and third metacarpal bones normally align within 10 degrees of each other, as seen on the lateral view.

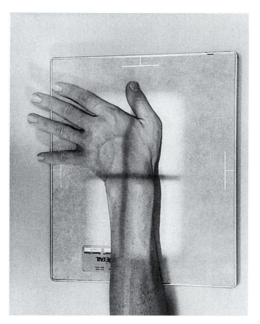

FIGURE 12–34. Patient position for ulnar deviation view of the wrist.

CLINICAL OBJECTIVES

1. Trace the first metacarpal and the trapezium.
2. Trace the distal radius and ulna.
3. Trace the radius, lunate, and capitate.
4. Measure the volar tilt of the radius.

OPTIONAL WRIST VIEWS

Ulnar Deviation (Figs. 12–34, 12–35)

This PA view of the wrist is made with the hand positioned in *ulnar deviation* to view the scaphoid and adjacent opened radial intercarpal spaces. The scaphoid normally appears elongated in this projection because of rotation of its distal pole toward the ulna. This elongated appearance verifies normal articulation to the adjacent carpals and excludes scapholunate dislocation.[18]

Radial Deviation (Figs. 12–36, 12–37)

This PA view of the wrist is made with the hand positioned in *radial deviation* to view the ulnar side carpals and adjacent opened ulnar intercarpal spaces. The lunate, triquetrum, hamate, and pisiform are best shown. Note the foreshortened appearance of the scaphoid. The distal pole of the scaphoid has rotated toward the palm to clear the radial styloid and now is seen end-on.[19]

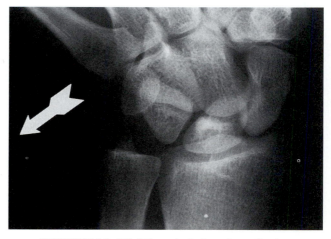

FIGURE 12–35. Ulnar deviation view of wrist.

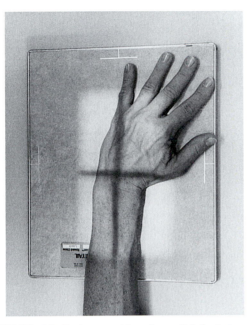

FIGURE 12–36. Patient position for radial deviation view of the wrist.

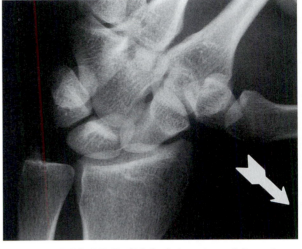

FIGURE 12–37. Radial deviation view of the wrist.

TRAUMA

Fractures of the hand are probably the most common fractures in the skeletal system.[20] The distal pha-langes, being the most exposed portion of the hand, account for more than half of all hand fractures. The mechanism for the majority of hand fractures is direct blows or crushing type injuries.[21] Radiographic evaluation of hand fractures is generally complete on the routine PA, lateral, and oblique plain film projections. Individual fingers may also be evaluated if they are the specific area of interest. A finger examination is also comprised of PA, lateral, and oblique projections (Fig. 12–38).

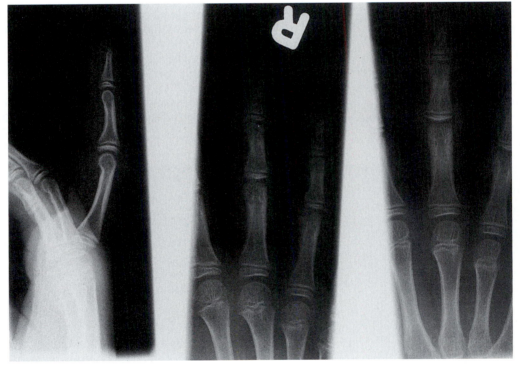

LATERAL   OBLIQUE   PA

FIGURE 12–38. Examination of an individual digit. The routine examination of an individual digit includes lateral, oblique, and PA projections as demonstrated above in the evaluation of the third digit, or middle finger, in this 9-year-old boy.

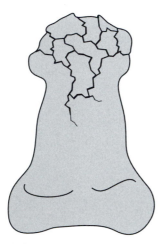

FIGURE 12–39. Crush injury to the distal phalanx.

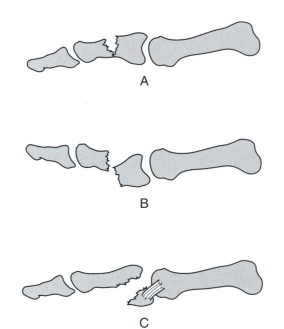

FIGURE 12–41. Fractures of the middle and proximal phalanges are classified as (*A*) stable, (*B*) unstable, or (*C*) intra-articular.

The wrist is also a frequently fractured area of the upper extremity. The distal radius is the most commonly injured bone at the wrist, followed by the scaphoid. The mechanism for the majority of wrist fractures is a fall on an outstretched hand.[22] Radiographic evaluation of distal radius and carpal fractures is generally complete on the routine projections and the optional ulnar and radial deviation projections presented previously.

Fractures of the Hand

PHALANGEAL FRACTURES

The distal phalanges are most often injured by a crushing mechanism that results in comminution of the distal tuft (Figs. 12–39, 12–40). Generally, significant displacement does not occur, owing to the presence of fibrous tissue septa radiating from the bone

into the soft tissues. Healing by fibrous rather than bony union usually takes place within a few weeks. Radiographic evidence of complete bony union may not be evident for several months.[23]

Fractures of the middle and proximal phalangeal shafts may be classified as *stable, unstable, or intra-articular* (Fig. 12–41). Stable shaft fractures are undisplaced and treated conservatively with immobilization (Fig. 12–42). Unstable shaft fractures are displaced and may exhibit angular or rotational deformities. Treatment usually consists of closed reduction followed by

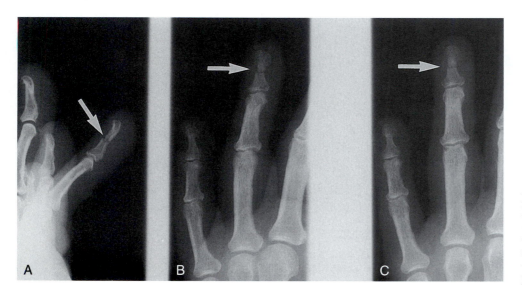

FIGURE 12–40. Distal phalanx fracture. These (*A*) lateral, (*B*) oblique, and (*C*) PA views of the fourth digit demonstrate a complete, transverse fracture of the midshaft of the distal phalanx (arrows).

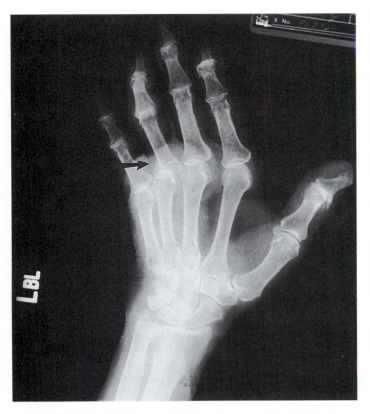

FIGURE 12–42. Proximal phalanx fracture. On this PA view of the hand, an impacted, incomplete fracture on the ulnar side of the base of the fourth proximal phalanx is present (arrow). The distal fragment is angulated ulnarly. Note the soft tissue swelling in the palm and along the extent of the fourth digit. Note also the osteoarthritic changes at all of the interphalangeal joints, including joint narrowing, subchondral sclerosis, and osteophyte formation.

immobilization. Internal fixation is sometimes necessary, especially in long oblique fractures of the proximal phalanx. Intra-articular fractures may be avulsion-type fractures, with the dorsal aspect of bone disrupted at the attachment of the extensor tendon, or the lateral or volar aspect disrupted at the attachment of the collateral ligament. Intra-articular fractures may also involve one or both condyles, or exhibit comminution. Most large-fragment and comminuted intra-articular fractures require internal fixation to maintain anatomic reduction.[24,25]

METACARPAL FRACTURES OF THE FINGERS

Metacarpal fractures are classified by location as fractures of the *head, neck, shaft, or base* (Fig. 12–43). Fractures of the metacarpal *neck* are common. Angular deformity that causes the metacarpal head to protrude into the palm is a serious consequence of this fracture, and treatment is aimed at restoring alignment. Likewise, fractures of the metacarpal *shafts* can cause angular deformities and must be adequately reduced to prevent painful protrusion into the palm and preserve functional grasp ability. Fractures of the metacarpal *bases*, along with severely angulated shaft fractures, are often associated with carpometacarpal dislocations.[26,27]

THUMB METACARPAL FRACTURES

As the thumb is a unique digit, fractures of the first metacarpal are distinctly different from fractures at the other metacarpals. The majority of thumb metacarpal fractures occur at or near the *base* and are divided into intra-articular and extra-articular types. The two intra-articular fracture patterns seen are commonly known by the eponyms *Bennett's fracture* and *Rolando's fracture*.

FIGURE 12–43. Metacarpal fracture. (*A*) This oblique of the hand demonstrates a midshaft fracture of the fifth metacarpal (arrow). The fracture line is complete, transverse, with dorsal angulation of both fracture fragments. (*B*) After closed reduction and casting. Note the configuration of the cast, which has placed the fifth finger in extension in order to prevent the motion of finger flexion, which would act to distract the fracture fragments and prevent union.

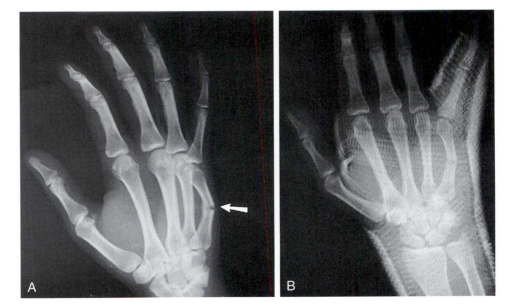

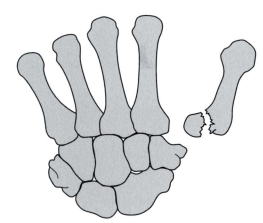

FIGURE 12–44. Bennett's fracture is a fracture-dislocation injury at the first carpometacarpal joint. An axial blow to a partially flexed thumb dislocates the metacarpal base and avulses a fragment of bone from the anterior aspect of the base.

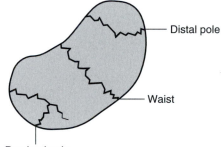

FIGURE 12–46. Possible fracture sites of the scaphoid. The majority of fractures occur through the waist.

Fractures of the Carpals

Fractures of the scaphoid account for more than 60 percent of all carpal injuries. The scaphoid is susceptible to fracture due in part to its location, where it (1) acts as the principal block to excessive wrist dorsiflexion, (2) accepts compressive forces from the capitate and the thumb axis, and (3) serves as a link between the carpal rows, pushing or pulling the proximal row into position during wrist motions.[33] Fractures of any of the remaining carpal bones occur infrequently and are considered uncommon.

Scaphoid fractures occur at three levels: the distal pole, the midportion or *waist*, and the proximal pole (Fig. 12–46). The majority, 70 to 80 percent, occur at the waist. Rates of healing, lengths of treatment immobilization, and complications vary between the fracture locations due to the differentiated vascularity of the scaphoid. The major blood supply of the scaphoid enters through the distal pole (Fig. 12–47). Thus heal-

Bennett's fracture is actually a fracture-dislocation resulting from an axial blow to the partially flexed metacarpal (Fig. 12–44). The base of the metacarpal dislocates, and an avulsion fracture occurs at the anterior lip of the base where strong ligamentous attachment to the trapezium is located. Treatment methods are widely varied, ranging from closed reduction with numerous types of immobilization suggested, to open reduction with internal fixation.[28–30]

Rolando's fracture is a Y- or T-shaped intra-articular fracture with an anterior fragment, as seen in Bennett's fracture and additionally a dorsal fragment (Fig. 12–45). The comminution present in this type of fracture makes reduction difficult. Rolando's fracture is the least common of adult metacarpal fractures.

Extra-articular fractures are the most frequently seen fracture pattern at the thumb. The fracture line is usually transverse and, less often, oblique. Treatment is usually successful with closed reduction and cast immobilization.[31,32]

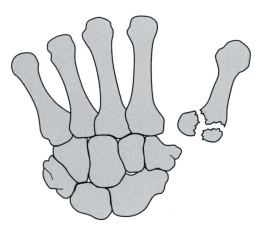

FIGURE 12–45. Rolando's fracture describes a comminuted fracture at the base of the thumb metacarpal.

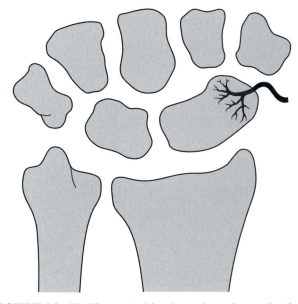

FIGURE 12–47. The major blood supply to the scaphoid enters through its distal pole, rendering the proximal end of the scaphoid vulnerable to avascular necrosis if the fracture line occurs across the midportion, or waist, of the scaphoid.

ing of fractures located across the waist or at the proximal pole is rendered less certain, and avascular necrosis of the proximal pole is a common complication.[34-37]

Fractures of the Distal Radius

The most frequent fracture seen at the distal forearm is well known by the eponym *Colles' fracture* (Fig. 12–48). The classic Colles' fracture is described as an extra-articular fracture located about 1½ inches proximal to the end of the radius with dorsal angulation or displacement of the distal fragment (Fig. 12–49). Other variations in alignment of the fragments may be seen, including impaction, lateral displacement, or lateral displacement with radial angulation.[38] Fracture of the ulnar styloid is a frequently associated injury (Fig. 12–50). Some authors also include under this type of fracture an intra-articular extension of the fracture line and associated fracture at the distal end of the ulna.[39-41]

Treatment ranges from closed reduction with cast immobilization to open reduction and internal fixation. Possible complications are many, including radioulnar or radiocarpal instability owing to ligamentous injury, median or ulnar nerve injury, inadequate reduction causing deformity and posttraumatic arthritis, soft tissue adhesions, reflex sympathetic dystrophy, and nonunion.[42,43]

Radiographic examination on the lateral view identifies the amount of fracture fragment angulation relative to the normal volar tilt of the distal radial articular surface. The "dinner fork" deformity sometimes resulting from this fracture is apparent on the lateral films. The PA view may identify *radial shortening*, caused by overlap of the fracture fragments. Postre-

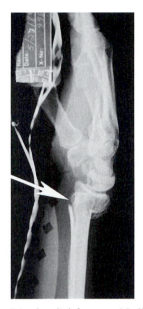

FIGURE 12–49. Distal radial fracture (Colles' fracture). This lateral view of the wrist demonstrates a complete, impacted fracture of the distal radius with a volar apex of the fracture site and dorsal angulation of the distal fragment (arrow). An incomplete, longitudinal fracture line is also seen extending along the volar aspect of the radial shaft distal to the primary fracture site.

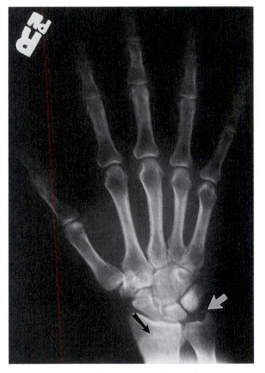

FIGURE 12–50. Colles' fracture. This PA view of the hand demonstrates a complete transverse fracture of the distal radius (black arrow) and an avulsion fracture of the tip of the ulnar styloid (white arrow). This is the most frequent fracture seen at the distal forearm. It is typically sustained in a fall on an outstretched hand and is commonly known by the eponym *Colles' fracture.*

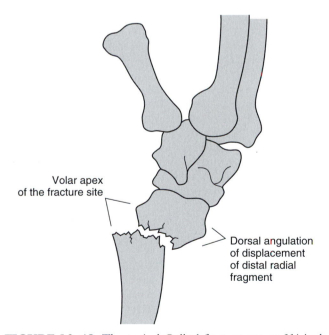

Volar apex
of the fracture site

Dorsal angulation
of displacement
of distal radial
fragment

FIGURE 12–48. The typical Colles' fracture occurs 1½ inch proximal to the distal end of the radius.

duction films should verify that the dorsal displacement of the distal fragment and radial shortening have been corrected. Restoration of normal volar tilt will help ensure a preserved radiocarpal articular relationship.[44]

ABNORMAL CONDITIONS

Degenerative Joint Disease

Degenerative joint disease (DJD) or *osteoarthritis* is commonly seen in the small joints of the adult hand after the fifth decade. The proximal and distal interphalangeal joints of the fingers and the carpometacarpal joint of the thumb particularly are affected.

Radiographic evidence of DJD in the hand, like other larger joints, is hallmarked by a (1) decrease in the radiographic joint space, (2) sclerosis of subchondral bone, and (3) osteophyte formation at joint margins (Fig. 12–51). The resulting joint deformities, when present in the distal interphalangeal joints, are known as *Heberden's nodes*. Similar deformities present in the proximal interphalangeal joints are known as *Bouchard's nodes* (see Fig. 12–42 for example).[45]

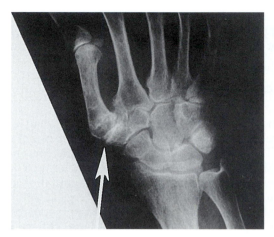

FIGURE 12–52. *Basal joint arthritis.* Severe osteoarthritic changes including joint space narrowing, sclerosis, and osteophyte formation, noted at the first carpometacarpal joint and adjacent joints. Degenerative changes involve the trapezium and its surrounding articulations, including the first metacarpal, second metacarpal, trapezoid and scaphoid articulations. (From Richardson and Iglarsh,[6] p 681 with permission.)

Degenerative joint disease occurring in the first carpometacarpal joint and other adjacent joints at the base of the thumb is sometimes referred to as *basal joint arthritis* (Fig. 12–52). It occurs most commonly in adults with no prior history of major trauma, but also is seen as a sequel to fracture or injury in this area, or in patients with rheumatoid arthritis. Arthritic involvement of the thumb base is a painful condition that can seriously impair hand function. The degree of joint damage has been graded radiographically and clinically as:[46]

Stage 1: Ligamentous laxity of the thumb carpometacarpal joint is demonstrated on stress views, whereby the metacarpal base subluxes dorsally and laterally as the tips of the thumbs are pressed together.
Stage 2: Chronic subluxation is present at the thumb carpometacarpal joint, and definite radiographic evidence of osteoarthritis is present in the thumb carpometacarpal joint.
Stage 3: Osteoarthritis is evidenced radiographically in adjacent joints, not only the trapezium-first metacarpal joint but also the trapezium-second metacarpal, trapezium-trapezoid, and trapezium-scaphoid articulations.
Stage 4: Osteoarthritis of the thumb metacarpophalangeal joint is present.

Treatment of DJD in the hand and thumb is dependent on the degree of involvement present. Early stages are often treated with pain management, splinting to prevent or reduce deformity, therapeutic exercise to maintain motion, and joint protection education. Later stages may require joint fusion or joint replacement to preserve a pain-free, functional hand.[47,48]

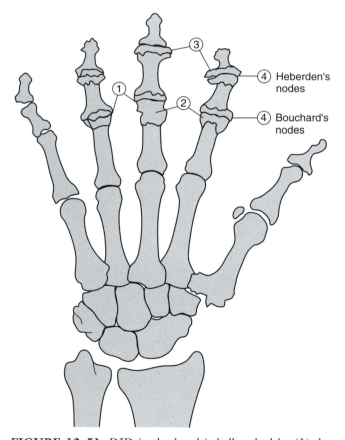

FIGURE 12–51. DJD in the hand is hallmarked by (1) decreased joint spaces, (2) sclerosis of subchondral bone, (3) osteophytes at joint margins, and (4) joint deformities. Deformities at the distal interphalangeal joints are known as *Heberden's nodes*. Deformities at the proximal interphalangeal joints are known as *Bouchard's nodes*.

Rheumatoid Arthritis[49–52]

Rheumatoid arthritis is characteristically manifested in the small joints of the wrist, the metacarpophalangeal joints, and the proximal interphalangeal joints. Radiographic evidence of rheumatoid arthritis in the hand, similar to the larger joints, is hallmarked by (1) periarticular soft tissue swelling, representing effusion, edema, and tenosynovitis; (2) diffuse symmetric narrowing of the radiographic joint spaces; (3) periarticular, localized osteoporosis; (4) articular erosions, without evidence of reparative processes such as sclerosis or osteophyte formation as seen in degenerative osteoarthritis; (5) synovial cysts and pseudocysts located close to the joint; and (6) joint deformities (Figs. 12–53, 12–54).

Advanced stages of rheumatoid arthritis in the hand exhibit multiple joint subluxations and dislocations. Characteristically the fingers ulnarly deviate at the metacarpophalangeal joints, and the wrist radially deviates at the radiocarpal joint. Metacarpophalangeal dislocations may cause an apparent shortening or "telescoping" of the phalanges. Rupture of the scapholunate ligament causes an abnormally wide space between the scaphoid and lunate. A rare finding in advanced

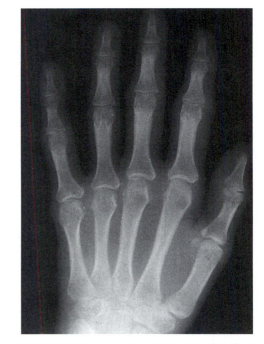

FIGURE 12–54. Rheumatoid arthritis, plain film findings. The characteristics of early-stage rheumatoid arthritis are demonstrated in this patient's hand by the soft tissue swelling of the proximal interphalangeal and metacarpophalangeal joints, thinning of the radial cortices of the metacarpal heads, and osteopenia of the periarticular cancellous bone. Findings such as this represent the pre-erosive changes commonly seen in rheumatoid arthritis. (Reprinted from the Clinical Slide Collection on the Rheumatic Diseases, © 1991. Used by permission of the American College of Rheumatology.)

rheumatoid arthritis, but which, when present, is often encountered in the midcarpal joints, is bony ankylosis (see Fig. 2–44).

Treatment, similar to that of DJD, depends on the degree of involvement and ranges from conservative measures to joint arthroplasties, as noted earlier.

Finger Deformities[53–56]

Two common deformities of the fingers are known as *swan-neck deformity* and *boutonnière deformity* (see Fig. 2–14). These deformities, most often seen as a consequence of rheumatoid arthritis, can also be present as a result of other inflammatory arthritides, traumatic tendon avulsions, contractures, or nerve injuries (see Fig. 12–14). When associated with rheumatoid arthritis, these deformities are related, in general, to imbalances caused by capsular laxity, intrinsic muscle contracture, flexor tendon synovitis, and extensor problems.

The configuration of the swan-neck deformity is hyperextension of the proximal interphalangeal joint and flexion of the distal interphalangeal joint. In the boutonnière deformity, the configuration is reversed, with hyperextension at the distal interphalangeal joints and flexion at the proximal interphalangeal joints.

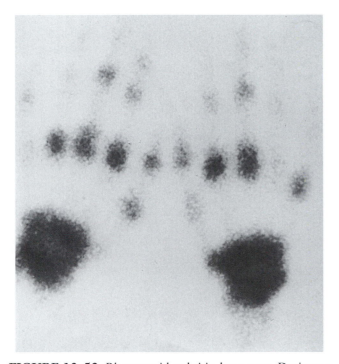

FIGURE 12–53. Rheumatoid arthritis, bone scan. During an initial work-up on a young woman with complaints of bilateral hand joint pain, plain films were negative for pathologic changes, and laboratory findings were inconclusive. A bone scan was done to further narrow the differential diagnosis. The radiopharmaceutical technetium was injected 2 hours before the scan. Note the marked uptake of technetium in both wrists, metacarpal joints, and the interphalangeal joints of the thumbs, index fingers, and middle fingers. These findings were determined to represent an inflammatory phase of early-stage rheumatoid arthritis.

Summary of Key Points

1. The routine radiographic evaluation of the hand includes three projections:
   - **The posteroanterior:** Demonstrates the phalanges, metacarpals, carpals, and joint spaces of the hand.
   - **Lateral:** Demonstrates the hand and wrist in profile.
   - **Oblique:** Demonstrates the lateral aspects of the shafts of the long bones of the hand without the superimposition seen in a true lateral view.
2. The routine radiographic evaluation of the wrist includes the same views and positioning as the hand routine, but the x-ray beam is now centered over the midcarpal joint, whereas in the hand routine the beam is centered over the third metacarpophalangeal joint.
3. Three common optional projections of the wrist are the:
   - **Ulnar deviation view:** Demonstrates the scaphoid and adjacent opened intercarpal spaces.
   - **Radial deviation view:** Demonstrates the ulnar side carpals and adjacent intercarpal spaces.
   - **Carpal tunnel view:** Demonstrates the arched arrangement of the carpals on the palmar aspect of the wrist.
4. Fractures of the hand are probably the most common fractures of adults. The distal phalanges most often sustain crush type fractures. Fractures of the remaining phalanges and metacarpals are described by their location at the head, neck, shaft, base, or intra-articular region, including avulsive type fractures at the attachment sites of tendons and ligaments.
5. Fractures of the metacarpals of the hand occur most frequently at the neck of the shaft.
6. Fractures of the metacarpals of the thumbs occur most frequently at or near the base of the shaft, and are divided into intra- and extra-articular types. Bennett's fracture is the eponym for a dislocation of the first metacarpophalangeal joint combined with an intra-articular avulsion fracture at the anterior lip of the base.
7. The scaphoid bone is the most frequently fractured carpal bone. The majority of scaphoid fractures occur through the waist of the bone. The entrance of the blood supply through the distal pole puts fractures occurring at the waist or proximal pole at risk for satisfactory healing. Avascular necrosis of the proximal pole is a common complication.
8. The distal radius is the most frequently fractured bone of the wrist. The eponym Colles' fracture generally refers to an extra-articular fracture located about 1½ inches proximal to the distal end of the radius, with dorsal angulation of the distal fragment. Associated fractures of the ulnar styloid are often present.
9. Degenerative joint disease is common in the small joints of the hand after the fifth decade in life. Joint deformities resulting from DJD present in the distal interphalangeal joints are known as Heberden's nodes. The same deformities in the proximal interphalangeal joints are known as Bouchard's nodes.

REFERENCES

1. Netter, FH: The Ciba Collection of Medical Illustrations, Vol 8, Part I, Musculoskeletal System. Ciga-Geigy Corporation, Summit, New Jersey, 1978, pp 68–72.
2. Nordin, M and Frankel, VH: Basic Biomechanics of the Musculoskeletal System, ed 2. Lea & Febiger, Malvern, PA, 1989, pp 265–266, 277–278.
3. Meschan, I: An Atlas of Normal Radiographic Anatomy. WB Saunders, Philadelphia, 1960, p 54.
4. Fischer, HW: Radiographic Anatomy: A Working Atlas. McGraw-Hill, New York, 1988, pp 17–19.
5. Bontrager, KL: Textbook of Radiographic Positioning and Related Anatomy, ed 3. Mosby, St. Louis, 1993, pp 99–145.
6. Wicke, L: An Atlas of Radiographic Anatomy, ed 5. Lea & Febiger, Malvern, PA, 1994, p 76.
7. Greenspan, A: Orthopedic Radiology: A Practical Approach, ed 2. Raven Press, New York, 1992, p 6.25.
8. Weissman, B and Sledge, C: Orthopedic Radiology. WB Saunders, Philadelphia, 1986, p 116.
9. Grenspan, p 6.4.
10. Weissman, p 116.
11. Greenspan, p 6.1.
12. Ibid., p 6.12.
13. Ibid., p 6.4.
14. Weissman, p 120.
15. Greenspan, p 6.25.
16. Weissman, p 118.
17. Ibid, p 118.
18. Ibid., p 117.
19. Ibid., p 117.
20. Rockwood, CA and Green, DP (eds): Fractures in Adults, ed 2, Vol 1. JB Lippincott, Philadelphia, 1984, p 316.
21. Rockwood, p 316.
22. Greenspan, p 6.14.
23. Weissman, p 87.
24. Ibid., p 93.
25. Rockwood, p 326.
26. Weissman, p 94.
27. Rockwood, p 343.
28. Ibid., p 356.
29. Weissman, p 94.
30. Richardson, JK and Iglarsh, ZA: Clinical Orthopaedic Physical Therapy. WB Saunders, Philadelphia, 1994, p 292.
31. Rockwood, p 356.
32. Weissman, p 94.
33. Rockwood, p 454.
34. Greenspan, p 6.14.
35. Richardson, p 291.
36. Weissman, p 133.
37. Rockwood, p 454.
38. Greenspan, p 6.6.
39. Weissman, p 125.
40. Richardson, p 289.
41. Rockwood, p 423.
42. Ibid., p 433.
43. Richardson. P 289.
44. Weissman, p 125.
45. Greenspan, p 12.8
46. Weissman, p 100.
47. Greenspan, p 12.8.
48. Weissman, p 100.
49. Greenspan, p 13.4.
50. Weissman, p 102.
51. Richardson, p 307.
52. Cailliet, R: Hand Pain and Impairment, ed 4. FA Davis, Philadelphia, 1994, p 89.
53. Richardson, p 309.
54. Greenspan, p 13.5.
55. Weissman, p 102.
56. Cailliet, p 219.

SELF-TEST

Chapter 12

REGARDING FILM A:

1. Identify the <u>projection</u>.
2. A surgical procedure has been done to alleviate the pain and limitation of <u>osteoarthritis at the first carpometacarpal joint</u>. Which <u>carpal</u> has been resected?
3. The <u>palmaris longus</u> has been coiled into the resected area in order to preserve joint space. How is this soft tissue secured in place?

REGARDING FILM B:

4. Identify the <u>projection</u>.
5. The bony findings are normal. The location and expanse of the soft tissue swelling (*arrows*) suggest that what structures are involved?

6. If the patient's history and clinical findings narrowed the possibilities to trauma caused by repetitive mechanical stresses, what is a likely diagnosis?

REGARDING FILM C:

7. Identify the <u>projection</u>.
8. What radiographic findings suggest that a <u>disease</u> state exists?

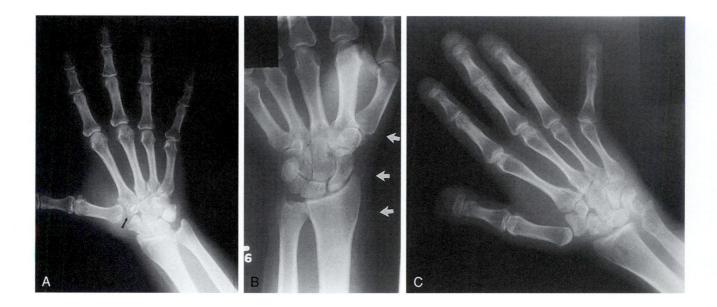

Answers to Self-Test Questions

Chapter 1

1. Low contrast is present, as there is little variation between the soft tissue and bone radiographic densities.
2. This is a chest film, as the low contrast makes the soft tissues of the lungs and heart more visible.
3. Yes. The film is positioned correctly for viewing the patient in anatomic position. The shadow of the heart to the patient's left side verifies this.
4. No. The film is *not* being viewed as if the patient is in anatomic position. The shadow of the heart should appear to the patient's left.
5. The small oval-shaped area of increased density is likely to be of metallic composition, as can be inferred by its solid white radiographic density.
6. No. Without a lateral projection made at right angles to this AP projection, the depth of the location of the foreign object in the body cannot be determined. The object could represent a bullet lodged

in a thoracic vertebra, or just as well represent a harmless medallion on a necklace resting on the skin.
7. A barium contrast study of the gastrointestinal tract.
8. The technician forgot to have the patient empty his pockets. Fortunately, the area of interest was not obscured by the metallic key, so a repeat study was not necessary.
9. A cat.
10. The cat swallowed its owner's pierced earring! The missing jewelry is visualized in the cat's stomach. Note that because of the small part-thickness of this animal, the necessary technical adjustments in mAs and kVp produce a radiograph that demonstrates bony anatomy as well as the soft tissue anatomy. The heart, liver, stomach, and intestines are easily identifiable.

Chapter 2

1. AP projection of the right femur.
2. The bone density of the distal femoral shaft is abnormally uneven. There is loss of a distinct cortical shell and no interface between the cortex and the medullary canal. The external architecture of the distal shaft is also uneven and deformed. These gross changes in mineralization are indications of a pathologic state.
3. No. The upper half of the femoral shaft and the pelvis do not show the bony changes as listed in answer 2. However, the neck of the femur does exhibit osteopenia and thinned cortical margins. This could be related to disuse atrophy.
4. No. The evidence of previous surgical intervention

is revealed by the regularly spaced radiolucent lines representing the removal of sideplate fixation screws.
5. No. The hip joint is decreased, a radiographic sign of degenerative joint disease.
6. AP projection of the right distal femur.
7. See answer 2.
8. Neoplasm. The most obvious reason is that the pathology has not crossed the joint space. Tumors may extend to the margin of the joint but do not cross the joint space. Infections and inflammatory processes usually involve the joint space and both articulating surfaces.

Chapter 3

1. A lateral projection and an AP projection of the left lower leg.
2. The fracture is located at the midshaft of the tibia.
3. The fracture is complete because the fracture line extends through all of the cortex of the shaft.

4. The distal fragment is displaced laterally and anteriorly. There is minimal angulation, and some overriding of the fragments is present.
5. The fracture line is transverse with comminution.

Chapter 4

1. The lateral projections are A and C. The oblique projections are B and D.
2. The intervertebral foramina of the cervical spine are best demonstrated on the oblique projection.
3. Patient C/D exhibits the greater degree of intervertebral disc space narrowing, or degenerative disc disease, at all intervertebral segments.
4. Patient C/D exhibits the greater degree of facet joint space narrowing, or degenerative joint disease, at all intervertebral segments.
5. C5-C6 and C6-C7 exhibit decreased disc height and spurs.
6. C4-C5 intervertebral foramen appears the most constricted; thus, the C5 nerve root may be impinged by foraminal encroachment. (Remember, however,

the appearance of degenerative changes on film does not always correlate with the severity of clinical symptoms.)
7. Because of the greater amount of degenerative changes, including joint space narrowing and spondylosis, it would seem likely that patient C/D suffers a greater loss of cervical spine range of motion. Again, however, remember that the appearance of degenerative changes on film does not always correlate with the severity of clinical symptoms. Other factors, for example, soft tissues or mechanical joint dysfunction, can restrict or alter joint motion either acutely or chronically. Patient A/B may just as well have restricted range. The correct answer is that it is not possible to determine.

Chapter 5

1. This is an AP projection of the posterior left ribs, below diaphragm.
2. The symmetrical position of the spinous processes between the equally spaced pedicles of the thoracic vertebrae tells you that this is an AP view, as does the image of the pairs of ribs attaching to the vertebrae. Furthermore, you know you are viewing posterior ribs because they must be closest to the film plate in order to be so well visualized, as is true in an AP projection. (If this were a PA projection, the costocartilaginous portions of the anterior rib cage closest to the film plate would image much differently.) The left side ribs of the patient are being evaluated, obvious by the area exposed by the central ray. Below diaphragm is known because you can see the lumbar spine (possessing no rib attachments) and can then identify the lower thoracic vertebrae and ribs by number. Ribs 8 through 12 are well-demonstrated.

3. AP projection or the thoracic spine.
4. All thoracic vertebrae, T1 through T12, are visible. The attachment of the first ribs is also visible at T1. L1 and L2 of the lumbar spine are visible. They are identified by their lack of rib attachments. (Note, however, that this is not always foolproof. T12 may lack ribs, or L1 may have ribs.)
5. A right major thoracic curve is present, seen in the long right-side convexity extending from T1 to T12 or L1.
6. Without viewing the entire lumbar spine, it cannot be said if a secondary or minor compensatory curve exists in the lumbar spine or not. (Likewise, identifying a compensatory curve above the thoracic curve requires cervical spine films.)
7. Erect AP lateral flexion projections of the entire spinal column, taken at the end ranges of sidebending right and sidebending left, would reveal the amount of flexibility present.

Chapter 6

1. This is a lateral projection of the lumbar spine.
2. L4-L5 and L5-S1 disc spaces are narrowed.
3. L5. If you trace lines along the anterior and posterior vertebral bodies, you will find that L5 disrupts the continuity of these two curving parallel lines with a sharp step-off.
4. There appears to be a retrolisthesis of L5.
5. Osteophyte or spur formation is present along the margins of the anterior vertebral bodies. Spondylosis deformans describes the condition whereby anterior protrusion of the intervertebral disc nucleus elevates the anterior longitudinal ligament and leads to spur formation. Traction spurs describe spur formation due to tension at the sites of attachment of the anterior longitudinal ligament on the

vertebral bodies. Note the different configurations of the spurs. AT T12-L1, the claw-like spurs have bridged together. At L3, a claw-like spur is present on the inferior margin, and a sharp spur is present on the superior margin. Some authors feel the claw-type spurs are related to disc degeneration, whereas the sharp-type spurs are related to traction.
6. This is a lateral projection of the lumbosacral junction, or an L5-S1 spot film.
7. An abnormal fusion is present between the bodies of L4 and L5, noted by the lack of an intervertebral disc space and malformation of the diameter of the bodies. This congenital anomaly is known as a block vertebrae. Because of lack of motion at this segment, compensatory excessive motion may be present at

adjacent segments, possibly accelerating degenerative joint changes. Another consequence of this anomaly is that the bodies may have developed asymmetrically and contributed to a scoliosis. Additional films are necessary to fully visualize the anomaly.

Chapter 7

1. This is an AP projection of the pelvis.
2. The heart-shaped pelvic inlet is generally attributed to men. However, the wide flared expanse of the greater pelvis is generally attributed to women. The angle of the pubic arch is not visible, nor is the soft tissue outline of the genitalia. Therefore the correct answer is, because of individual variations, it is not possible to determine the sex of the patient by this film.
3. The bilateral hip joint spaces exhibit severe concentric narrowing. Some regions appear to be bone-on-bone.
4. The femoral heads have migrated superiorly and medially into the acetabulum. This can also be described as axial migration.
5. Acetabular protrusio describes the out-pouching of the medial wall of the acetabulum in response to axial migration of the femoral head.
6. Both processes are evident. Signs present that are characteristics of rheumatoid arthritis include the bilateral, symmetrical involvement of the joints, the concentric joint space narrowing, and the acetabular protrusio. Signs present that are characteristics of DJD include sclerotic repair and spur formation. Both processes can exist simultaneously; degenerative processes can proceed while the joints are in a remission from RA.

Chapter 8

1. A—intercondylar notch or tunnel view of the knee; B—lateral view of the knee; C—tangential view of the patellofemoral joint.
2. The object lies within the joint capsule. The location of the object cannot be determined by the AP view alone. By consulting the lateral view, it is obvious the object is not anterior or posterior to the joint; it is thus being obscured within the joint.
3. Possibilities include an osteochondral fragment.
4. The medial compartment and the patellofemoral compartment show mild degenerative changes.
5. Degenerative changes present include subchondral sclerosis and joint space narrowing.

Chapter 9

1. This is an AP or dorsoplanar projection of the foot.
2. Hallux valgus. This term describes a condition whereby the first metatarsal is deviated medially and the first phalange is deviated laterally.
3. A bony exostosis or bunion is present on the medial aspect of the metatarsal head.
4. The great toe and second toe are crossed over each other.
5. This is an AP projection of the bilateral ankles.
6. There appears to be gross inversion and pronation of the ankles and feet, although complete collapse of normal bony architecture would also describe this deformity. Bilaterally, the joints of the ankle, hindfoot, and midfoot appear to be fused. This severe condition represents the burned-out stage of rheumatoid arthritis.

Chapter 10

1. This is an AP projection of the left shoulder.
2. Abnormal findings include the following: the humeral head has been completely resorbed and the surgical neck has migrated superiorly into the joint space; no lytic lesions are present in the humerus but demineralization is evident; the minimal soft tissue shadows indicate gross muscle wasting.
3. This is an AP projection of the right shoulder.
4. The acromioclavicular joint is stabilized via internal fixation.
5. This is an AP projection of the left shoulder.
6. A severely comminuted fracture pattern is present.
7. A gun shot wound, or any other high velocity trauma that would leave the tell-tale metal shards as seen on this film.

Chapter 11

1. All three are AP projections of the left elbow.
2. A—10 year old; B—30 year old; C—5 year old.
3. The presence of open epiphyseal plates tells you that patients A and C are the children. The younger child is determined by noting the smaller size and thus earlier stage of development of the epiphyses, especially the epiphyses for the radial head and medial epicondyle, which have just begun ossification.

Chapter 12

1. This is an PA or dorsoplanar projection of the hand.
2. The trapezium has been resected.
3. A metallic device is visible at the trapezoid. This mytex suture anchor secures the soft tissue to bone. (This procedure has been dubbed the anchovie procedure, as the palmaris longus is coiled into the resected space like anchovies packed in a can.)
4. This is a PA or dorsoplanar projection of the wrist.
5. The soft tissues present at this location are the tendons and muscles of the extensor pollicis brevis and the abductor pollicis longus.
6. Tenosynovitis of the first dorsal compartment of the wrist, also know as DeQuervain's disease.
7. This is a PA or dorsoplanar projection of the hand.
8. Abnormal findings include resorption or malformation of the distal radius, distal ulna, and distal phalanges of all the digits. Additionally there are irregularities in the density of all the bones. The shafts of the phalanges are sclerotic while the proximal ends of each phalanx are demineralized. There also is rarefaction of the metacarpal heads. The trabeculae of the carpals appear sparse and distinct. This young adult had been diagnosed years earlier with osteogenesis imperfecta.

Index

An "f" following a page number indicates a figure; a "t" following a page number indicates a table.